Emergency Medical Services

Emergency Medical Services
Behavioral and Planning Perspectives

Edited by

John H. Noble, Jr., Ph.D.

Henry Wechsler, Ph.D.

Margaret E. LaMontagne, M.S.N.

Mary Anne Noble, D.N.Sc.

Behavioral Publications
New York
1973

ABIGAIL E. WEEKS MEMORIAL LIBRARY
UNION COLLEGE
BARBOURVILLE, KENTUCKY

Library of Congress Catalog Number 73-9940
ISBN: 0-87705-117-8
Copyright © 1973 by Behavioral Publications

All rights reserved. No part of this work may be reproduced
or utilized in any form or by any means, electronic or
mechanical, including photocopying, microfilm and recording,
or by any information storage and retrieval system without
permission in writing from the publisher.

BEHAVIORAL PUBLICATIONS, 52 Fifth Avenue
New York, New York 10011

Printed in the United States of America
This printing 10 9 8 7 6 5 4 3 2 1

Library of Congress Cataloging in Publication Data
Noble, John H   1923-   comp.
  Emergency medical services.
  CONTENTS: Foreword. pt. I. The emergency medical care system. 1. DuVal, M. K. The hidden crisis in health care. 2. Skudder, P. A., McCarroll, J. R., and Wade, P. A. Hospital emergency facilities and services, a survey. 3. King, B. G. and Sox, E. D. An emergency medical service system: analysis of workload. [etc.]
  1. Emergency medical services. I. Wechsler, Henry, joint comp. II. Title. [DNLM: 1. Emergency health services—U. S. 2. Hospital emergency service. WX215 N749e 1973]

RA975.5.E5N6   362.1'1   73-9940

To E. Richard Weinerman, M.D., M.P.H. (July 17, 1917—February 21, 1970), clinician, medical care planner, health consultant, researcher, and teacher, whose contributions to the understanding of the dynamics of systems of emergency health care will long endure.

Contents

Foreword ix

PART I. THE EMERGENCY MEDICAL CARE SYSTEM

Introduction 3
1. The hidden crisis in health care 9
   Merlin K. DuVal
2. Hospital emergency facilities and services, a survey 17
   Paul A. Skudder, James R. McCarroll, and Preston A. Wade
3. An emergency medical service system: analysis of workload 37
   Barry G. King and Ellis D. Sox
4. Emergency medical services, a systems approach 73
   William R. Gemma, Daniel E. Strayer, Robert C. Chase, and Martin D. Keller
5. The social system of emergency medical care 85
   Geoffrey Gibson

PART II. PATTERNS OF EMERGENCY ROOM UTILIZATION

Introduction 129
6. Variations among emergency room populations: a comparison of four hospitals in New York City 135
   Paul R. Torrens and Donna G. Yedvab
7. The types of families that use an emergency clinic 165

Joel J. Alpert, John Kosa, Robert J. Haggerty, Leon Robertson, and Margaret C. Heagarty

8. Social class and medical care: indices of nonurgency in use of hospital emergency services   181
Marvin A. Lavenhar, Robert S. Ratner, and E. Richard Weinerman

9. Problems of communication, diagnosis, and patient care: the interplay of patient, physician and clinic organization   207
Irving K. Zola

10. Help?: the hospital emergency unit as community physician   227
David G. Satin and Frederick J. Duhl

11. Staff perceptions of patients' use of a hospital outpatient department   253
Jerry Solon, Cecil G. Sheps, Sidney S. Lee, and Maeda Jurkowitz

PART III. TRANSPORTATION AND COMMUNICATIONS

Introduction   275

12. An analysis of the demand for emergency ambulance service in an urban area   281
Carole A. Aldrich, John C. Hisserich, and Lester B. Lave

13. Variations in visits to hospital emergency care facilities: ritualistic and meteorological factors affecting supply and demand   305
John H. Noble, Jr., Margaret E. LaMontagne, Carole Bellotti, and Henry Wechsler

14. Cost-effectiveness analysis for evaluating alternative emergency medical care recovery systems   329
Erik Hanitzsch and William Hall

15.	Ambulance service size and level of service Dunlap and Associates, Inc.	345
16.	Analyzing the role of the helicopter in emergency medical care for a community Arthur R. Jacobs and Curtis P. McLaughlin	373
17.	Simulation study of a hospital emergency command system Stephen A. Levine	389
18.	Mobile emergency medical care E. B. Struxness	425

PART IV. STANDARDS AND POLICIES

Introduction		435
19.	Community-wide emergency medical services	441
	Committee on Acute Medicine of the American Society of Anesthesiologists	441
20.	Survey discovers what is wrong with hospitals' emergency service J. Cuthbert Owens	469
21.	Moonlighting policy: the hospital proposes but the chief disposes *Resident Physician*	479
22.	What it takes to organize for service Robert H. Kennedy	491
23.	Here are ways to use facts about E. R. to build good public and press relations Lee Feldman	501
24.	Hospital emergency service and the open door Leonard S. Powers	511
25.	Planning community emergency health care services: fitting together the fragments Martin D. Keller and William R. Gemma	561
Index		577

Foreword

This important compendium of papers brings to bear on emergency medical care expert knowledge from an appropriate variety of disciplines. It combines in one useful volume the essential historical and recent observations which are basic to the improvement of the system of providing emergency medical care within the larger system of medical care in America.

Those physicians who practice emergency medicine will read again that emergency medical care is the "weakest link" in the chain of medical care. They can see their link in a new perspective as Dr. DuVal concerns himself with the other links in the chain and as Dr. Keller points out that the weak link concept is influenced by the orientation of the individual conducting the study.

Without design, emergency departments have taken on, in addition to their traditional role, the buffering function of regulating the imbalance of the over-all health care system. They offer an escape valve for the socially deprived, a convenience service for those who require it, and serve as the interface between the community and hospital in all those conditions perceived to be urgent. They account for nearly five percent of all the patient visits to physicians. They do the important work of providing an entry into the medical care system and endeavor through medical staff support and other resources to provide continuing and comprehensive aftercare.

If tomorrow the emergency departments of the country were to filter out and reject all those cases determined by physicians not to be urgent the reverberations would be enormous. This implies that they serve their buffering function at least tolerably well. Fortunately this rejection will not occur for humanitarian, and, as Powers makes plain, for legal reasons. Nevertheless, Gibson shows that under sufficient impact, hospital emergency departments would find their capacity for hemostasis tested beyond their limits. Such a force might easily be the advent of national health insurance without first providing more system entries than now exist.

Throughout the volume you will learn from unbiased observers that there is much to be viewed with alarm and little in which to take pride. Though not a polemic, the political ramifications are worthy of sober study. The emergency medical specialist is concerned with the entire range of emergency treatment: detection, first-aid and transportation to the hospital, the functions and procedures of the emergency room; he also must be concerned with emergencies arising within the hospital. Organizing emergency treatment programs requires that the planner bring all these fragments together within the over-all medical system. Anyone involved with such programs will do well to be familiar with the core material that Noble and his colleagues have assembled.

Here, then, is the considered work of 48 authors who have concern for the socioeconomic ramifications of emergency medical care, who have demonstrated predictive capabilities, and whose input will be important in the broad-based solutions we require.

James D. Mills, M.D.
President
American College of Emergency Physicians

Part I

The Emergency Medical Care System

INTRODUCTION

The generally increasing use of hospital emergency care facilities for treatment of nonemergent conditions has been the subject of extended study and commentary. Attempts to interpret and explain this trend almost invariably lead to discussion of the nature of the "system" that is creating this profound health care problem. The articles in this section present different yet complementary definitions of the emergency medical care system with their authors' individual perspectives and beliefs as to "what is wrong." Cumulatively, they provide insights into the behavioral and organizational complexities of a system that has the considerable burden of drawing together the appropriate manpower and technologies needed to respond effectively to a "call for help."

The first article, by DuVal (1972), analyzes and describes the emergency medical care problem as part of the general "crisis in health care" involving "the increasing lack of accessibility of health care for the American consumer." DuVal attributes the neglect of emergency medical care problems to the tendency of both government and the medical profession to invest in "the more exciting and glamorous aspects of medicine." He cites studies that show the effects on the nation's health of both underinvestment and uneven investment in emergency medical care facilities and services. With respect to properly manned ambulance service in urban areas, evidence suggests that the nation may even have retrogressed since pre-World War II days. DuVal's prescription for solving the current crisis is, first, to recognize that there is no single problem requiring a single solution, and, second, that relatively advanced existing technologies should be applied in an integrated fashion to the solution of various problems.

The next group of articles present extensive data on varying aspects of the emergency medical care system, such as information on the variability between sites and facilities in policies, staffing, equipment, and procedures. To our knowledge, the survey of hospital emergency facilities and services reported by Skudder, McCarroll, and Wade (1961) is the only existing nationally representative study. It has significance not only for its baseline data on hospital emergency facilities and services in the late 1950's, but also for the stimulus it gave to many local communities and hospitals to conduct studies of their own immediate situations. The large volume of literature now available in this field is a result. Undoubtedly, some of our current discontent and concern about the adequacy of available emergency medical services is due to what represents years of accumulated findings.

Skudder, *et al.* found by indirect measures that the quality of medical care offered by hospital emergency facilities in the United States was deficient in one-fifth to two-thirds of the sites—depending upon the dimension of care considered. For example, one-fifth of the hospitals posted no sign showing the entrance to the emergency area; one-quarter permitted physicians to bill patients whom they had not treated after only a telephone conversation with a house officer or nurse; and while three-quarters of the hospitals used tetanus toxoid routinely in treatment of the open wounds of unimmunized patients, only one-fifth provided the patients with a written record for future use. Interestingly, Skudder, *et al.* thought that education of the public about the "appropriate" use of emergency care facilities could stem the tide of nonemergent use, estimated at the time of their study to be 42 percent of total usage.

Insight into the operations and characteristics of demand on an "integrated" system combining specialized staff, equipment, facilities, and transport within a communications network capable of coordinating the several components, is offered by King and Sox (1967) in their survey and analysis of the emergency medical service workload in San Francisco. As the first known systems analysis of an emergency medical care system, it is still among the best. It is also one of the few studies to give a complete picture of the place and circumstances of the emergency, describing how the patient is managed at the scene and during transport to the hospital, what equipment is used or needed, and what changes in the patient's condition occur due to either proper management or poor handling and delay. The apparent success of San Francisco's integrated emergency care system in reduced morbidity and mortality from accidents and sudden illness offers encouragement to other communities to make a similar investment on behalf of their citizens.

The last two articles in this section represent different approaches to systems analysis. Gemma, Strayer, Chase, and Keller (1972) present a systems analytic model that considers all pertinent variables in a community emergency health service system—from the point at which an emergency occurs and is detected to the point of treatment in an emergency medical facility. Their model is designed to simulate the operations of an emergency medical care system under varying resource availability conditions by means of a computer using real or estimated data. Input data provides description of available emergency medical facilities for a given area, probable number and types of emergency patients, and delay times involved in detection, communications, transportation, and treatment. Output is produced in the form of extensive information about the functioning of the system during specified time periods. The model's utility lies in its ability to help the decision-maker grasp the complexity of the total emergency medical care system while simulating what would happen if alterations were made in one or more of the system's components. In doing so, it allows "consideration of new, untried methods of providing emergency medical care, without the financial cost and social risk of premature implementation."

Gibson's article (1972) on the social systems of emergency medical care uses a "living system" analogy to explore the meaning of certain well-documented trends here in the United States and in the United Kingdom. He compares the emergency medical care system with other systems in terms of their shared generic properties and functions, zones of predisposition, and the expressive processes of information flow. While abstract at times, Gibson's systems analogy is valuable for its many insights and several testable hypotheses. The notion that emergency medical services can be isolated from other health care services is rejected in Gibson's convincingly argued point that "the problems of hospital emergency departments are almost entirely attributable to imbalances elsewhere in the system, and thus these problems are only solvable ... by broad-scale reforms in the wider health care system." Gibson's thesis that simple internal reorganization of the emergency medical subsystem will not suffice, while not denying the validity of narrower studies and analyses, does raise questions about the relevance of many proposed solutions.

Because hospital emergency rooms cannot, for a number of reasons, fend off nonemergent use by patients who lack access to the wider health care system, they have come to serve as "escape valves" for the wider system—enabling the system to adjust to imbalances resulting from the maldistribution of physicians, the unavailability of physicians at night and on weekends, and the decline in private health care resources within many inner-city areas.

None of the articles in this section suggest that emergency medical services are part of a "nonsystem" defying our understanding. The message is just the opposite. We are informed about the dimensions of an emergency medical care system that is considerably overburdened. While it is difficult to foretell which of the insights into the behavioral and organizational complexities of the emergency medical care system will be found most useful in defining solutions to its problems, the articles in this section offer us some of the "raw ingredients" with which to begin.

1. The Hidden Crisis in Health Care
Merlin K. DuVal, M.D.

Nearly three years ago President Nixon expressed concern about an impending "crisis in health care," with one of the major manifestations of this crisis being the increasing lack of accessibility of health care for the American consumer. It is now becoming more and more apparent that nowhere is this lack of accessibility more crucial and yet more widespread and profound than in the area of emergency care. Any description of our current emergency medical services becomes a litany of inadequacy and neglect.

One of the first documentations of this developing crisis in emergency care was a survey of 782 traffic deaths occurring in rural and urban California counties during 1961, when it was convincingly demonstrated that persons injured in rural counties were almost four times as likely to die of their injuries as those injured in urban counties. It might be postulated that accidents in rural areas on open highways occurred at higher speeds and therefore led to more severe injuries. Surprisingly, the opposite was found to be true: accidents occurring in rural counties tended to be single vehicle accidents which resulted in *less* severe injuries, while those in urban counties tended to be two-vehicle and multiple vehicle accidents resulting in more serious injuries. Although the anatomic distribution of injuries was the same for both urban and rural accidents, people dying in rural accidents more often died at the scene of the accident, died sooner after injury, and died of less serious injuries than did those injured in urban accidents.

Ten years later, in 1971, we find little change in highway fatality rates, and a widespread lack of improvement in ambulance services, except for those areas with an active Highway Safety Program. The University of Vermont recently reported that a study of 163 highway fatalities in Vermont revealed that 23 percent died of injuries that were either definitely or possibly survivable. A University of Michigan review of autopsy protocols from 159 patients dying in motor vehicle accidents suggested that 18 percent might have been salvaged and restored to their previous state of health had they received adequate care at the scene, or en route to the hospital, with another 6 percent listed as possibly salvageable. A 1968 University of Iowa study was probably typical of most of the country in revealing that approximately 60 percent of the ambulance services in the State were dispensed by undertakers. Since only half of these services required any first aid training for their ambulance attendants, it is not surprising that nearly half administered no first aid at all in severe injuries. More than half of the vehicles involved carried no splints, and less than half of the operators bothered to clean the medical equipment after each use.

Tragically, further investigation reveals that the American patient fails to find adequate emergency care even if he survives the accident and the ride to the hospital. Again we find that this is not a recent phenomenon, since a review of therapeutic failures in a group of seriously injured soldiers, who arrived at civilian hospitals alive and were seen by a physician in a three-year period, 1957-1959, showed that at least one out of six would have had an excellent chance of survival had prompt diagnosis been made and adequate treatment instituted. An additional one-sixth of the cases had such limited treatment that an appreciable number could probably have been salvaged. In other words, in spite of multiple other deficiencies in our current health system, none seem quite so profound or as obvious as the deficiencies in our emergency medical services. It seems appropriate, to me, that we identify this problem as the real crisis in health care.

However, thus far we have merely outlined *what* the problem is. To stop with only a definition and identification of the chief complaint is to complete only a part of the total work-up; indeed, we would be guilty of neglect unless we also tried to determine *why* the problem developed.

Problems in emergency medical services were not especially outstanding during the preceding centuries or the first half of this century. Significantly, records of the Cincinnati General Hospital indicate that they used a vehicle to transport patients prior to 1865, although Bellevue Hospital in New York City claims to have used "the world's first ambulance" in 1869. By the end of the 19th century, there began the gradual motorization of ambulance vehicles, with one of the first semi-horseless ambulances being an electric auto used by the Presbyterian Hospital in New York (a horse was also stabled on the hospital grounds to pull the vehicle up the hills that had a significant incline). The first autonomous automobile ambulance, capable of speeds up to 16 mph, was operated by the Michael Reese Hospital in Chicago in February, 1899.

This pattern of hospital-based ambulances remained the precedent in urban areas until the onset of the Second World War. With the loss of personnel to the wartime effort, many hospitals turned their ambulance service over to a volunteer group or to an agency capable of operating a motor vehicle. With thousands dying weekly on the beaches of the South Pacific and in the forests of Europe, no one seemed aware, much less concerned, about a few extra deaths on the home front.

With ambulances being operated strictly by volunteers, whether members of the Red Cross, the Y.W.C.A., or the P.T.A., whatever levels of skill and care had been achieved during the previous decades declined and, by the end of the War, both the public and the health professions had become accustomed to thinking of the ambulance as a transport vehicle, a horizontal taxi. With the end of the War in 1945, the Nation failed to translate its newly learned military lessons in emergency-rendered care into civilian advance and, instead, permitted itself to be captured by the more exciting and glamorous aspects of medicine, exemplified during the 40's by the first blue-baby heart operations and the first miraculous successes of penicillin. At the same time, the Federal Government became infected with this enthusiasm and began to budget millions for basic medical research.

Hospitals, which had borne the burden of red-ink ambulance services before the War, concentrated on the lucrative possibilities of research within their own walls. Even the few hospitals that maintained ambulance services were unable to utilize any of this new Federal largesse in the area of emergency medical services. As a result, the problem of emergency medical transport was left virtually unattended and unsupervised.

Because hospitals had been operating ambulances before the War at a level that was quite compatible with medical standards of the time, no further standards or regulations seemed to be required, nor were they developed. During the succeeding decades, it was entirely possible for an individual or an organization with a station wagon or other similar vehicle to install red lights and a siren and initiate an ambulance service. Unfortunately, both the public and the medical profession assumed that the post-War ambulance system was as adequate as the pre-War ambulance system. Both were deluded.

This neglect of emergency problems went beyond ambulance services. As physicians assumed increasing duties in research laboratories and on patient wards, the problems of first-aid and emergency care outside the hospital disappeared from the curricula of medical schools and post-graduate training programs. In retrospect, today's deficiencies in emergency care could be said to have been predictable.

On the other hand, there has not been a total absence of either Federal or private efforts as regards the problems of emergency medical services since the Second World War. In fact, there have recently been some highly sophisticated attempts to tackle the problems of emergency transport by the use of helicopters, and the problem of intensive hospital treatment with the use of very sophisticated trauma centers. Yet, none of these efforts has produced a dramatic change in the problems of emergency medical services, for the good and sufficient reason that there is no single problem in emergency care: there are numerous problems, and they require numerous solutions. It is this concept of multiple factors, in an interrelated chain of events, which offers the best key to understanding emergency medical services.

The *first* links in this chain are PREVENTION and public education; without this link no attempted solution can be truly complete. The *second* link seems more obvious; it is the actual OCCURRENCE of an emergency incident (such as an automobile accident, with multiple trauma and a surgical emergency; or a myocardial infarction and a medical emergency). Once the incident has occurred, the *next* link must be DETECTION of the incident, either by the patient himself, if he is still responsive, or by a passer-by if the patient is unconscious. Following this comes the *next* link in the chain, NOTIFICATION of the proper authorities that an emergency has occurred. These authorities must then complete the *next* link in the chain and DISPATCH an ambulance or other emergency vehicle to the scene as quickly as possible. The *next* link is completed when the personnel of this vehicle accomplish on-the-scene TREATMENT, extrication if necessary, and stabilize the patient with splints or other necessary supplies. The patient is then ready for the *next* link in the chain, the continuing care and supervision during TRANSPORT to a medical facility. The ambulance generally concludes its portion of involvement in this chain of events by delivering the patient to the *next* link; in most instances the EMERGENCY ROOM of a nearby hospital. If the patient has a substantial emergency medical problem, however, delay in the emergency room should generally be minimal before he is transferred to the appropriate inpatient INTENSIVE CARE unit, the *next* link in the chain. Once the patient's condition has stabilized and improved sufficiently in the intensive care area, he then moves to the *next* link, RECUPERATION in a general hospital ward or graded-care facility. Then, finally, comes the *last* link in this chain: appropriate REHABILITATION with return to his family and his job.

With all of these steps viewed as interconnecting links in a continuing chain of events during an emergency medical problem, one can see why even the most dedicated, but limited, efforts may not succeed. To concentrate solely on a single link in this chain of eleven separate links offers no more hope for long-term success than does the focusing of attention on only one or two players on a football team. Although isolated progress may be achieved by focusing on some of the weakest of these links, the most significant progress will be achieved when all links are adequately strengthened and integrated.

I would reason that it is precisely because emergency medical services constitute an aggregation of separate and distinct efforts, each of which may be subject to separate professional, political, and fiscal persuasions; and because we Americans are singularly poor at thinking in terms of totally integrated systems; that it should come as no surprise that, as a nation, we have failed to mount a successful attack on the problem of emergency medical services. Indeed, most of our greatest scientific, as well as philosophic, advances have come about as the consequence of individual, or small group, contributions. Only when we decided to land on the moon did we undertake a concerted and integrated effort—with notable success. And, while it has been argued that in our current concern for a cure for cancer we are stretching the individual technologies past the states of their respective arts, I would submit that such an observation does *not* hold true with respect to emergency medical services. On the contrary—each of the links in the chain has marked a point of considerable development—what we lack is their integration.

The time is now. Personally, I am committed to using the full force of my office to stimulate the several departments of government that have a stake in this effort to full performance. I am also counting on you*—and groups like yours—to match this Federal effort with an equivalent regional or local concern and investment.

The average citizen today considers it a tragedy when a relative dies of cancer in a hospital. He must also develop the same concern for one who dies of acute myocardial infarction or of accidental injury outside the hospital. It is only when every American has access to first-rate emergency care that we will eliminate the most crucial portion of our current crisis in health care and guarantee to the consumer the most basic health-right of all: the right to *life,* first and foremost, and then liberty and the pursuit of happiness.

*Second National Conference on Emergency Health Services, Bethesda, Maryland, December 2-4, 1971.

2. Hospital Emergency Facilities and Services: A Survey*

Paul A. Skudder, M.D.

James R. McCarroll, M.D.

Preston A. Wade, M.D.

In recent years the soaring costs of hospital care and the accompanying criticism of these costs by the public have prompted a series of critical self-analyses by hospitals of all aspects of their services. In this process of self-analysis few hospital departments have fared as badly as the emergency unit. Justly or unjustly, emergency services have been characterized in such well publicized statements as "the weakest link in the chain of hospital care,"[1] and "a frequent source of inferior patient care, and a prolific breeder of much adverse public relations."[2]

These and similar statements by respected medical leaders have been used by many lay publications as evidence that hospitals are failing to meet one of their principal obligations. This criticism ignores the fact that the functions and responsibilities of the hospital emergency service have been radically altered and expanded during the last 15 years. What was once the

*Reprinted from *American College of Surgeons Bulletin,* March-April 1961.

"accident room," designed to handle acute emergency problems in trauma, is now regarded, at least by the general public, as the appropriate initial source of medical care for a wide variety of medical, surgical, pediatric, and even psychiatric problems. The resulting increase in emergency room visits has been shown to exceed 400 percent in many hospitals and, in some, to exceed prewar levels by 600 percent.[3] It is obvious that this increased use of emergency facilities by the general public indicates a basic shift in patterns of medical care. Many of the reasons for this change are obvious, and both the medical profession and the hospitals themselves must share the responsibility for directly or indirectly encouraging these trends.

Although the increased utilization of hospital emergency facilities has been well documented, the charges of a decrease in the quality of emergency medical care have not been similarly substantiated. In an effort to determine the actual quality of medical care given in hospital emergency facilities, the Cornell Trauma Research Group joined with the American College of Surgeons and the American Hospital Association to carry out a nationwide investigation.

Initially, it was decided that the quality of medical care afforded an accident victim could best be judged by the actual result of the patient's treatment, including complications and residual disabilities. Only by following a consecutive series of patients treated in a hospital emergency department from the time of injury to the final outcome could such an evaluation be made directly.

Accordingly, a pilot study of this type was carried out in the emergency department of a large metropolitan hospital. As this study progressed, it became apparent that although this method of investigation yielded valuable information on the emergency department at hand, it was far too demanding in terms of time and personnel to serve as a suitable tool for a major investigation of a large number of institutions. Nevertheless, this method is recommended for those hospitals having a trained and interested emergency department physician with sufficient time to carry out such a project.

Since this direct approach proved impractical for surveying a large number of emergency departments, an indirect approach was devised. This was based on the physical plant and equipment of the emergency department and on the organization and staff in relation to the demands placed upon them, the premise being that deficiencies in these areas would probably reflect similar deficiencies in patient care and thus indirectly mirror the quality of medical care afforded by a given hospital.

To obtain a representative sample of all hospital emergency facilities, a two-stage sampling plan was employed. Representation (Table 1) from both urban and rural areas was required, as was geographic distribution based upon population density. As the proportion of emergency care rendered by different hospitals in a city varies, all hospitals within each sample city were included so as to obtain a picture of the total facilities provided. In each of the four major geographic regions used one major metropolitan area was selected for survey representation. All short-term, nonfederal, general hospitals in each of these major metropolitan areas were included in the survey.

In addition to these major urban complexes, a number of minor metropolitan areas were also selected from each of the four geographic regions.

Since the demands upon emergency services in most urban areas vary with the number of facilities available, all hospitals in each major and minor met-

Table 1
Geographic Areas Used in Survey of Emergency Facilities

Region	Number of Hospitals	Major Metropolitan Areas*	Number of Hospitals	Minor Metropolitan Areas**	Number of Hospitals	Rural Area† Hospitals
1. New England and Northeastern States	65	Pittsburgh	41	Altoona	4	13
				Lawrence	3	
				Atlantic City	2	
				Waterbury	2	
2. Southeastern and South Central States	103	Houston	26	Macon, Georgia	4	47
				Tampa-St. Petersburg	13	
				Durham	3	
				Little Rock	5	
				Wichita Falls, Texas	4	
				Gadsden, Alabama	2	
3. Midwestern and Plains States	86	Minneapolis-St. Paul	28	Kalamazoo, Michigan	3	36
				Hamilton-Middleton, Ohio	4	
				Des Moines, Iowa	4	
				Toledo, Ohio	8	
				Racine, Wisconsin	3	
4. Mountain and Pacific States	75	San Francisco-Oakland	51	Albuquerque	5	16
				Spokane	3	
Total	330		146		72	112

*City and suburban complex numbers over 1,000,000 persons
**From 50,000 to 1,000,000 persons
†Population of 50,000

ropolitan area were included. In addition to these urban groups, a random selection of hospitals in rural areas was also included.

This combination of stratified and random sampling techniques offered the best possibility for obtaining an accurate, representative sample for this survey. It took into account the relative population density of various geographic regions as well as the urban-rural balance in each area; and the interdependence of hospitals in metropolitan areas, recognizing this by including all hospitals where more than one provided emergency care. The sample totaled 330 or six percent of the 5,364 short-term, nonfederal, general hospitals in the United States.

A questionnaire covering all aspects of emergency room care was submitted to the 330 hospitals surveyed. A total of 90 questions was put to all hospitals, and six additional questions were put only to hospitals in rural areas. These six concerned the population served and the radius from which patients were drawn.

Response to the questionnaire (Figure 1) was excellent, with 87 percent or 286 of 330 hospitals cooperating. Of this group 21 stated that they had no emergency facilities, leaving 265 hospitals in the sample group.

Response from hospitals in the various geographic regions and population groups was remarkably uniform, encouraging the belief that a truly representative sample of the short-term, nonfederal, general hospitals was obtained. Additional evidence for this belief is provided by the similarity of the survey group to the total number of short-term, nonfederal general hospitals in several respects. Table 2 shows the similarity of hospitals in the survey group to all other hospitals when compared by type of control.

Table 2
Type of Control: Comparison of Hospitals Surveyed With All Short-Term Nonfederal Hospitals

Control	Hospitals Surveyed	Percent	All Hospitals	Percent
Voluntary	191	67	3,259	61
Government	60	21	1,215	23
Proprietary	35	12	890	16
Total	286	100	5,364	100

Almost all of the hospitals responding—93 percent—stated that they operated an emergency department, but many of those with negative responses also indicated that they provided care for many accident victims.

In one of the major metropolitan areas, San Francisco and Oakland, a regional agreement exists

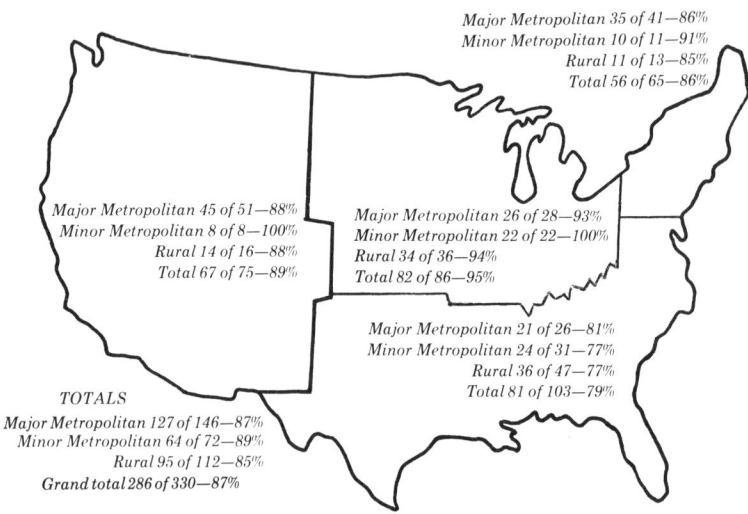

Figure 1. Response to survey of hospital emergency facilities and services is shown according to the four geographic areas covered. Of the 286 hospitals which replied to questionnaire, 21 stated they had no emergency facilities, leaving 265 institutions in the sample group.

whereby certain hospitals are designated as "emergency hospitals" for specific areas. Although all emergency cases within these areas are supposed to be brought to these emergency hospitals, other hospitals there nevertheless must provide a certain amount of emergency care to patients who come to them. Such difficulties in the execution of regional plans are probably inevitable, but they can be lessened by publicity. Less than a quarter of the hospitals in the major and minor metropolitan areas had arrangements for dividing responsibility.

Of the rural hospitals surveyed, many stated that some patients came to their emergency rooms from over 25 miles away, and one hospital stated that patients came from as far as 400 miles. Half of the rural hospitals stated that the majority of their patients traveled over 10 miles to the emergency unit. Such distances make first aid and transportation of victims of acute illness and injury of vital concern in these areas.

Only a very few hospitals (six percent) in the survey group operated their own ambulance service. The major part of ambulance service is provided by organizations not under the control of the local hospital, such as fire and police departments, and private, volunteer, and commercial groups. Since hospitals have little responsibility for or control over ambulance attendants, it is not surprising that only 65 percent of hospitals responding stated that the agencies providing ambulance service require attendants to be trained in first-aid procedures, and virtually never are significant first-aid data recorded by ambulance attendants. The groups providing ambulance service vary widely in different geographic areas. In general, commercial ambulance services tend to operate primarily in urban areas, whereas in rural areas such service is provided principally by police and fire departments, volunteer groups, and morticians. Morticians were the single group most commonly mentioned by hospitals as providing ambulance care, and their services were used by nearly half of all hospitals in major metropolitan areas as well as by institutions with fewer other organizations on which to rely.

The crucial gap between time of injury and arrival at a hospital emergency department offers one of the principal opportunities for improvement of present methods in the management of trauma and acute illness. Although the assignment of physicians to ambulance duty may not be defensible on economic or practical grounds, the obvious responsibility of the medical profession for the training and supervision of ambulance attendants should not be ignored. Certainly, principles of first aid and transportation of the injured should be taught to all persons routinely serving on an ambulance team, and the practicing physicians of an area are the logical individuals to supervise this training. The medical profession should also have an active voice in the type of vehicle used for ambulance work, and in its equipment.

Two-thirds of the responding hospitals indicated that the physical plant of their present emergency unit was inadequate and that some structural changes were contemplated. However, most of these changes were planned by the larger metropolitan institutions, which presumably include a larger proportion of the older hospital construction. Only one-fifth of the rural area hospitals, which presumably include much of the recent hospital construction, plan changes for their emergency units. A check of such obvious aids as signs indicating the entrance to the emergency area shows none in one-fifth of the hospitals surveyed. In 37 of the 265 hospitals the emergency department was not even accessible from the street.

Each hospital was requested to submit a floor plan of its emergency department. Some of the essential features obtained from the plans submitted by 70 percent are listed in Table 3.

A thorough review of equipment, supplies, and ancillary facilities was made. Items commonly found and deemed important are listed in Table 4. Not all of these were kept in the emergency department, but they were available in the hospital, particularly in smaller hospitals where the supply area was readily available to the emergency department. A simple but important procedure is to post the location of all

Table 3
Basic Physical Components
of Hospital Emergency Departments

1. Well illuminated entrance from street
2. Space for loading, unloading, and turning around of vehicles
3. Ramps and platforms for unloading patients
4. Registration area for incoming patients
5. Waiting room with toilet facilities, public telephones, adequate seating, and public information brochures
6. Patient examining units which can accommodate emergency equipment; and sufficient in number to accommodate the average patient load
7. Doctors' and nurses' station
8. Call room for doctors
9. Nearby x-ray facilities
10. Facilities for treatment of fractures
11. Minor surgery operating room facilities, including lighting and scrub sinks, operating table
12. Storage facilities for emergency equipment strategically located and conspicuously labeled
13. A hospital page or call system

equipment and supplies in some central and readily visible area in the emergency room. One-quarter of all hospitals questioned had no such central list of equipment and supplies.

Seventy-one percent of all hospitals studied replied that the function of an emergency department should be restricted to the care of patients with actual emergency conditions. The remainder indicated that the emergency department could legitimately serve other functions such as a screening or general clinic, either full time or when the outpatient department is closed.

Table 4
Supplies for Emergency Use

Oral airways of all sizes	Plaster of all sizes
Pressure dressings	Sphygmomanometers
Surgical dressings of all sizes	Ophthalmoscopes
	Otoscopes
Positive pressure resuscitation equipment	Surgical suture equipment of good quality
Intravenous equipment	Catheterization equipment
Stomach tubes	Pharmaceuticals for emergency use
Oxygen equipment	
Suction equipment	Sterile gloves and drapes
Plasma or plasma expanders	Elastic bandages
	Flashlights
Intravenous solutions	Head mirrors
Splints	Nasal speculi
Tourniquets	Sterile packing of all sizes
Tracheotomy tubes	Syringes and needles of all sizes
Wheelchairs	
Stretchers	Sterile irrigating solutions
Litters	Suture material of various sizes
Crutches and canes	
Chest suction equipment	Thermometers
	Antidotes for specific poisons

In actual practice, however, only half of these hospitals were able to restrict their care to true emergency patients. Half of the hospitals stated their emergency departments routinely performed such functions as caring for hospital personnel or serving as a general clinic. As many hospitals in this survey do not have an outpatient department, the emergency department is forced to assume additional functions.

ALL ASPECTS OF MEDICAL PRACTICE REPRESENTED

Since the demands on emergency facilities now represent all aspects of medical practice, including medicine, surgery, pediatrics, obstetrics, and psychiatry, it is logical that supervision of an emergency service should be vested in a committee representing all clinical services, the hospital administration, and the nursing department. Only one-third of the hospitals had such a committee, and in rural areas the percentage fell to 17 percent. Nevertheless, the activities of individuals working in the emergency department were relatively closely regulated. Nearly half of the urban hospitals placed some restriction upon practitioners performing certain procedures. Only 31 of 114 urban hospitals permitted general practitioners to practice in the emergency department without some restriction of their activities. In rural areas, however, only one-third restricted activities of general practitioners. In only one-fifth was the direct professional responsibility for the supervision of the emergency department assigned to one individual. In the remaining hospitals this responsibility was assumed by the chief of surgery, or assigned on a rotating basis.

Coverage in most hospitals was supplied by rotation of house officers or attending physicians. Screening of the patients to determine which specialty physician should be called was done, in most instances, by a nurse or clerk in those institutions without interns.

Another simple but important matter affecting the smooth functioning of an emergency facility is the posting in the emergency area of a roster of all physicians on call in the various specialties. In this survey, 27 percent neglected to do this.

An emergency department manual is useful in outlining simple procedures to be followed and in serving as a reference source for newly assigned personnel. Only one-third of the hospitals questioned have prepared such a manual, and many neglected to include location of vital equipment and supplies.

A cross-check of the actual functions of the emergency department in the surveyed hospitals was provided by a series of questions on clinical procedures routinely performed in the emergency area. More than half of the hospitals stated such major procedures as the treatment of open fractures and the repair of tendon and nerve injuries were regularly carried out in the emergency department. For such major procedures hospital emergency facilities designed primarily for minor surgical procedures can rarely substitute effectively for a regular hospital operating room.

In addition to the use of hospital emergency units for major procedures, two-thirds of all hospitals questioned routinely permit the performance of elective minor surgery, and four-fifths use this area for nonemergent diagnostic purposes.

The widespread use of emergency facilities for nonemergent purposes can occur only at the expense of decreased efficiency in the care of actual emergencies. One-third of the hospitals surveyed have major operating facilities in the emergency room. In general, major operating facilities in emergency units are found to be impractical and inefficient, but the authors believe that a complete minor operating unit is an essential part of every emergency department. High standards of asepsis, lighting and equipment, and sterile technique should be rigorously maintained, and include surgical preparation of operative fields and the use of sterile gloves and masks. Most hospitals indicated that they adhered to these standards. One-third permit the administration of general anesthesia in the emergency room. Three-fourths are prepared both physically and philosophically to perform thoracotomy and cardiac massage in the emergency room.

An encouraging indication that principles of prevention of disease are being incorporated into routine procedures is the fact that three-fourths of hospitals initiate active immunization with tetanus toxoid as a routine part of the treatment of open wounds in unimmunized individuals. Arrangements are made for completion of this series by virtually all hospitals, but unfortunately the advantage is considerably dissipated by the fact that only one-fifth of all hospitals give the patient a written record of this immunization.

It is interesting that only 77 percent of hospitals relied on desensitization in individuals with open wounds who had never been immunized against tetanus and were sensitive to equine antitoxin. The remaining hospitals stated that such patients were treated with bovine or human antitoxin, antibiotics, tetanus toxoid, or a combination of these agents. Only a small number mentioned adequate wound care as being important in the management of such individuals.

Of all hospitals surveyed 88 percent permit attending physicians on call by the emergency department to submit bills to patients who come there for care and have no private physician. Although such an arrangement seems equitable for the physician, it may lead to misunderstanding by the patient, who may assume that the hospital charge covers all his professional care. This points up the need in emergency departments for brochures containing information for the public.

One-quarter of all hospitals permit physicians to bill patients whom they have not seen, following a telephone conversation with a house officer or nurse. This procedure is undoubtedly misunderstood by many patients and thus contributes to poor public relations for the hospital. Relatively few—32 of 244—of the hospitals questioned charge a separate professional fee for house staff services. This question was probably misinterpreted, as most of the hospitals answering affirmatively were not approved for internship training.

Few circumstances create more criticism of the medical profession than the patient's inability to obtain a physician when an emergency arises. Nearly half (43 percent) of the hospitals surveyed stated that the medical profession through the local medical society or other agency assumed some responsibility for providing emergency care, in addition to that provided by the hospital. This is usually a panel of physicians on call or an agreement for rotation on duty by the physicians of a community. In actual practice the success of such arrangements has been extremely uneven. Of the 30 hospitals commenting on the effect of such local arrangements on emergency department visits, it was discouraging to note that two-thirds felt there was no change in the number of visits due to this arrangement. Only five hospitals noted a definite decrease in emergency department visits, which they thought represented the response to this service; and five hospitals stated that visits were actually increased by the existence of a panel of physicians on call for emergency services.

EMERGENCY DEPARTMENT VISITS DOUBLED

The increase in the use of hospital emergency facilities in recent years was one of the principal factors in undertaking this study. Statistics on emergency services for the nation as a whole were not available until 1954. In the succeeding four years hospital emergency department visits doubled to a total of 17 million in 1958. For hospitals in this survey, the increase between 1945 and 1958 was 120 percent (Figure 2). This increase in emergency department visits did not occur at the expense of outpatient departments,

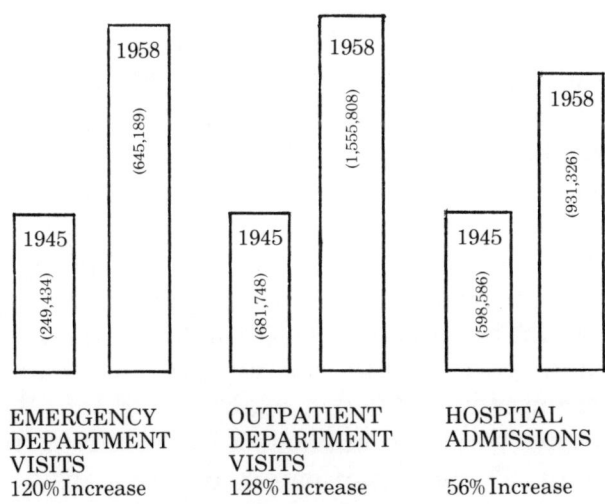

Figure 2. Increase in emergency unit visits as compared with outpatient department visits and hospital admissions is shown.

for the same hospitals reported an exactly equal increase in visits to their outpatient departments during the same period. Nevertheless, emergency department visits accounted for one-third of the total outpatient visits. In contrast to the increase in outpatient visits, the total number of hospital admissions during the same period rose only 56 percent. This disproportionate use of hospital outpatient facilities may represent a substitution, to some extent, of the services formerly performed in the physician's office. This trend is undoubtedly encouraged by physicians who refer patients to the hospital emergency department for care and physicians who use the emergency department instead of their office. This practice is understandable because in most instances facilities for diagnosis and treatment are better in the emergency department than in the doctor's office, particularly for care of acute, serious illness and injury.

Each hospital in the survey was requested to keep a running tabulation of all emergency unit visits for a period of one week. The compilation of these reports showed several interesting aspects of emergency unit care. A breakdown by specialty of 29,300 emergency unit visits at 197 hospitals during one week shows the types of cases seeking emergency care to be as follows: general surgery, 27 percent; medicine, 27 percent; pediatrics, 14 percent; orthopedics, 14 percent; and other, 18 percent. The foregoing confirms the impression of many authorities that the spectrum of emergency care is widening to include all specialties, and that the relative proportion of trauma cases is declining. In this study only 30 percent of emergency unit visits were the result of trauma. These facts have far-reaching implications in terms of physical facilities and coverage by physicians representing all specialties.

It was also noteworthy that the average daily loads were remarkably uniform with only a slight increase on week-ends, although the staff is usually smaller then.

Of all patients visiting the emergency department, 42 percent were considered to have nonemergency problems, and 18 percent were subsequently admitted to the hospital as inpatients.

A breakdown of visits by shifts showed that the day and evening staffs carry the responsibility for the majority of cases: day shift, 47 percent; evening shift, 40 percent; and night shift, 13 percent. Although the case load during the evening shift is almost as great as during the day, personnel is considerably reduced during evening hours.

Although only 14 percent of the patients were pediatric cases, 29 percent were under the age of 15. It was of interest that the increase of 22 percent in Saturday and Sunday visits was due almost entirely to children and adolescents. Adult visits showed no significant increase on week-ends.

The present survey indicates that the increasing number of visits to hospital emergency departments represents a change in function of these facilities rather than a simple increase in visits for accidental injuries. Since two-thirds of all emergency room visits are for conditions other than accidental injuries, the public obviously looks to the hospital emergency department for medical care for a wide variety of illnesses. Actually, 42 percent of all emergency visits were considered by hospital personnel to be nonemergent. Despite this evidence of widespread use of emergency facilities for routine medical care, nearly three-fourths of all hospitals surveyed thought that their emergency facilities should restrict activities to the care of true emergency problems. These conflicting concepts of emergency room function are obviously responsible for many of the problems in emergency department administration, and in relations with the public. Some of these difficulties could be resolved by the formulation of an acceptable definition of emergency department responsibility and function by the medical profession and the hospitals. Once the responsibilities of both of these groups have been delineated, the public should be educated in the proper use of hospital emergency facilities.

Another problem arising from these trends and lack of agreement concerning function is providing coverage in the emergency department, particularly in hospitals without a house staff. This problem has been solved in many hospitals by permitting attending physicians to bill patients they see in the emergency department. Other hospitals pay a stipend to physicians covering the emergency department.

Another possible solution, already used in many areas, is to designate certain hospitals as emergency receiving centers with responsibility for providing emergency care for a specific geographic region. The success of this plan depends primarily upon widespread, repeated publicity aimed at the general public. As occasional patients will still present themselves to hospitals other than those designated, some provision must be made for emergency care in all hospitals. Nevertheless, the saving in expensive physical equipment and in the time of skilled personnel outweighs the practical difficulties.

The most critical period in the treatment of trauma is generally acknowledged to be the time between the accident and the victim's arrival at a medical facility. Unfortunately, medical care during this critical period is frequently given by an individual with inadequate first-aid training. If this situation is to be corrected, the medical profession must assume full responsibility for directly or indirectly supervising the training of ambulance attendants, policemen, and other individuals called upon to render emergency care.

Finally, an important part of the immediate care of the accident victim includes the recording of pertinent observations and a brief description of the treatment rendered. This information should be given to the emergency department physician and become a part of the patient's permanent hospital record.

REFERENCES

1. Kennedy, Robert H. Our Fashionable Killer. Bull. Am. Coll. Surgeons, Mar.-Apr., 1955, 40:73.
2. Hawley, Paul R. Emergency Care, Hospitals, Feb. 16, 1956, 30: 53.
3. Shortliffe, E. C., Hamilton, T.S., and Noroian, E. H. The Emergency Room and the Changing Pattern of Medical Care. N. Eng. J. M (ed.,) Jan. 2, 1958, 258: 20.

# 3. An Emergency Medical Service System: Analysis of Workload*

Barry G. King, Ph.D.

Ellis D. Sox, M.D., C.P.H.

Knowledge of the population, nature and distribution of emergencies, and geography and physical environment of a community is a basic requirement for setting up an emergency medical system and can be used to evaluate existing or proposed systems and facilities. But there have been no such data with which to work. The San Francisco study was undertaken to accumulate samples of these data.

The San Francisco Study

San Francisco has many advantages as a subject of a systems analysis of an urban emergency medical service because of the organization of services and the interest of the department of public health, which operates the emergency hospitals and their ambulances.

A 1963-64 study by the San Francisco Department of Public Health and the Injury Control Program,

*Reprinted from *Public Health Reports,* Vol. 82, No. 11, November 1967.

Public Health Service, was undertaken to develop methodology and data as a partial basis for improving timeliness and adequacy of emergency care systems. The study is concerned with the initial phases of emergency care—from the time the patient is discovered until he leaves the emergency hospital. While the information gathered has certain values unique for San Francisco, the intent has been to obtain data broadly applicable for systems analysis.

The study had five specific objectives.

1. To determine the nature and distribution of emergencies and the workload of the emergency medical services system.

2. To determine the sequence of times from occurrence of injury to discharge of the patient from the system.

3. To analyze the cases of patients who were dead on arrival.

4. To derive a general, predictive mathematical model of the operation of an emergency medical system.

5. To evaluate the method with respect to future studies.

This paper discusses background information and the findings concerning the first objective.

Method and Sample

Staff members of the Injury Control Program were assigned to the San Francisco health department to accumulate reports on emergency patients treated by the San Francisco emergency medical service. The study group was headed by Dr. Walter Clowers, a now-retired medical director, Public Health Service.

For the study, emergency patients were persons treated at emergency clinics, including out-patients, and all ambulance patients. The report forms were filled out by personnel of the emergency services system. Separate forms were used for ambulance and nonambulance patients.

The report on ambulance patients had four sections. Section a, completed by the ambulance steward, recorded home station of the ambulance, site of the emergency, time and circumstances of the run, acquisition of the patient, and transport or reason for nontransport of the patient. Section b, completed by the steward or driver, included personal data on patient, type of emergency, state of consciousness, aid given prior to arrival of ambulance, and action taken by the crew at the the scene and on returning to hospital. Section c, completed by the emergency room nurse, recorded time of emergency and discharge and disposition of the patient. Section d, completed by the physician, called for provisional diagnosis, treatment, condition of patient, and judgment on the urgency for treatment and use of ambulance. The report on nonambulance patients included only sections c and d.

Reports were deposited in a box at each hospital and retrieved by study group personnel who reviewed them onsite and attempted to obtain missing data and verify questionable responses. The census tract in which the emergency occurred was determined and the reports numbered sequentially for each participating hospital. Data reduction and subsequent analysis were done by Public Health Service staff in Washington. Data were collected for 13 months, April 1963— April 1964. The 13th month was included because of omissions and inappropriate responses in the early part of the study. Data were collected from four participating emergency hospitals; Mission Emergency, the emergency station of the San Francisco General Hospital, was not included.

Mission Emergency is not only a unit of the emergency medical system, but also an admission unit for San Francisco General Hospital. To use reports from Mission in this study, it would have been necessary to change the system to separate the receiving and emergency admissions functions.

It has been questioned whether data reported from the four other emergency units were representative of the San Francisco emergency service workload or if the portion of the total emergency calls, about 16 percent, that went to Mission differed in nature from those received by the other four units. While direct evidence concerning differences between the nature and distribution of the workload imposed by the Mission district population and that of the rest of the urban population was lacking, those concerned with the operation of the ambulances and the emergency stations believe that if such differences did exist, they were not meaningful as far as this study is concerned.

Emergency Medical Services System

The 1960 census listed the urban population of San Francisco as 740,316 persons, the San Francisco-Oakland areas as 2,395,098, and the Standard Metropolitan Statistical Area (San Francisco-Oakland) as 2,783,359 (1). Emergency patients of the San Francisco emergency medical service were principally from the urban population. Each health department emergency unit was staffed by a physician, a nurse, and ambulance crews of a medical steward and ambulance driver. There were 51 persons and 16 ambulances. The emergency services operated in an area of 50 square miles at all times. In 1964, the population served by the medical services system included 753,000 residents and 199,000 transients.

Mission Emergency had immediately adjacent supporting facilities. The other four emergency hospitals —Central, Harbor, Alemany, and Park—did not have X-ray or other major medical and surgical facilities required for definitive care. They were not really hospitals, but rather emergency aid stations.

The total cost of operation to the city and county was approximately $1,100,000 per year or just under $1.50 per person in the urban population. No charge was made to persons using this service.

Characteristics of Emergencies

There were 18,350 reports on ambulance patients and 39,470 reports on nonambulance patients from participating hospitals. The 20 percent sample used, every fifth report from each hospital, included reports on 3,431 ambulance runs involving 3,670 patients. Reports on 147 patients dead on arrival were limited to the notation D.O.A. Data on more than 400 additional records were limited because the patient refused treatment or was referred to a private physician. In 98 ambulance runs the patient left before the arrival of the ambulance. Patients were transported in approximately 70 percent of the runs, and items relevant to transport and delivery were not applicable for the other 30 percent. Thus the base number is less than 3,670 for various factors analyzed.

There were 7,894 reports in the 20 percent sample of the nonambulance patients. Data were provided on more than 95 percent of the patients.

Race, Sex, and Age Distributions. The proportion of white emergency patients was nearly equal to the proportion of white persons in the urban population. The proportion of Negroes was more than 1.4 times

Table 1
Ambulance and Nonambulance Patients, by Area of Residence and Race
San Francisco Emergency Medical Service

Area of residence and race	Total		Ambulance				Nonambulance			
			Male		Female		Male		Female	
	Number	Per cent	Number	Per cent	Number	Per cent	Number	Per cent	Number	Per cent
All areas[1]	10,765	100.0	1,846	100.0	1,203	100.0	5,243	100.0	2,473	100.0
White	8,822	82.0	1,492	81.0	951	79.1	4,357	83.1	2,022	82.0
Negro	1,431	13.3	244	13.2	173	14.4	668	12.7	346	14.0
Oriental	338	3.1	66	3.6	58	4.8	136	2.6	78	3.2
Other	174	1.6	44	2.4	21	1.7	82	1.6	27	1.1
Urban San Francisco[2]	9,498	100.0	1,467	100.0	1,054	100.0	4,713	100.0	2,264	100.0
White	7,684	81.0	1,157	79.0	826	78.0	3,875	82.2	1,826	81.0
Negro	1,343	14.1	214	14.5	157	14.9	634	13.5	338	14.9
Oriental	317	3.3	61	4.2	54	5.1	128	2.7	74	3.3
Other	154	1.6	35	2.4	17	1.6	76	1.6	26	1.1
Other[3]	1,267	100.0	379	100.0	149	100.0	530	100.0	209	100.0
White	1,138	90.0	335	88.4	125	83.9	482	91.0	196	93.8
Negro	88	6.9	30	7.9	16	10.7	34	6.4	8	3.8
Oriental	21	1.6	5	1.3	4	2.7	8	1.5	4	1.9
Other	20	1.5	9	2.4	4	2.7	6	1.1	1	.5

[1] Race of 230 patients unknown. [2] Race of 199 patients unknown. [3] Race of 31 patients unknown.

their representation, and that of "others," principally Indians, was four times as great as their representation. Orientals constituted 7.9 percent of the urban population but only 3.3 percent of the emergency cases (Table 1). Among white persons, the percentage of ambulance patients was slightly less than the percentage of nonambulance patients.

The differences in proportion of males and females were less than 1 percent for both white and nonwhite ambulance patients, and not greater than 1.5 percent for nonambulance patients for the races reported. The racial composition of a population may be significant in estimating the workload on the medical system and the location of emergency facilities.

The distribution of emergencies by age of patients showed somewhat more marked differences between ambulance and nonambulance patients (Table 2). Except for persons in the age groups 15-24 years, persons from under 1 year to 35 years constituted a smaller percent of ambulance cases than their representation in the San Francisco urban population. The differences at ages 15-19 and 25-34 are small. The percentage of total cases involving persons 35-84 years was from 1 to 2.6 percent greater than their representation in the population.

The percentages of nonambulance patients in age groups 1-44 years were greater than their representation in the total population; for persons 45-84 years the situation was reversed, with a relatively rapid falling off of nonambulance emergencies.

Types of Cases. Information on the type of emergency was provided by the ambulance crew and for the nonambulance emergencies by a nurse at the emergency hospital. More than 66 percent of 11,000 persons suffered accidental injury, more than 6 per-

Table 2
Urban San Francisco Population and Emergency Patients,
by Age, San Francisco Emergency Medical Service

Age group (years)	San Francisco population		Ambulance patients		Nonambulance patients		Total emergency patients	
	Number	Percent	Number	Percent	Number	Percent	Number	Percent
Total	740,316	100.0	2,950	100.0	7,837	100.0	10,726[1]	100.0
Under 1	12,098	1.6	21	0.7	70	0.9	91	0.8
1-4	47,053	6.4	81	2.7	818	10.4	899	8.4
5-9	50,374	6.8	82	2.8	684	8.7	766	7.1
10-14	47,815	6.5	89	3.0	571	7.3	660	6.2
15-19	42,080	5.7	179	6.1	705	9.0	884	8.2
20-24	49,075	6.6	280	9.4	775	9.9	1,055	9.8
25-34	97,926	13.2	380	12.9	1,233	15.7	1,613	15.0
35-44	101,136	13.7	424	14.7	1,145	14.6	1,569	14.6
45-54	105,875	14.3	461	15.6	896	11.4	1,357	12.7
55-64	93,274	12.6	448	15.2	548	7.0	996	9.3
65-74	63,046	8.5	329	11.1	243	3.1	572	5.3
75-84	26,115	3.5	176	6.0	88	1.1	264	2.5
85 and over	4,449	.6	0	—	61	.8	0	—

[1] Does not include 61 nonambulance patients age 85 and over.

Table 3
Ambulance and Nonambulance Patients, by Type of Emergency,
San Francisco Emergency Medical Service

Type of emergency	Total patients		Ambulance patients		Nonambulance patients	
	Number	Percent	Number	Percent	Number	Percent
Total sample	11,000	100.0	3,184	100.0	7,816	100.0
Assault	641	5.8	183	5.7	458	5.9
Suicide or attempted suicide	100	.9	84	2.6	16	.2
Accidental injury	7,272	66.1	1,707	53.6	5,565	71.2
Traumatic	7,071	64.3	1,637	51.4	5,434	69.5
Motor vehicles	1,279	11.6	838	26.3	441	5.6
Falls	2,090	19.0	582	18.3	1,508	19.3
Other accidents	3,702	33.7	217	6.8	3,485	44.6
Poisoning	201	1.8	70	2.2	131	1.8
Illness	2,987	27.1	1,210	38.0	1,777	22.7
Psychiatric	37	.3	21	.7	16	.2
Alcoholic	300	3.0	79	2.5	221	2.8
Obstetric	51	.5	44	1.4	7	.1
Medical	2,411	22.0	1,040	32.7	1,371	17.5
Not further classified	188	2.0	26	.8	162	2.1

cent were victims of assault or were suicides or attempted suicide, and more than 27 percent were ill. For 5 percent of the total sample, the type of emergency was not stated (Table 3).

Perhaps the most striking features of the distributions were the high proportion of accidental injuries reported for both the ambulance and nonambulance patients and the considerable differences between the proportion of various injuries among ambulance and nonambulance patients. The reports did not list the type of injury or probable cause of death for persons dead on arrival.

Nature of Emergencies. A provisional diagnosis was entered for the 10,361 persons seen by a physician at one of the emergency hospitals (Table 4). Of these patients, 73.7 percent were injured, more than 90 percent of these in accidents. Lacerations and open wounds were the most frequent injuries, with contusions and crushing the second most frequent; together these amounted to more than 40 percent of total injuries. Fractures ranked third. Emergencies resulting from mental, psychoneurotic, and personality disorders, including alcoholism which was responsible for four-fifths of these cases, ranked fourth. Head injuries (excluding facial injuries) were fifth. For 32 percent of the ambulance patients with diagnoses involving alcohol, there were multiple diagnoses with mention of alcohol, and for another 2 percent there were "possible" or "probable" multiple diagnoses with mention of alcohol.

Distribution of Workload. The workload was fairly evenly distributed throughout the week with some increase over the weekend for both ambulance and nonambulance emergencies (Table 5). If the reports in

Table 4
Selected Diagnoses Among Ambulance and Nonambulance Patients,
San Francisco Emergency Medical Service

Diagnosis	Total patients		Ambulance patients		Nonambulance patients	
	Number	Percent	Number	Percent	Number	Percent
All cases	10,361	100.0	2,482	100.0	7,879	100.0
No apparent illness or injury	179	1.7	75	3.0	104	1.3
Injuries	7,632	73.7	1,626	65.5	6,006	76.2
Fractures	686	6.6	303	12.2	383	4.9
Dislocations, strains, sprains	473	4.6	112	4.5	361	4.6
Head injury, except face	612	5.9	210	8.4	402	5.1
Lacerations and open wounds	3,230	31.2	461	18.6	2,769	35.1
Contusions and crushing	1,024	9.9	262	10.6	762	9.7
Foreign body in orifice	437	4.2	5	.2	432	5.5
Burns (except sunburn)	240	2.3	16	.6	224	2.8
Superficial injury	534	5.2	110	4.4	424	5.4
Poisoning	252	2.4	96	3.9	156	2.0
Gas inhalation	26	.3	15	.6	11	.1
Overdose of medicine	159	1.5	63	2.5	96	1.2
Other (including food)	67	.6	18	.7	49	.6
Other injuries; other external causes	144	1.4	51	2.1	93	1.2

Table 4 (Cont.)
Selected Diagnoses Among Ambulance and Nonambulance Patients,
San Francisco Emergency Medical Service

Diagnosis	Total patients		Ambulance patients		Nonambulance patients	
	Number	Percent	Number	Percent	Number	Percent
All cases	10,361	100.0	2,482	100.0	7,879	100.0
Illness						
Allergic, metabolic, nutritional	2,550	24.6	781	31.5	1,769	22.5
Mental, psychoneurotic personality, excluding alcoholism	235	2.3	30	1.2	205	2.6
Alcoholism	652	6.3	167	6.7	485	6.2
Nervous system; sense organs, excluding vascular lesions and convulsions	522	5.0	110	4.4	412	5.2
	389	3.8	139	5.6	250	3.2
Vascular lesions (CNS)	60	.6	51	2.1	9	.1
Convulsions	85	.8	68	2.7	17	.2
Circulatory system	156	1.5	96	3.9	60	.8
Respiratory system	194	1.8	51	2.1	143	1.8
Digestive system	265	2.6	68	2.7	197	2.5
Other	659	6.4	230	9.3	429	5.4

Table 5
Percent Distribution of Workload by Day of Week,
San Francisco Emergency Medical Service

Patients	Sunday	Monday	Tuesday	Wednesday	Thursday	Friday	Saturday	Unknown
Ambulance patients	14.9	13.4	13.1	13.1	14.4	14.0	16.1	1.0
Nonambulance patients	16.1	13.1	13.1	13.7	13.5	14.6	15.9	0
Alcohol mentioned:								
Ambulance patients	10.0	18.2	17.3	12.7	9.1	14.5	17.3	.9
Nonambulance patients	15.5	14.8	14.1	13.6	13.3	14.1	14.6	0
Ratio of injuries to disease among ambulance patients	4:2	2:2	2:2	2:2	2:7	3:4	3:1	—

which alcohol was mentioned are considered separately, the distribution started building up Friday and continued through Tuesday; for the ambulance emergencies, however, Sunday was an exception and showed the second lowest percent in the week. The maximum difference in daily workload for all cases was about 3 percent; the maximum difference for ambulance cases in which alcohol was mentioned was about 4 percent.

The composition of the caseload changed with day of week, with the ratios of injury to disease among ambulance patients highest for the weekend (Table 5).

About 30 percent of all ambulance calls and nonambulance emergency admissions occurred between midnight and noon. The same percent applied to the ambulance patients with alcohol mentioned in their diagnoses. About 40 percent of nonambulance patients involved with alcohol were admitted between midnight and noon. Calls and admissions increased at 4 p.m. to 6 p.m. and reached a peak for ambulance calls between 10 p.m. and midnight, with an earlier peak between 6 p.m. and 8 p.m. for nonambulance admissions (Table 6).

Ambulance Runs

In addition to transporting emergency patients, ambulances were used to transport non-emergency patients and distribute supplies and equipment. Transfer runs, not considered in this study, amounted to an average of 24 calls a day in 1963-64. Further, an ambulance stands by at large fires and during events attended by many people.

Emergency Workload. The average number of ambulance responses per day for the four emergency hos-

Table 6
Percent Distribution of Average Weekly Workload,
by Time of Day, San Francisco Emergency Medical Service

Patients	A.M.							P.M.					
	12:00-1:59	2:00-3:59	4:00-5:59	6:00-7:59	8:00-9:59	10:00-11:59	12m.-1:59	2:00-3:59	4:00-5:59	6:00-7:59	8:00-9:59	10:00-11:59
Ambulance patients	6.7	5.3	2.3	3.7	6.5	7.5	11.1	9.2	13.3	9.6	8.9	15.9
Nonambulance patients	5.8	4.4	2.0	2.1	6.3	10.0	10.7	11.9	12.3	13.6	11.9	8.9
Alcohol mentioned:												
Ambulance patients	5.4	4.5	.9	6.4	9.1	6.4	9.1	7.3	10.0	7.3	13.6	20.0
Nonambulance patients	10.7	7.3	3.2	3.9	7.0	9.2	6.1	6.1	9.0	9.9	16.0	11.6

pitals was at least 43. Central ranked first and Harbor second in the number of runs. The distribution of runs and the reported number of patients per run are shown in Table 7.

Two ambulances stationed at Central for transfer runs were available for reassignment to pick up and transport patients during peak workloads. One of the Central ambulances was available for special assignments and was dispatched to work out of another emergency hospital from 4 p.m. to midnight when needed.

Notification and Dispatch. The notification initiating an ambulance run was received at an emergency hospital for 91 percent of total runs. In about 2 percent the ambulance was dispatched by two-way radio while enroute. Less than 1 percent of the notifications were received at other institutions and 6 percent at other places.

Of the 3,431 runs, the point of origin was the home station about 85 percent of the time and other emergency hospitals 6 percent of the time. Both crew and ambulance were reported available for dispatch without delay in 99 percent of the runs. In 97 percent of the 3,063 runs for which time was recorded, dispatch occurred within 1 minute.

The distances from place of origin to the place of emergency was reported for 2,208 ambulance runs. In more than 55 percent of the runs the distance was less than 1 mile; in 85 percent, less than 2 miles. The distance exceeded 4 miles in less than 2 percent of the runs. In runs of 3 miles or less for which the time is known, approximately 18 percent reached the scene of the emergency within 4 minutes after dispatch, 70 percent within 5 minutes, and more than 99.5 percent within 15 minutes. Detailed consideration of time sequences for the total operation is beyond the scope of this report.

Right-of-way. Information on use of siren, emergency lights, and overriding of traffic controls is known for approximately 3,400 runs. En route to the emergency no signals were used or traffic lights overridden in about two-thirds of the runs. All resources were exercised in about 23 percent of the runs, lights only in 8 percent, and lights and siren in about 3 percent. Use of these devices was not related to distance traveled.

When transporting a patient to an emergency hospital no right-of-way was exercised in more than 92 percent of the runs. All resources were used in less than 3 percent, lights only in about 5 percent, and siren only in less than 1 percent of the return trips.

Table 7
Patients Carried on Each Ambulance Run,
by Home Station of Ambulance,
San Francisco Emergency Medical Service

Patients carried per run	Total runs reported		Number of patients by home station			
	Number	Percent	Central	Harbor	Alemany	Park
All runs	3,431	100.0	1,429	826	539	637
0	979	28.5	353	219	208	199
1	2,218	64.6	995	555	289	379
2	162	4.7	54	38	31	39
3	36	1.0	15	7	6	8
4	19	.6	7	2	2	8
Not stated	17	.5	5	5	3	4

Place of Emergency. There are 3,095 ambulance reports stating the place the emergency occurred. Of these, 35 percent cite the home as place of emergency, 43 percent the street or highway, and 22 percent public buildings, resident institutions, industrial premises, schools, parks, and elsewhere. The percent of runs not completed because of wrong or inadequate address is negligible.

In only a few emergencies were rescue operations by the ambulance crew required to gain access to or free the patient.

Situation at the Scene. The type of emergency, based on information given the crew by the patient, police, other officials, friends, relatives, and people who had witnessed the accident, and upon judgments of the crew, was stated in 3,184 reports (Table 4).

Not less than 9 percent of the patients were either gone when the ambulance arrived or refused service. The condition of the patient when the ambulance arrived was stated for 2,570 persons (approximately 80 percent of the emergencies in which the patient remained at the scene). Of these, 90 percent were reported to be conscious, 6 percent unconscious, and about 2 percent judged dead. Approximately 5 percent of the patients were referred to a private physician.

Time spent on patients not carried by the ambulance is part of the workload. The crew must survey the situation, reassure the patient and others in attendance, and make phone calls when warranted. In about 6 percent of all emergencies, the coroner or a private physician was notified, and his instructions were carried out.

In 67 percent of the emergencies in which the 252 telephone calls were made, the time spent at the scene was 15 minutes or more; in 25 percent, 5 minutes; and in 8 percent, less than 4 minutes. For the 3,106 other emergencies for which the time at the scene is known, nearly 40 percent of the reports showed 15 minutes or more; 30 percent, 5 minutes; and the other 30 percent, less than 4 minutes. If an ambulance remained at the scene longer than 15 minutes, the crew reported to the home station that they were temporarily out of service and confirmed their location.

Patient Management. Three percent of all patients present when the ambulance arrived received emergency care, guidance, and reassurance but required no further treatment and were not transported.

There were 75 patients (about 3 percent) who were transported with no injury or illness apparent and no emergency measures at the scene indicated who did not require any treatment at the emergency hospital (Table 4).

For persons whose treatment at the scene and provisional diagnosis upon arrival at the hospital is known, the most frequent injuries were lacerations and open wounds, head injuries, contusions and crushing, superficial injuries, and fractures of limbs, nose and jaw, skull except face, and spine and trunk. Relatively few instances of illness treated at the scene with subsequent provisional diagnosis are reported; the most frequent are psychoneurosis or psychoses, alcohol, and heart disease.

The listing of emergencies for which a provisional diagnosis was made subsequently at the emergency hospital (Table 4) demonstrates the variety of principal medical conditions with which the ambulance crew may be confronted.

Equipment Used or Needed. The medical equipment and supplies normally carried on the San

Francisco ambulance are listed (Table 13). Queries on the ambulance report called for information on equipment used, missing, or needed but not routinely carried. The question excluded blankets, pillows, poles, and stretchers. Use of equipment or supply items was reported for 781 emergencies (Table 8). Only two reports listed equipment missing—one a pressure bandage, the other a crowbar. Most responses concerning

Table 8
Frequency of Equipment and Supply Use at Scene and En Route to Hospital, San Francisco Emergency Medical Service

Equipment used	Times used	At scene	En route	At scene and en route
Number of patients[1]	781	528	47	187
Wheel chair	1	1	0	0
Emesis basin	3	1	2	0
Oxygen tank	89	12	29	48
Medications	15	11	0	4
Gauze	379	337	3	39
Adhesive	6	5	0	1
Bandage	479	424	3	52
Splint, not otherwise specified	4	3	0	1
Splint, arm	20	19	0	1
Splint, leg	63	55	0	8
Pulmotor	1	0	0	1
Obstetrical equipment	4	3	0	1
Other	69	26	10	33

[1]Number of times equipment used is greater than number of patients because more than 1 piece of equipment could be used per patient.

Table 9
Frequency and Location of Specific Actions Taken by Ambulance Crew, San Francisco Emergency Medical Service

Action taken	Times action taken	At scene	En route	At scene and en route
Number of patients[1]	765	529	47	189
Drugs administered	2	0	0	2
Delirium tremens mix	16	3	0	13
Internal medications or nourishment or both	13	7	0	6
Bandage or dressing applied	439	377	3	59
Splints applied	86	76	0	10
Artificial respiration	5	2	0	3
Heart massage	16	3	3	10
Airway inserted	3	0	2	1
Oxygen administered	112	12	28	72
Put to bed, made comfortable	22	3	0	19
Delivery or assisted at delivery	5	4	0	1
Gave advice to patient or family	68	31	0	37
Supportive care	2	5	3	4
Treatment for or prevention of shock	8	1	1	6
Elevated body or part of body	3	1	2	0
Quieted or restrained patient	4	1	1	2
Treatment attempted, could not be completed	2	1	1	0
Aroused or attempted to arouse patient	1	1	0	0
Cleared mouth of mucus, blood; kept airway open	7	3	1	3
Other	52	24	2	26

[1]Number of specific actions taken are greater than the number of patients because more than 1 action could be taken per patient.

the need for equipment not routinely carried were negative. The affirmative responses which were given in about 1 percent of the cases noted different items such as resuscitators, an inhalator, demerol, and special stretchers. Only one item was mentioned in more than two reports—the resuscitator was mentioned in eight. The number of times that ambulance crews took certain actions and the place where these actions were taken is shown in Table 9.

If an ambulance crew attending an emergency requires supplies or equipment, they radio or phone Central and an ambulance is dispatched with the required items.

Delivery of the Patient. Patients were transported in about 72 percent of ambulance runs, covered by 73 percent of the reports. One patient was carried in about 65 percent of the runs, two patients in about 5 percent, and more than two in about 2 percent (Table 7).

There were 2,253 patient-carrying runs of 3 miles or less for which the time from the site of the emergency to the hospital is known. In 11 percent of the runs, the elapsed time was less than 4 minutes, in 56 percent within 5 minutes, and in 98.5 percent within 15 minutes.

Two-thirds of the runs carrying patients from the scene of the accident returned to their home station (Table 10). Mission was the first alternative to home station and Central the second. The straight line distance from Mission to Central is less than 2 miles, and from Mission to Alemany, Harbor, or Park is 3 miles or less. Delivery to an alternate station nearer to the site of emergency than the home station may be elected in urgent cases. Park and Harbor are within less than 2 miles straight line distance from Central and deliver there as an alternative. Direct delivery to

Table 10
Place to which Patient was First Transported, by Home Station of Ambulance,
San Francisco Emergency Medical Service

Patients transported to—	Total runs		Central		Harbor		Alemany		Park	
	Number	Percent	Number	Percent	Number	Percent	Number	Percent	Number	Percent
All runs	2,455	100.0	1,076	100.0	604	100.0	336	100.0	439	100.0
Home station	1,630	66.4	693	64.4	417	69.0	212	63.1	308	70.2
Mission	432	17.6	232	21.6	72	11.9	93	27.7	35	8.0
Other emergency hospitals	251	10.2	110	10.2	88	14.6	12	3.6	41	9.3
Other	62	2.5	15	1.4	7	1.2	7	2.1	33	7.5
Not stated	80	3.3	26	2.4	20	3.3	12	3.6	22	5.0

Mission may be made when there is some urgency and delivery to the nearest hospital is indicated or when the nature of the injury indicates that the facilities of a general hospital will be needed. In the majority of emergencies the distance will not exceed 4 to 5 miles.

Change in the Patient's Condition. The attempt was made to determine any change in the patient's condition because of handling or management or because of time intervening between injury and obtaining adequate medical care. The report form called for information from the steward concerning care given the patient prior to arrival of the ambulance and for judgment concerning any change in condition of the patient observed at the time of delivery to the hospital. The physician was asked to evaluate early management and judge the influence of elapsed time.

In the 1,825 reports (for about 75 percent of the persons transported) in which the effect of patient management prior to delivery at the hospital was stated, 85 percent had no mention of observable effect of the action taken on the patient's condition. Management having a favorable effect included careful handling of about 8 percent of the patients; bandage or tourniquet applied, 2 percent; splint applied, 1 percent; and all other acts such as assisting respiration, inducing vomiting, and administering drug, less than 1 percent. Unfavorable effects were reported for less than 1 percent of the patients. These resulted from the patients' delay in seeking treatment, rough handling, unnecessary moving, and the like.

The relation of state of consciousness and type of accident was reviewed with respect to change in the patient's condition. No change was observed in 80 percent of the 2,318 patients about whom this information was reported, improvement in about 20 percent, and some deterioration in about 1 percent. A greater percent of those who were unconscious (134 persons) showed a worsening of condition than of those who were conscious (by a factor of 5).

Thirty-five of the 36 persons judged to be dead and transported to the hospital by the ambulance were pronounced dead by the hospital physician. Others judged dead were picked up by the coroner.

The type of injury or illness did not appear to have an important influence on change of condition. From 66 to 75 percent of the patients underwent no change in condition before reaching the hospital. Those patients who improved en route ranged from about 10 percent of those who attempted suicide to about 29 percent of those who were poisoned. Those patients who deteriorated ranged from about 1 percent of those involved in motor vehicle-pedestrian accidents and falls to about 3 percent of the obstetrics patients.

Time Spent at the Hospital. The duration of hospital stay was recorded for 72 percent of the ambulance patients. Approximately 4 percent remained 5 minutes or less; 17 percent, 15 minutes or less; and 30 percent, a half hour or less. About 40 percent of the patients remained from 45 minutes to 12 hours—approximately half for more than 2 hours and 10 percent from 9 to 12 hours. An additional workload was imposed by patients referred to Mission Emergency with its more extensive medical facilities for further emergency care. This type of referral involved not less than 5 percent of the ambulance patients.

Patient Disposition. Forty-five percent of the ambulance patients for which both disposition and provisional diagnosis were reported were sent to their homes upon discharge. About 46 percent were referred for further care and of these, 18 percent were sent to the San Francisco General Hospital for hospitalization or further care, 18 percent to private hospitals, and 10 percent to their own physicians. Six percent were discharged to the police and less than 1 percent each went back to work or were discharged to the coroner.

The referrals were about equally distributed between injury and illness. The patients sent to San Francisco General for hospitalization were predominantly those who were ill, while most sent to other hospitals for hospitalization or further treatment were injured.

The type of transportation by which 2,400 ambulance patients left the hospital is known. Of these, approximately 12 percent left by public ambulance, 12 percent by private ambulance, 6 percent by police vehicle, and 70 percent by other means.

Nonambulance Patients

An average of 143 persons per day were admitted to the four hospitals—100 nonambulance and 43 ambulance patients. This average was essentially in agreement with the average of 148 per day for the four reported in 1962 (2).

Approximately 10 percent of the nonambulance patients arrived in police vehicles; of these, 65 percent were injured (Table 11). Ninety percent arrived by other means, such as walking, public transportation, taxi, or private car. Only four patients arrived by private ambulance.

Of the 7,671 patients for which the information was reported, 87 were judged to have needed an ambulance. Eighteen of these were transported by the police and 67 by other means. The method of arrival was

Table 11
Means of Arrival of Nonambulance Patients, by Nature of Emergency, San Francisco Emergency Medical Service

Nature of emergency	Total		Police vehicle		Private ambulance		Other	
	Number	Percent	Number	Percent	Number	Percent	Number	Percent
Patients	7,847	100.0	778	100.0	4	—	7,065	100.0
No apparent illness or injury	103	1.3	15	1.9	0	—	88	1.3
Injury	5,975	76.1	502	64.5	3	—	5,470	77.4
Illness	1,754	22.4	257	33.0	1	—	1,496	21.2
Dead on arrival	4	—	1	.1	0	—	3	—
Not seen by physician	11	.1	3	.4	0	—	8	.1

not stated for two such patients. More than 70 percent of the patients who arranged their own means of arrival were accompanied by friends, relatives, or the police.

More than two-thirds of the patients for whom time spent in the emergency hospital was given remained for 15 minutes. About 80 percent of all patients were discharged in 15 minutes or less (Table 12). The patients who were referred for further care showed similar patterns but at lower percentages with the distribution shifting to somewhat longer durations.

Three percent of the patients spent 12 hours or more at the emergency hospital. Of the 37 diagnostic categories shown for those spending 12 hours or more, those applicable to more than five persons are laceration and open wounds, 69 patients; alcoholism, 23 paients; contusion and crushing, 20 patients; fractures, strains, sprains, and foreign body in the eye, 13 patients each; superficial injury, 15; head injury except facial, 9.

Seventy percent of the nonambulance patients were sent home and about 20 percent referred for further care. Other dispositions were reported for the remaining 10 percent (Table 12). Of those referred for further care, about 62 percent were sent to their own physicians, 20 percent to the San Francisco General Hospital either for further emergency treatment or for hospitalization, and 18 percent to another hospital.

Discussion

The San Francisco study is the first attempt to do a systems analysis of the operation of an emergency medical service system known to the authors. The intent was to investigate an established system in terms of its components and their interrelations as a basis

Table 12
Time Spent in Emergency Room and Disposition of Nonambulance Patients,
San Francisco Emergency Medical Service

Elapsed time from arrival to discharge	All patients		Patients sent home		Patients referred for further care		Other patients	
	Number	Per cent	Number	Per cent	Number	Per cent	Number	Per cent
Total	7,689	100.0	5,417	100.0	1,492	100.0	780	100.0
5 minutes or less	989	12.9	752	13.8	143	9.6	94	12.0
15 minutes	5,211	67.7	3,748	69.2	931	62.5	532	68.2
30 minutes	752	9.8	490	9.0	184	12.3	78	10.0
45 minutes	235	3.0	144	2.7	69	4.6	22	3.0
1 hour	94	1.2	49	.9	39	2.6	6	.8
1¼ to 2 hours	106	1.4	47	.9	45	3.0	14	1.8
2¼ to 3 hours	21	.3	14	.3	6	.4	1	—
5 hours	28	.4	17	.3	8	.5	3	.4
9 hours	22	.3	10	.2	8	.5	4	.4
12 or more hours	231	3.0	146	2.7	59	4.0	26	3.3

for a general description, such as a mathematical model, suitable for analysis and evaluation of other existing or contemplated emergency medical care systems. Of course, the findings per se are more pertinent to large urban than to rural communities, and considerable caution is essential in generalizing from data specific for San Francisco.

In San Francisco, the workload did not vary greatly by day of the week. The peak loads which occurred on Saturdays and Sundays involved an average of 160 patients for the four emergency hospitals combined. On Tuesday, when the minimum workload occurred, the average was 131 patients. The average of the ambulance runs by day of week did not vary by more than 10. About half the runs for a single day were made between 4 p.m. and midnight.

The crews, ambulances, equipment, and central support personnel constituted one of two principal subsystems within the total emergency medical service system. In operation, however, it interacted with and actively participated in the operation of the second subsystem—the emergency hospital.

The central communication station served all emergency hospitals and performed services for them in addition to receiving emergency calls and dispatching ambulances.

In about a third of the runs, no patient was delivered. When first aid was adequate or action limited to surveillance pending the arrival of a private physician, the ambulance subsystem acted as an extension of the emergency hospital by dealing with a part of its workload. At the hospital, ambulance stewards who are registered nurses serve as nurses, and others serve as aides in the emergency clinic.

In planning or improving community emergency medical services, certain aspects of the San Francisco

Table 13
Standard Equipment Carried by Ambulances

General equipment

1 fire axe	6 towels	1 Thomas splint
1 fire extinguisher, Ansul	4 pieces sheet wadding 6 in. x 2 yd.	4 padded arm-shaped splints
1 crowbar	1 sheet	4 padded, leg-shaped splints
4 stretchers	1 life preserver and 100 ft. rope	1 emesis basin
4 stretcher poles	1 battery lantern	2 restraint straps
4 blankets	2 road flares or fusees	2 oxygen tanks, D-size
2 pillows and cases	2 molded splints	1 oxygen regulator, hose, mask

Maternity grip

1 sterile sheet	Sterile umbilical tape	Coramine, 2 amps.
4 sterile towels	Silver nitrate 1 percent solution, 2 amps.	Montrazol, 2 amps.
1 pair sterile gloves, size 8	Alcohol 50 percent, 4 oz.	1 sterile 2-cc. luer, 2 needles 25 × 5/8
4 peripads	Pituitrin, 2 amps.	4 hemostats
1 hot water bag	Ergotrate, 2 amps.	1 sterile surgical scissors

Antidote grip

Universal antidote, 4 oz.	Ammonia, 4 oz.	Megimide, 1 amp.
Alcohol 95 percent, 4 oz.	Chalk, 4 oz.	Dimercaprol, 1 amp.
Olive oil, 4 oz.	Milk of magnesia, 4 oz.	1 lavage tube

Table 13 (Cont.)
Standard Equipment Carried by Ambulances

Starch, 4 oz.	Metrazol, 2 amps.	1 medicine glass
Acetic acid, 4 oz.	Coramine, 2 amps.	1 tongue forceps
	Sodium pentothal, 1 amp.	1 jaw expander

General grip

1 holocaine ointment	Aminophyllin, 2 amps.	4 eye pads
1 yellow mercuric oxide ointment	Adrenalin, 6 amps.	Gauze 2 x 2; 4 x 4
	Sterile water, 2 amps.	Bandages, 1 in., 2 in., 3 in.
Pyrol, 8 oz.	Nitroglycerin 1/100, 24 tablets	Swabs
Ampojel, 4 oz.	Grade 5 aspirin, 50 tablets	Tongue blades
Peroxide, 4 oz.	1 sterile 2-cc. luer	Adhesive ½ in.; 1 in.
Ringer's solution, 4 oz.	2 sterile needles ⅝ in. x 25 gauge	4 sterile hemostats
Merthiolate, 4 oz.	1 sterile intracard needle, 20 gauge x 3 in.	1 band scissors
Nitrite amyl, 6 amps.	1 tongue clamp	1 sterile surgical scissors
Ammonia, 6 amps.	1 tourniquet	1 sterile bayonet forceps
Metrazol, 2 amps.	1 eye dropper	1 sterile scalpel
Coramine, 2 amps.	1 thermometer	1 intubation tube
Caffeine, 2 amps.	1 sterile tracheotomy set, threaded sutures	

operation warrant consideration from the viewpoint of economy and effectiveness. The single system serves patients with injuries and those who are ill. The combined resources of the system provide flexibility in use of equipment and personnel for emergency calls, transfer runs, and patient management at the scene, en route, and at the emergency hospital; the organization offers career opportunities for personnel and retains most of the benefit of their initial and continued training. Ambulance personnel also stand by at fires and public gatherings, transfer equipment, supplies, and patients, and make vehicle maintenance and repair runs.

Most illnesses and injuries are common to many, if not all, communities and can be predicted from general medical knowledge. Thus, special studies are not needed to determine content for comprehensive training courses. Some conditions, such as extreme heat and cold, venomous reptiles, and various types of industrial or farm hazards are associated with specific environments.

While the proportion and rate of occurrence of the common emergency conditions may be fairly similar in urban and rural communities, such an assumption should be carefully examined in considering a particular community. In applying mathematical models for establishing a community emergency service system, it is desirable to have input data from a number of urban and rural areas to establish similarities and differences.

Determining the training required for an ambulance crew in a given community involves a number of considerations. Civil authorities and local medical societies must consider the community's emergencies in relation to distances, terrain, and location of emergency hospitals or clinical facilities in establishing what ambulance crews will be authorized to do and what training they need to provide the authorized measures.

In remote locations, where acquisition and transport of the patient requires considerable time, more far-reaching authorization may be warranted. Equipment and supplies must be adequate to enable the crew to carry out authorized measures.

Ambulance stewards, however experienced, cannot be expected to be diagnosticians. The emergency care they provide should be the minimum needed to sustain the patient until the physician can take over. Hence, their training should instill judgment of emergencies so that handling of patients will minimize their possible deterioration and reduce suffering. Quite different emergencies may fall within a single category. For example, acute heart failure and head injury may cause difficulties in breathing and make it necessary to transport the patient in a sitting position.

The crew may receive information concerning the condition of the patient from the patient himself as the great majority are usually conscious, as well as from police and others. Such information must, however, be evaluated and does not substitute for the stewards' judgments. The significant number of alcoholics with and without injuries require special caution and a high degree of judgment by the crew. The high proportion of injuries among emergency patients is especially important for community planning in locations lacking specialized facilities staffed with physicians experienced in treatment of trauma.

The priority of communications equipment in the ambulance should be considered with respect to access to a specialized dispatching system and the availability of telephones and of police and fire communication networks. In certain locations direct communication may be essential for en route dispatch, calls for help, obtaining instructions, or alerting clinics or facilities. In urban areas such as San Francisco there is less need for a communication system to dispatch ambulances en route or notify an established emergency hospital to expect an emergency since police-fire emergency networks or public telephones are usually adequate in limited emergencies. In a metropolitan area, however, the toll of injuries may be high in a single emergency and the police and fire network may become overloaded with other emergency control communications and official notifications. A separate channel for emergency medical communications is necessary for such situations so that ambulance personnel can request supplies, reassign equipment, and notify other hospitals to supplement emergency facilities. Radiotelephone equipment is also needed to maintain continuous surveillance over the vehicles within the system.

Not unexpected was the finding that in only a few cases was there evidence of deterioration of patients during transport. Staffing by a professional, full-time crew and the relatively short time spent in acquisition and transport undoubtedly contribute to the satisfactory patient maintenance.

The accumulation of information on cases of individual patients provides input data for developing computer simulation studies on distribution of the workload in the emergency hospital and in other parts of an emergency medical service system. Such data are useful for determining for a moment, or any given period of time, how many people are being transported, waiting for treatment, being treated, or being discharged. If a system has bottlenecks, proposed methods of correction can be tested by computer simulation.

REFERENCES

1. U.S. Bureau of the Census: California, 1960: General population characteristics. PC(1)-68. U.S. Government Printing Office, Washington, D.C., 1961.
2. San Francisco Hospital Conference: Master plan for hospital system operated by city and county. San Francisco, June 1964.

4. Emergency Medical Services: A Systems Approach*

William R. Gemma, M.H.A.

Daniel E. Strayer, M.B.A.

Robert C. Chase, M.S.

Martin D. Keller, M.D.

The problems confronting emergency medical services (EMS) have been the subject of much recent comment across the nation. Ambulance personnel are often insufficiently trained and many ambulances are equipped below the minimum standards recommended by the National Academy of Sciences—National Research Council. Recent publications indicate that less than five percent of the ambulances and equipment meet minimum requirements.[1] Despite the proliferation of health-planning agencies, there is as yet little evidence of success in community planning for emergency medical care. This is partly due to the lack of clear federal guidelines and the lack of coordination between the federal agencies that have program responsibilities in emergency medical services.

*Presented at the Annual Conference on Engineering in Medicine and Biology in Las Vegas, Nevada, in November, 1971.

There has been little evaluation of the many government-funded programs that are now in operation. When such programs have been successful, little effort has been made to adapt proven techniques and capabilities to other communities for the improvement of their emergency medical service systems.

This situation exists despite increased concern on the part of providers and administrators in both the public and private sectors. Federal support for emergency medical programs through the Department of Health, Education and Welfare amounted to approximately $7.7 million in 1970 for programs related to accidental injury, acute illness, poisoning, and hazardous environmental situations.[2] Benefits from this and previous investments in the area of emergency medical services have not been fully realized because of the emphasis on the study of specific cases of trauma, with little attention to the important general problems. What actually constitutes emergency medical care? How can its quality be measured? Further difficulty is introduced by studies of emergency medical services that concern themselves with single elements of the system. Studies focusing on methods for detecting the emergency event, transportation systems, communications systems, and emergency care, tend to fragment over-all consideration of the system. The individual conducting the study and the discipline he represents influence the designation of one component as the "weakest" link in the system. This can result in the recommendation of a variety of partial remedies that may even conflict with one another.

It has become apparent that new methods must be developed to permit a comprehensive, systematic approach to the solution of the problems of management of emergency medical services. In the past, analysis has been hindered by the lack of a conceptual framework and appropriate techniques to examine the data that may be gathered in EMS systems. The lack of uniformity and reliability of these data have indicated the need for improving the reporting procedures.

There is little value in providing improved detection of emergency events and rapid communication and transportation of the patient, if the emergency rooms cannot rapidly deliver the required treatments. All of these elements must be considered simultaneously if we are to have a proper picture of the system. Simulation techniques offer an approach of great flexibility and power for the analysis of these complex and interdependent systems.

A model for the systematic analysis of emergency medical services offers a mechanism for entering information in an organized manner and for analyzing the response of the system to changes in the relevant variables. It can also serve as a tool in decision-making and the planning processes. The present paper describes: (1) the use of a simulation model in the analysis of emergency medical services; (2) the general form of the logic on which the simulation model is based; (3) the character of the input data required; and (4) enumeration of some of the benefits the model provides for health care planners and administrators.

THE MODEL

The simulation model, EMSS II, was developed by Operations Research, Inc. of Silver Spring, Maryland, under contract with the Department of Health, Education and Welfare.[3] It is a complex model that has not yet been tested with real data in an actual community context. EMSS II is a closed, stochastic, event-based simulation. It offers a format for the introduction of data from the moment a call for help is received by a designated community response agency, through the entire process of emergency medical services, to the outcomes of the services. The model divides the emergency medical care delivery system into the following components: 1. Detection and communication: police; fire; other. 2. Transportation: police; fire; other. 3. Treatment: at site; in transit; in treatment facility.

Using real data, or estimates, the model generates patient data; dispatches ambulances to bring patients to the emergency medical facilities; supplies treatments; and allows patients to be admitted to the hospital or discharged, as appropriate in relation to the information entered. Figure 1 presents an abstract of the emergency medical service sequence simulated by the model.

Since EMSS II is a stochastic simulation, based on events that occur through time, it generates outcomes based on probabilities entered into the model. It represents the manner in which the given emergency medical system responds to the demands placed upon it. By design the model provides great flexibility in specifying the geographic and demographic characteristics of the regions served by an EMS system.

Since this simulation model is highly descriptive, it requires entry of real data in a general context.[4] This is true even for a model intended for general utilization, such as EMSS II. For this reason the Columbus Metropolitan Area was selected for preliminary investigation. This community in central Ohio is typical of many middle-size cities in the United States.

LOGIC AND INPUT DATA

Initial specifications of the model divide the system into five subsystems:
1. Patient Generation
2. Detection

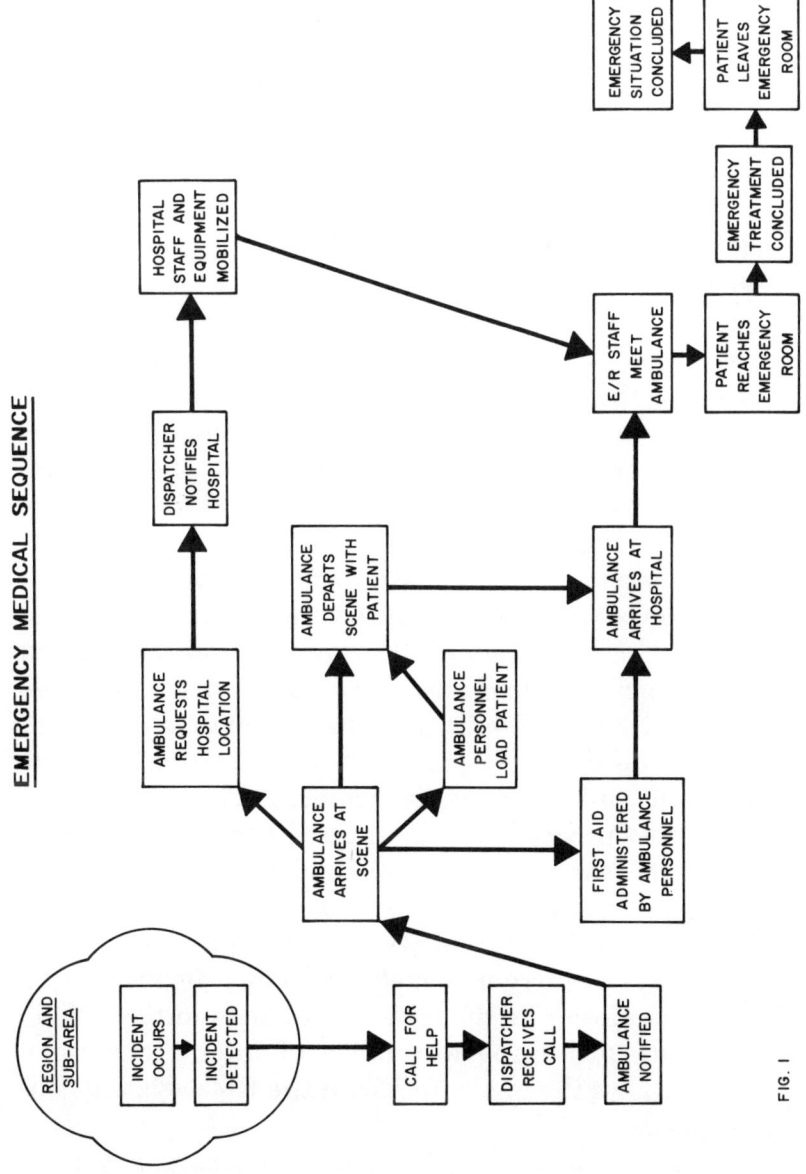

FIG. 1

3. Communication
4. Transportation
5. Treatment

"Patient generation" concerns itself with the factors affecting the demand for emergency medical services. This is determined by experience in the geographic area under consideration. Once the regional emergency medical services characteristics have been specified and the probable number and type of emergency patients estimated, the model can generate demand data. The detection process is simulated by the assignment of random "delays" from the time of the event to the request for assistance, as part of the communication subsystem. Demands are imposed on the transportation subsystem and result in the dispatch of ambulances. The ambulances proceed at "probable speed" to the scenes of the events. Time is then spent at the scene and treatments are administered, as a function of the nature of the emergency medical situations. The ambulances then proceed to designated emergency medical facilities, again at a probable speed. Other possibilities include ambulances returning to the dispatch point, when a decision is made that the ambulance is not required. The ambulances may also proceed to a morgue, if the patient is pronounced dead. These actions and lapsed times simulate the actual operation of the system and indicate the utilization and capacity of the system. Patients arriving at an emergency medical facility demand treatment in relation to the nature of their conditions. This addition to the above complex of interrelated functions allows the model to mirror the EMS system conceptually.

When a stochastically generated emergency of a specified type occurs in a given geographic location, the model of the EMS system must respond with a series of resource commitments. If these resources are not provided promptly, the model indicates that the outcome is unfavorable. The time frame within which the patient must receive designated services is generated as each emergency enters the system. These time decisions are based on estimated means and standard deviations of time for each step until unfavorable results occur. Thus, once entered into the system, the patient and his demands become a parameter for which the various components of the system must provide designated resources within given times. After the transportation subsystem has delivered the patient to the facility, the model compares the patient's demands with the resources available at the given emergency medical facility. Since the operating policies of the facility have a great impact on the delivery of care, the model provides for specification of these policies. In effect, the operating policies are constraints on the ability of a given emergency medical facility to deliver the required services within periods specified.

Required care is defined for each "patient class" as a "treatment description package." The treatment description package (TDP) includes the following information:
1. The patient's priority for treatment.
2. The type of personnel needed and at what stage of the treatment their services are required.
3. The time required to form the treatment team.
4. Additional treatment capability that may be required should the patient's condition deteriorate.
5. Such delays as may be permitted at each stage, without compromising the outcome.

The treatment description package establishes a set of resource requirements specifically tailored for each patient class. The model constructs requirement vectors dealing with treatment capabilities and specifies the operational procedures in the emergency medical facilities. Entry of up to 200 patient classes (cardiac, URI, etc.), eight stages (each requiring a different set of resources to deliver appropriate treatment), and up to 8 "treaters" plus seven additional specialists are permitted by the model.

Upon specification of the patient-care requirements and the resources available in the community to meet these requirements, the model compares the two vectors and generates a "patient history." Resources of manpower are specified in the periodic input data as

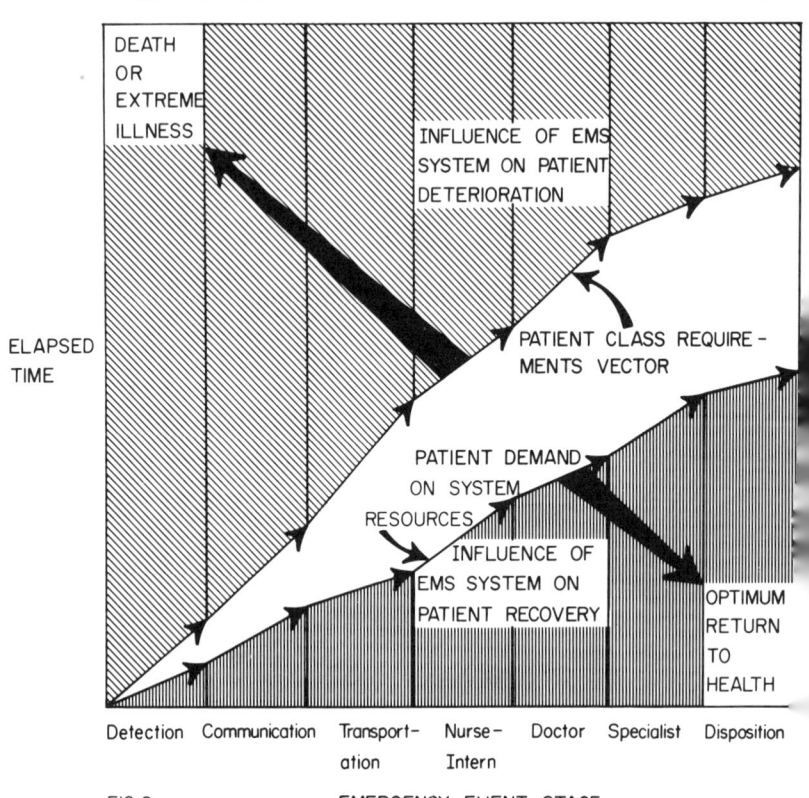

FIG. 2

being "immediately available," "unavailable," or "on call." If treatment personnel or specialists are on call, the model provides for their arrival within specified or stochastically established times. Figure 2 presents a graphic summary of the logic of the model.

The model employs two restrictions in the treatment logic. The first is that each emergency medical facility in the community establishes and maintains similar operating procedures and policies. The second is that all of the patient care resources perform with equal effectiveness. In this sense the model does not realistically portray the provision of health services. What is represented is the availability of health care resources in different component arrays, over varying periods of time. The output data produced by the model will, nonetheless, provide the health planner with an analytical tool of unusual flexibility. In the Columbus Metropolitan Study, the above restrictions are being removed by entry of specific information on the policies and capabilities of each facility.

POTENTIAL OUTPUT

The model produces output information and data which describe the functioning of the community EMS system for a specified period of time. The following classes of output can be obtained from the model:
1. Case Classification
2. Ambulance Utilization
3. Emergency Medical Facility Utilization
4. Sequence of Events in Patient Care
5. Sequence of Events in EMS System

These sets of data may be changed or expanded into other categories, to meet the requirements of various applications of the model.

The total number of patients by case classification

are shown for the chosen time period. This information includes the time-related circumstances surrounding the emergency event and the complex of activities through the treatment at the emergency medical facility and the ultimate disposition of the case.

The ambulance utilization output data include the hours and percentage of use in terms of time spent waiting for assignments, responding to emergencies, transportation of patients, engaging in nonemergency tasks, and standing-by during special emergency situations.

A similar utilization report is prepared for each emergency medical facility specified in the model. Such utilization data include: the number of patients admitted; the number of hours that each medical specialist was present during the reporting interval; and the time spent in the actual treatment of patients. The number of patients who are dead on arrival at the emergency medical facility and the number that may suffer serious consequences from the lack of supportive care while awaiting treatment are also identified in the output data.

The sequence of events in the patient-care category of output is a chronological listing of the events from detection to hospital admission or discharge. This listing allows the tracing of an emergency event through the system and the comparison of the model logic to the investigation of actual events in the community.

The output of the category of sequence of events in the EMS system further identifies circumstances surrounding the emergency event. The location of the emergency situation is indicated in terms of geographic coordinates, and the time delay to the arrival of an ambulance is shown in the output data. The time of occurrence, the type of emergency, and whether the ambulance requirement was met are also included in this category of output information.

The delivery of emergency medical services involves a complex system. Difficulties in studying this system arise in part from the fact that most of the analytical tools available deal with relatively limited problems such as queuing, or inventory of existing resources, or are restricted to single components of the larger system. Because of the importance of this system to our society, more incisive tools are required for evaluation and decision-making. The simulation model discussed herein offers a useful approach to decision-making in emergency medical systems and their components, allowing:

1. Consideration of the environment and its impact on the structure and process of emergency medical care delivery.
2. Rapid analysis of alternative combinations of medical and allied capabilities.
3. Evaluation of alternative methods of organization, supervision, and management of existing human resources and facilities.
4. Consideration of new, untried methods of providing emergency medical care, without the financial cost and social risk of premature implementation.
5. Provision of comprehensive data for evaluation of emergency medical care systems.

In planning future EMS systems, a simulation model allows assessment of the potential impact of such changes as new ambulance bases; relocation of emergency medical facilities; redistricting the area to be covered by one system; alterations of staff capabilities; introduction of new equipment; etc. For the administrator monitoring and managing the system, the simulation model allows assistance in such day-to-day decisions as the purchase of equipment;

changes in staffing of ambulances and facilities; changes in the communication system; and procedural changes in the operation of emergency medical facilities. When major changes are to be introduced into the system the simulation model allows projection of probable outcomes. These can serve as evaluation criteria against which accomplishments can be measured. It is with these possible benefits in mind that a study of EMSS II is being undertaken in the Columbus Metropolitan Area. The information gathered in this study will be generalized for application in other communities concerned with similar problems.

REFERENCES

1. Final report of the Surgeon General's Steering Committee on Emergency Health Care and Injury Control. June 1970. Paul Q. Peterson, M.D., Chairman.
2. Material for the May 27, 1970 Meeting of the Surgeon General's Steering Committee on Emergency Health Care and Injury Control. Paul Q. Peterson, M.D., Chairman.
3. Operations Research, Inc.: Model for the analysis of emergency medical services systems. Division of Emergency Health Services, U. S. Public Health Service, 1970.
4. Van Horn, R. L.: Validation of simulation results. Management Science 17:247, 1971.

5. The Social System of Emergency Medical Care

Geoffrey Gibson, Ph.D.

Introduction: The System Model

When discussing health services today, it is increasingly popular to speak of health care as being organized into a system and to use the "systems" analogy to imply that the various units of medical care are or should be interconnected. The degree of sophistication in using this analogy ranges from a flat assertion that health care at present is a "nonsystem" to the most complex application of modern cybernetic and information theory to health services use. Whatever the level of description, systems analysis has a number of distinct advantages in understanding the network of health services. It is an effective device for integrating knowledge about a particular substantive area and in taking the vital step from mere description of discrete units to theoretical explanation of a set of units interacting to achieve some viable kind of balance or equilibrium. Systems analysis may also provide a much needed theoretical and methodological "market place" and common meeting ground where researchers interested in a particular subject matter but coming from different and increasingly divergent disciplines can each apply their own perspective in a way that refines their own contribution while improving collective understanding.

It is much more theoretically useful to consider a system in general terms rather than limiting it to a specific set of circumstances, such as the provision of health care. A system, then, is a set of units interacting in such a way that over time an equilibrium is achieved such that change in certain system units results in changes in others. This equilibrium can, of course, be either stable or dynamic. Referring to the units as a set implies that they have certain shared characteristics.

A system depends on bringing matter-energy into the system, transforming it through internal processes, and returning the changed matter-energy back into the surrounding environment. In addition to this instrumental process, each system has a high reliance on a parallel expressive process that must bind the system units into a cohesive integrated whole if a viable equilibrium is to be maintained and the system survive. Similarly, every system has an external structure which controls and mediates the relationship between system units and the external environment. This is paralleled by an internal structure oriented towards coordinating the system units as they perform their task functions.

The Health Care System and the Emergency Medical Service Subsystem

The purpose of this article is to attempt to apply this generalized, theoretical systems concept to emergency medical care services, considered as a separate system apart from the provision of all health care services. The emergency medical system is an open system of interrelated units which interact in such a way as to maintain a dynamic equilibrium while also performing general functional necessities for the health care system as a whole. This close interrelatedness between emergency medical services and the wider health care system appears to be an obstacle both to understanding the present burden being carried by hospital emergency departments and to predicting the impact on this sector of proposed changes and existing trends in the total United States health care system. As obvious as this claim seems to be, it is in fact diametrically opposed to the rationale that underlies much of the present thinking and strategies having to do with emergency medical services.

For far too long, emergency medical services have been conceptualized as a separate arena in isolation from other health care services. This implies that the problems of emergency medical services can be solved internally and without recourse to the wider health care system. The opposite is in fact the case: The problems of hospital emergency departments are almost entirely attributable to imbalances elsewhere in the system, and thus these problems are solvable not by internal reorganization of the emergency medical subsystem but only by broad-scale reforms in the wider health care system. The nature and degree of these problems will be delineated later and examples offered from a recently completed study of emergency medical services in the Chicago area.

At this point it is sufficient to indicate the major problem of increased visits to hospital emergency departments throughout the entire country. Table 1 shows that emergency department visits have more than quadrupled over the last 15 years, a greater increase than that experienced by any other unit of the health care system. Even when the population rise has been taken into account, the figures indicate that

Table 1
Utilization Data for Non-Federal, General Short-Term U.S. Hospitals, 1954-1970

	1954	1970	Percent Change
Number of Hospitals	5,212	5,952	14
Number of Inpatient Beds	553,068	864,774	56
Number of Inpatient Admissions	18,391,657	29,370,467	60
Number of Inpatient Days	143,455,065	202,056,026	41
Total Outpatient Department Visits	50,408,617	124,287,646	147
Referred	10,850,922	37,297,792	244
Clinic	26,405,125	44,297,093	68
Emergency Room	9,418,755	42,692,761	353
Emergency Department Visits:			
as a percent of all O.P.D. visits	19%	34%	
per admission	0.5	1.4	
per bed	17	49	
per inpatient day	0.06	0.21	
per hospital	1,807	7,172	
per 1000 population	58	212	

Source: American Hospital Association, *J.A.H.A.*, Guide Issues, Volume 29, Number 8 (1955) and Volume 45, Number 15 (1971).

while in 1954 there were only 58 visits to hospital emergency departments per 1000 population, by 1970 this had risen to 212.

Although this increase in visits related to population is a truly substantial one, it must be remembered that emergency room visits comprise a small proportion of *all* physician visits in the United States, about five percent. As the following data indicate, however, emergency room visits are a major source of health care for certain segments of the U.S. population. Table 2 reports data available from the Health Interview Survey of the National Center for Health Statistics. Unfortunately, the Health Interview Survey does not distinguish hospital clinic visits from hospital emergency room visits by demographic characteristics although the total of 77.3 million visits to hospital clinics and emergency rooms is acknowledged to comprise 20 million emergency room visits and 57.3 million clinic visits.

Table 2 shows that while on average only nine percent of physician visits over-all take place in a hospital clinic or emergency room, for nonwhites the proportion is a quarter. For families with less than $3,000 annual income it is 14 percent; for separated persons, 20 percent; and for individuals with less than five years formal education, 14 percent. Clearly, when these characteristics are combined, the proportion of all physician encounters which take place in a hospital emergency room increases even further, particularly when coupled with residence in a large city. The population of several inner-city areas in Chicago receives well over two-thirds of its ambulatory health care in hospital emergency departments.

Even if visits to hospital clinics are taken into account, it is apparent that these are not independent of the emergency room and in fact represent in large

Table 2
Percent Distribution of Physician Visits by Site of Visit

Characteristic	Mean Physician Visits per Year	Site of Visit				
		Office	Home	Hospital Clinic/ Room	Company/ Industry Health Unit	Telephone	Other/ Unknown
All persons	4.3	71.8	3.3	9.3	0.8	11.3	3.4
Sex							
Male	3.8	70.4	2.9	10.1	1.5	10.9	4.1
Female	4.8	72.8	3.5	8.7	0.3	11.7	2.9
Age							
Under 5 yrs.	5.7	60.0	2.4	10.0	*	23.4	4.2
5-14	2.7	65.6	2.5	11.5	*	16.8	3.5
15-24	4.0	71.7	1.3	10.1	0.9	9.6	6.4
25-34	4.4	74.3	1.3	10.7	2.4	8.7	2.5
35-44	4.3	77.8	1.4	8.9	1.1	7.8	2.9
45-54	4.3	76.8	2.7	9.3	*	7.5	2.8
55-64	5.1	77.4	4.2	7.4	1.5	6.8	2.6
65-74	6.0	76.4	8.0	6.2	*	6.9	2.3
75 and over	6.0	69.3	14.9	5.6	*	9.2	*

Table 2 (Cont.)
Percent Distribution of Physician Visits by Site of Visit

	Mean Physician Visits per Year	Site of Visit					
Characteristic		Office	Home	Hospital Clinic/ Emergency Room	Company/ Industry Unit	Company/ Industry Health Unit	Other/ Unknown
Family Income							
Under $3000	4.6	68.9	5.4	13.6	*	6.2	5.5
$3000-$4999	4.1	70.6	3.8	12.3	*	8.9	3.9
$5000-$6999	4.2	70.8	2.8	10.3	0.9	12.0	3.1
$7000-$9999	4.3	72.8	2.0	7.5	0.8	13.8	3.2
$10,000 and over	4.6	73.9	3.1	6.1	1.2	13.2	2.5
Race							
White	4.5	72.9	3.4	7.7	0.8	12.0	3.2
Nonwhite	3.1	60.3	2.2	25.8	*	4.0	6.3
Education of Head of Family							
Under 5 years	3.7	71.9	6.0	13.8	*	3.8	4.1
5-8 years	4.0	75.9	3.8	10.3	*	7.3	2.1
9-12 years	4.3	71.1	2.5	9.7	1.1	12.1	3.5
13 years or more	5.0	70.0	3.2	7.0	0.6	14.9	4.3

Table 2 (Cont.)
Percent Distribution of Physician Visits by Site of Visit

Characteristic	Mean Physician Visits per Year	Site of Visit					
		Office	Home	Hospital Clinic/ Emergency Room	Company/ Industry Health Unit	Telephone	Other/ Unknown
Marital Status (17+ yrs.)							
Married	4.8	77.0	2.9	8.1	1.3	8.3	2.4
Widowed	5.7	72.0	9.2	8.5	*	8.0	1.9
Divorced	5.1	72.2	*	8.9	*	9.2	*
Separated	5.8	62.1	*	20.1	*	*	*
Never married	3.7	70.3	3.3	10.2	*	7.3	7.7
Residence							
All metro areas	4.5	69.6	3.5	9.7			17.1
Large metro areas	4.7	68.3	4.5	10.3			16.8
New York	4.8	62.4	9.4	12.1			16.0
Los Angeles	5.1	79.3	*	4.8			14.2
Chicago	4.6	70.7	*	8.5			19.7
Philadelphia	6.2	64.7	5.8	10.3			19.3
Detroit	3.5	79.2	*	12.6			*

Table 2 (Cont.)
Percent Distribution of Physician Visits by Site of Visit

Characteristic	Mean Physician Visits per Year	Site of Visit				
		Office	Home	Hospital Clinic/ Emergency Room	Company/ Industry Health Unit	Telephone	Other/ Unknown
San Francisco	5.4	67.5	*	16.7			14.0
Boston	4.2	53.8	*	17.5			20.1
Washington	5.1	59.5	*	9.7			30.1
St. Louis	4.3	66.5	*	14.8			15.5
Other metro areas	4.3	71.3	2.2	8.9			17.5
Outside metro areas:							
Nonfarm	4.1	75.5	2.8	8.5			13.2
Farm	3.3	82.9	*	7.7			7.1

*Figure does not meet standards of reliability or precision

Source: National Center for Health Statistics, *Volume of Physician Visits: U. S. July, 1966—June, 1967,* Series 10, Number 49, Washington: United States Department of Health, Education and Welfare, November 1968.

measure follow-up care for a condition initially treated in the emergency room. In the city of Chicago, for example, no less than 60 percent of all hospital clinic visits were generated by emergency department referrals. Similar figures can be given for the impact of the emergency department on the inpatient ward of a hospital. Thus, for the 80 general hospitals in Cook County, Illinois, about one-fifth of all hospital inpatient admissions come through the emergency department. And since such emergency admissions have a length of stay half as long as other admissions (15 days vs. 10 days), the emergency room generates approximately one-third of all inpatient days.

From these initial data, it is apparent that emergency room visits are increasing at an extremely rapid rate, that for underprivileged segments of the population a substantial proportion of all physician visits take place in the hospital emergency room, and that the emergency room has emerged as a critically important entry point for the health care system in general and the hospital in particular. Why should this increase have occurred? Contrary to some suggestions, it is *not* because of an increase in emergencies *per se*. Indeed, a major related problem of the emergency room is precisely the increase in patients with nonemergency conditions.

One of the most significant findings from the Chicago Survey[1] is shown in Table 3. During interviews with about 4000 emergency department patients at the 80 hospitals in Chicago and suburban Cook County, the attending physician for each patient was asked to rate the clinical emergency represented by the case just treated. He was asked to rate in terms of the following categories:

A. Emergent: Requires immediate medical attention. Delay is harmful to patient. Disorder is acute. Po-

tentially threatens life or function.
B. Urgent: Requires medical attention within a few hours. Danger if not attended. Disorder is acute, but not necessarily severe.
C. Nonurgent: Does not require the resources of an emergency room. Disorder is minor or nonacute in severity.
D. Scheduled: Procedure planned in advance.

In the judgment of the attending physician, well over half of these patients did not represent clinical emergencies nor did they need the specialized resources of a hospital emergency department. Significantly, this proportion was higher in the city (50 percent) than in the suburbs (37 percent). In the ghetto areas of the city it rose even further to between 60 and 80 percent. Typically, for these 3,000 patients the precipitating incident was nontraumatic and care was not sought immediately. Only 15 percent came by ambulance while

Table 3
Distribution by Clinical Emergency Rating of Emergency Department Patients Interviewed

Emergency Rating by M.D.	Chicago		Suburbs		All of Cook County	
	Number	Percent	Number	Percent	Number	Percent
Emergent	191	10%	109	10%	300	10%
Urgent	803	40	580	53	1383	45
Nonurgent	809	40	293	27	1102	35
Scheduled	194	10	103	10	297	10
Total	1997	100%	1085	100%	3082*	100%

*excluding 686 no data cases
Source: Gibson, et al., *Emergency Medical Services in the Chicago Area,* Center for Health Administration Studies, University of Chicago, 1970.

47 percent drove themselves and fully 10 percent walked or came by public transportation. These are not the characteristics of severely traumatized patients nor even of those with clinical emergencies. Nor does the situation in Chicago seem to be atypical of other metropolitan areas. Kirkpatrick and Taubenhaus[2] reported that only 36 percent of the emergency department patients at Boston City Hospital were rated as emergencies by physicians. Lee, Solon, and Sheps[3] rated only seven percent of cases at the Beth Israel Hospital emergency room in Boston as emergencies, under 55 percent as "urgent," and 38 percent as "nonurgent." White and O'Connor[4] used the same categories as the Chicago Survey to rate 3957 emergency room patients at Saginaw General Hospital, Michigan and indicated that three percent were emergent, 57 percent urgent, 36 percent nonurgent, and three percent scheduled. At the Yale-New Haven Hospital, Lavenhar, Ratner, and Weinerman[5] categorized 2,028 consecutive registrations at the emergency room as seven percent emergent, 35 percent urgent, and 57 percent nonurgent. Clearly, whatever the reasons for increasing emergency room utilization, a rise in emergencies is not one of them—although the high proportion of nonurgent use is a useful insight in discovering the actual reasons as well as in delineating problems associated with increased use.

To clarify the reasons for increased emergency room use, let us utilize the concepts of system boundary and entry points. A system generically has a *boundary* with physical and social-psychological parameters which defines for both the entry points and the potential entrants the range of eligible conditions or statuses to be accepted. At various places on the boundary there are entry points or *ingestors* which select and bring into the system matter-energy from the environment. In the system we are discussing, the ingestor is the initial encounter in the emergency room, the matter-energy (or ingestee) is the potential patient, and the social-psychological parameters are the potential patient's attitudes and beliefs as to what constitutes an appropriate emergency room visit.

Associated with the system boundary, but outside of it, are what could be characterized as *zones of predisposition*. These are constituted by a set of factors such as the readiness of a particular patient to seek emergency room care should the need arise and the availability of an emergency room to him. This concept of zones of predisposition will be discussed separately from that of boundaries.

Boundaries

In discussing emergency room use, let us begin with the concept of system boundary. Generally, what is meant by boundary maintenance in a system is the process and properties that allow a set of interacting units to achieve internal cohesion by creating physical and nonphysical barriers between themselves and the external environment. The functional problem is that without such barriers to unrestricted entry to the system, the units may be overloaded by an excessive volume of client input or malintegrated by too great a range of heterogeneous input. Thus, an emergency department with its finite number of treatment rooms and of physicians may be faced with so great a number of patients seeking treatment that either the waiting time must be increased or the treatment time decreased to professionally unacceptable levels. Similarly, the range of conditions presented by patients may be so great, ranging from the trivial to the fatal, that the specialization and homogeneity upon which a physician and his setting depend for efficiency and quality of patient care are seriously threatened.

Although most systems are dependent in some sense on the environment, they vary greatly in their ability to generate resources internally and thus to be "resource autonomous" from the environment. The less the autonomy of a system in this sense, the more delicate the balance must be between controlling entry and facilitating the flow of resources into the system. As a system, hospital emergency rooms have very little autonomy. The double bind is, of course, that on the one hand emergency department resources function most efficiently with a highly specialized intake of clinical emergencies while, on the other hand, achieving this goal necessitates turning away nonemergencies, which in turn means forfeiting available environmental resources in the form of Medicare, Medicaid, and other third-party reimbursements as well as the possibility of law suits with the attendant loss of the hospital's license for refusing service.

In any system, boundaries must be defined so that clients are admitted to the system who are within the range of tolerance appropriate to the specialized system units. In the case of the emergency medical system, it ideally should be able to establish physical and nonphysical boundaries so that only appropriate medical emergencies are admitted. Then the system could maintain a stable and viable equilibrium operating at maximum efficiency. In order for this ideal to occur, the boundary must be such that a consensus exists between patients and physicians as to the limited range of medical conditions that make a patient an eligible candidate for entry to the emergency medical system. The resources of the system (ambulances, surgical residents, diagnostic equipment, etc.) are specialized and specifically prepared to deal with emergency conditions on an around-the-clock basis. The entry of nonemergency conditions which should have been coped with by the wider health care system imposes a severe environmental stress on emergency rooms.

Such a consensual boundary depending on shared norms and expectations rather than on physical boundaries or categorical eligibility is substantially more important to an emergency medical system than to most other systems because of one unique characteristic. The hospital emergency room cannot control its intake. Any patient may present himself for treatment in the emergency room and must be seen and examined for reasons of legal liability. This patient-determined entry does not characterize any other aspect of hospital activity nor any other treatment setting in the entire health care system. A person can only be admitted by a physician as an inpatient; as an outpatient he must either be referred by a physician or, in the case of a charity clinic, be evaluated for entry by a long interview to determine his financial eligibility and medical need. Similarly, most other service systems can control entry—even if it is to the limited extent of determining the hours of intake. A private doctor's office may delay an appointment for several days or refuse to take any new patients. Commercial service systems can insist on proof of the potential customer's ability to pay. Public Aid offices are only open between certain hours and operate with fixed criteria of eligibility. None of these options or restrictions are open to the hospital emergency room. It is open 24 hours a day. It may not insist on the potential patient's showing he can pay for the necessary treatment. It cannot defer the encounter nor impose geographic, social, or clinical standards of eligibility. Even the "queuing" option used by most service systems to adjust and space input to capacity has limited applicability since a true emergency may be overlooked. Any person at any time may enter the emergency medical system purely on his own initiative. In other words, boundaries to admit only appropriate cases to the emergency system do not exist. A consensus by patients and doctors as to the range of medical conditions for system entry has disappeared, if indeed it ever existed. As a result, no one with any knowledge of either systems analysis or present day health services could seriously suggest that the emergency medical system now exhibits a stable or even a viable equilibrium. Thus physicians accuse patients of abusing the emergency room by seeking treatment in it for relatively trivial complaints. Hospital administrators accuse doctors of abusing the emergency room by referring their private patients to it at night or on weekends rather than making house calls. Fiscal comptrollers of hospitals are critical of insurance companies for defining an emergency visit for reimbursement purposes as a visit for an accident only or within a narrow time range following the precipitating incident, thus depriving the hospital of revenue for noninsured conditions. Many hospital emergency rooms have prominent wall signs stating: "This is an emergency room, not a private doctor's office. Come here for emergencies but see your private doctor for nonacute conditions." Yet they allow private physicians to use the emergency room to see his regularly scheduled private patients. More often than not the extra expenses incurred by the hospital as a result (additional nurses, and coverage of X-ray and laboratory facilities) are not met by either these physicians or his private patients. Clearly, there is not a shared set of beliefs among patients, physicians, the hospital, and third-party payers as to the role of the emergency room and the definition of its appropriate utilization.

Zones of Predisposition

The preceding section indicated that the boundary of the emergency medical system is not well delineated. Indeed, Miller[6] argues that groups and systems of a higher order than cells and organisms "have no common matter-energy boundary at all beyond those of individual members," although he does concede that they do have a common information boundary. In view of this, it may well be that there is, for certain systems, an intermediate area between the environment and the system boundary. I believe that this is the case for the total health care system and for the emergency medical system in particular. It is this intermediate area that has previously been described as the zone of predisposition.

Although similar to some existing formulations of the illness referral system, the zone of predisposition is more than an amalgam of them. It is the sum total of beliefs held latently by an individual or group of individuals which come into play when a symptom occurs and which guide him to a particular entry point in the health care system. It constitutes a cognitive map of meanings and cues that enables a person to place a behavioral event into a conceptual set and to organize his perception of this event in such a way that it calls for specific action on his part.

Zones of predisposition vary from person to person and have other aspects as well. In general, they have two types of focuses: a symptom and a system entry point. Thus, there is a zone of predisposition associated with each type of symptom which cues a person as to the significance of that symptom and the immediacy with which he should seek professional care in response to it. Zones of predisposition with a symptom focus are well documented and their sources of variation (income, race, ethnicity, education, etc.) are known. This is not, however, true of the zones which are focused on particular system entry points (i.e., the set of beliefs as to the appropriate medical conditions that make one eligible for entry at a particular treatment site).

At a time when medical leaders are critical of so-called abuse and political leaders are debating the effect of national health insurance on utilization, it is as surprising as it is depressing that there should be so little research addressed to the problem of defining the parameters of perceptual boundaries for service units in the health care system. Many assumptions are made in health planning about appropriate or rational response by patients in seeking medical care for given symptoms, yet little is known about the validity of these assumptions. Of course, we know a great deal about whether a patient does or would seek a physician in response to particular symptoms. But much more specific information is needed with regard to zones of predisposition, including the medical setting in which a physician would be seen and the immediacy with which his help would be sought in response to a given symptom. The planning and location of supermarkets in this country depend on market research a great deal more sophisticated than asking a housewife if she would go shopping if her family were hungry. And yet this, for the most part, is the present state of knowledge about health shoppers.

Zones of predisposition have a second aspect. There is a whole set of physical characteristics of a person's environment that impel him into the emergency medical system. These characteristics constitute zones of structural predisposition (as opposed to the zones of perceptual predisposition previously outlined), and they include the following:

1. Environmental violence or such other aspects of an individual's environment that are likely to generate emergency medical incidents as exposure to automobile injuries, physical assaults, job injuries, home accidents, etc.
2. Access to alternative medical care other than a hospital emergency department. This includes such aspects of the environment as the availability of private physicians willing to treat emergencies by house calls, the ratio of general practitioners to specialists as an indicator of the availability of nonhospital-based primary care physicians, and the net influence of an individual's health insurance status in reimbursing him at various treatment sites.
3. The structural attachment of the individual to the general health care system, which includes such dimensions as whether the person has a stable relationship with a private family doctor or a hospital outpatient clinic.

Just as the zones of perceptual predisposition have two subdivisions—symptom and treatment site—the zones of structural predisposition may be delineated into those structural attributes of the physical environment which, first, influence the incidence of precipitating medical episodes and, second, influence the choice of the hospital emergency room over alternative treatment sites for the clinical care of the episode. Figure 1 clarifies this relationship and serves to summarize this discussion of zones of predisposition.

If these theoretic formulations concerning the use of hospital emergency rooms have any empirical validity, they ought to be able to predict statistically different levels of utilization among population subgroups. Indeed, in the face of the increasing number of visits to hospital emergency departments and the complex

Figure 1

Zones of Predisposition

	Zones	
	Structural	Perceptual
Symptom	1. Patient falls "sick" with a symptom	2. Patient's attitude toward seeking care for this symptom
Treatment Site	3. Availability of competing treatment sites	4. Treatment site appropriate for given symptom

pattern of differential use by segments of the population, this matter of predicting the number of visits from knowledge of basic population parameters in a community is one of the most important priorities in contemporary ambulatory health care planning. It is perhaps the one technique that would enable health agencies to move beyond the present practice of reacting to utilization changes after the event to planning for future changes. If, as suggested by our model, emergency department utilization is a function of: (1) the occurrence of precipitating medical incidents; (2) blocked access to treatment sites other than the emergency room; and (3) structural isolation from the private health care system, then the next step is to choose measurable indicators of these concepts and examine whether differences in these indicators are related to differences in emergency room utilization. Given the availability of U.S. Bureau of the Census data and the indications in the literature on health care, the following measures have been developed for each concept:

1. *Occurrence of Precipitating Medical Incidents:*
    a. percent of population under 18 years of age or over 65;
    b. percent of housing that is substandard;
    c. percent of households with more than one person per room.
2. *Blocked Access to Alternate Treatment Sites:*
    a. percent of population nonwhite;
    b. median family income per year;
    c. private physicians per 1000 population.
3. *Structural Isolation from Private Health Care System:*
    a. median years at school;
    b. percent of population living in a different house five years previously;

c. percent of emergency department patients with a private family doctor.

These measures are available from the 1960 Census and other sources for each of the 75 Community Areas in Chicago. Emergency room utilization rates have also been obtained for each area. Table 4 indicates utilization rates for these Community Areas ranked by quartiles on several of these measures and shows

Table 4
Quartile Rankings of 75 Chicago Community Areas and Hospital Emergency Department Utilization

Quartile Rankings	Mean for Ranking Variable	Emergency Room Visits per 1000 Population (1969)
Median Family Income (1959)		
1	$10,773	15.1
2	9,092	14.6
3	8,051	20.4
4	5,664	45.9
Percent Nonwhite (1960)		
1	33.8%	36.1
2	10.0	29.8
3	2.6	17.8
4	1.0	12.1
Percent over 65 years of age (1960)		
1	13.5%	17.9
2	10.5	21.8
3	8.8	25.0
4	5.4	38.8
Percent Substandard Housing (1960)		
1	83.3%	49.3
2	16.5	21.7
3	0.9	15.7
4	0.1	8.5

strong positive associations between family income, percent nonwhite, percent substandard housing, and utilization as well as a negative relationship with percent over 65 years of age. This negative relationship is due to the fact that residents of the Black communities are much younger on average and is not a true correlation with age. Unfortunately, variations in total utilization rates by quartile rankings of Community Areas is not entirely satisfactory because, first, it is a relatively weak statistical test and, second, it does not distinguish between urgent and nonurgent utilization.

Table 5 presents the Pearsonian correlations between similar measures and three types of emergency room utilization: total utilization, nonurgent utilization (the combination of physician-defined categories

Table 5
Correlation Matrix for 1969 Emergency Room Utilization Per 1000 Population of 75 Chicago Community Areas

Community Characteristic	Total E.R. Utilization Rate	Cook County Hospital E.R. Utilization Rates	Nonurgent E.R. Utilization Rate
Percent nonwhite	.86	.77	.82
Median family income	-.58	-.55	-.53
Percent of population under 18	.33	.36	.27
Percent living in a different house	.54	.47	.50
Median school years	-.29	-.37	-.31
Percent overcrowded households	.67	.66	.60
Private M.D.'s per 1000 population	-.08	-.02	-.06

of "nonurgent" and "scheduled procedures"), and utilization at Cook County Hospital (an inner-city public hospital used predominantly by low income and nonwhite population groups). With the exception of the last row of coefficients (private M.D.'s per 1000 pop.), all correlation coefficients are statistically significant at the .01 level. Clearly, percent nonwhite, family income, overcrowding in housing, and geographic mobility are powerful determinants of both total emergency room utilization and its nonurgent component. Percent nonwhite is such a powerful determinant with a known high association with the other causal variables that the independent effect of these other variables can only be seen by holding it constant as a control variable.

This is done in Table 6 which partials out the effect of race. The obvious result is that by doing so the influence of all other variables (with the exception of education) disappears so that from the seven predictor variables examined only race and education may be said to exert a substantial independent influence on emergency room utilization. This may be seen from the following predictive equations calculated by stepwise regression analyses of our 30 predictor variables:

1) Total Emergency Room Utilization =
   408.9 + 3.0 (% nonwhite) - 14.7 (school years) - 1.6 (% with family M.D.)
   s.e. 87.0   0.4   7.5   0.6
   t.   4.7   7.6   - 1.9   - 2.9
   $R^2 = 0.78$

2) Emergency Room Utilization at Cook County Hospital =
   295.9 + 2.2 (% nonwhite) - 34.3 (school years) + 1.7 (% white collar)
   s.e. 87.2   0.2   11.8   1.0
   t.   3.4   10.0   - 2.9   1.7
   $R^2 = 0.65$

3) Nonurgent Emergency Room Utilization =
   274.4 + 1.9 (% nonwhite) - 11.9 (school years) - 1.2 (% with family M.D.)
   s.e. 65.7   0.3   5.7   0.4
   t.   4.2   6.3   - 2.1   - 2.8
   $R^2 = 0.73$

In both Tables 5 and 6 the influence of M.D.'s per 1000 population (as a measure of private physician

Table 6
Partial Correlation for Emergency Room Utilization Controlling for Percent Nonwhite

Community Characteristic	Total E.R. Utilization Rate	Cook County Hospital E.R. Utilization Rates	Nonurgent E.R. Utilization Rate
Median family income	-.17	-.18	-.09
Percent of population under 18	-.09	.04	-.18
Percent living in a different house	.04	.01	-.008
Median school years	-.23	-.33	-.25
Percent overcrowded households	.02	.15	-.12
Private M.D.'s per 1000 population	-.009	.07	-.005

availability) on utilization was disappointingly negligible. Since the original concept this variable sought to measure was "blocked access to alternate treatment sites," it may be that a more appropriate measure is the balance between specialists and generalists among the physician population, or rather the availability of primary care physicians in alternate treatment sites for nonurgent conditions. Unfortunately, such measures are not available for the 75 Chicago Community Areas, although they are for the seven counties which make up the Chicago Standard Metropolitan Statistical Area. Table 7 indicates that the correlation between these variables and emergency room utilization for selected years is positive for the availability of specialists and negative for that of general practitioners. Interestingly, the availability of hospital-based physicians (which may be taken as a measure of the extent to which hospitals rather than pri-

Table 7
Correlations between Physician Availability and
Emergency Room Utilization per 1000 Population for
Seven Chicago S.M.S.A. Counties

Physician Availability Measures for Selected Years	1960	1965	1967
Total M.D.'s per 100,000 population	0.87**	0.92**	0.83**
Specialist M.D.'s per 100,000 population	0.58	0.77*	0.80*
Hospital-based M.D.'s per 100,000 population	0.93**	0.89**	0.81*
Percent General Practitioners	−0.40	−0.79*	−0.80*

*$p < .05$ **$p < .01$

vate physicians provide primary medical care) produces high positive coefficients with total utilization. In general, Table 7 confirms the model that emergency room utilization is in part a negative function of the availability of primary medical care from private physicians in contrast to hospital emergency departments.

Entry Points: Ingestors and Input Transducer

Thus far, boundaries and zones of predisposition have been described as generic features of systems and applied to the notion of an emergency medical system. Both features point to the process whereby the system takes input from the environment—in this case, how and why patients enter the emergency room portion of the health care system. From this discussion it is clear that key aspects of any system are those areas in the boundaries which allow this input to cross over from the environment (or rather that intermediate part of the environment called zones of predisposition) into the system. Such entry points may be categorized as either ingestors, which receive matter-energy input, or input transducers, which receive informational input.

Dealing first with matter-energy input, we might ask how patients enter the health system and what functions the hospital emergency room and the emergency medical subsystem play as entry points to the wider system. Thus, the entry point to the health care system may be said to include the following:
1. general practitioner's private office
2. specialist's private office
3. hospital (primary care) clinic
4. nonhospital ambulatory clinic
5. hospital emergency department.

At this point it is important to distinguish between ingestors and aids to ingestors. Ambulances and public health screening programs, for example, are aids to ingestors associated with entry points into the health care system. Their function is, of course, to act as agents of the ingestor in moving the patient from the boundary of the system into the immediate environment so that he is ready to be ingested. It should also be noted that hospital inpatient services and hospital outpatient referral clinics (to which a physician refers a patient for diagnostic tests) are *not* entry points in the contemporary U.S. situation.

Given separate entry points, the question arises of what difference it makes to the system and to the patient how he comes into the system. This involves characterizing the various entry points and is no mere academic typology but an important pragmatic exercise in evaluating the present health system and the suggestions being made for its reform. It is clear, for instance, from the greater number of entry points available to the American patient than to his British counterpart that Americans make different assumptions about the ability of the patient to seek out appropriate health care. While in many European countries a patient is on the "panel" of a general practitioner who is the "gatekeeper" to allow or deny him access to all other units of the health system, the American patient has a plethora of entry points. This has implications for both the patient and the system.

From the patient's viewpoint, appropriate treatment in the U.S. as compared with England requires a much greater degree of sophistication and knowledge as to the clinical significance of his symptoms since he must identify and locate the specialist and treatment site appropriate for that symptom. Studies have shown that from 80 to 90 percent of Americans have a family doctor. This doctor, however, is more and more likely to be a specialist with only a restricted scope of concern with the patient's potential range of conditions, rather than a general practitioner. In Great Britain, virtually everyone has a general practitioner.

Clearly, the complex model presented on the Zone of Perceptual Predisposition (site focus) as a cognitive map for patients determining an appropriate treatment site for a given symptom does not apply in countries with single entry points. This is not to say, however, that clinically-defined rational patient behavior is guaranteed by centralized systems with single entry points. Indeed, there is disturbing evidence emerging from the British National Health Service that the single gatekeeper approach does not entirely work. Structurally, one would expect, given the overwhelming proportion of British patients on the list of a general practitioner, the absence of financial barriers to utilization, the role of the general practitioner as a gatekeeper for the rest of the system, and the contracted requirement that G.P.'s make house visits and night calls, that British hospital emergency rooms would not be facing a problem of nonurgent utiliza-

The Social System of Emergency Medical Care   113

tion, and that, in fact, they would be concerned exclusively with clinical emergencies. Yet research in several London and provincial hospitals in 1971 indicate levels of nonurgent emergency room utilization in Britain entirely comparable with those documented in the Chicago Survey. Such evidence should give pause to those in this country who see structural reform—whether in the form of Health Maintenance Organization, family practice, or group practice prepayment plans—as the guarantor of appropriate patient utilization.

Multiple entry points also have implications for the organization of the system itself. It has been indicated that systems need to protect themselves by filtering environmental input according to specified selection criteria, and that the more specialized the system the more selective must be the input criteria if that system is to maintain an organizational balance at the desired level of specialization. This filtering may be achieved by boundaries, and by zones of predisposition. In part it may be achieved by the actual number of system entry points, and it is this strategy that is of particular importance in responding to and regulating increased external input. For example, the removal of financial barriers to health care utilization will result in sharply increased demand, and the location and number of available entry points will determine the health system's ability to absorb this increase with minimal disruption. Thus, the impressive ability of the British National Health Service in the immediate post-war period to respond to increased utilization without disruption was in large measure attributable to the sole entry point being the general practitioner who acted as a very effective entry filter. By contrast, the likely effect of National Health Insurance in the United States would be much more disruptive on the U.S. system with its multiple nonselective entry points. Despite the current enthusiasm for prepaid group practice and Health Maintenance Organization, present indications are that the major impact of National Health Insurance would be seen in very substantial increases in emergency department utilization and in severe systemic dislocations which would result.

At present this projection about the impact of National Health Insurance can be a guess only. The basis for it as well as an estimate of its implications are contained within the remarks that follow. In any event, the current prospect of health system reforms points to the importance of the selection criteria of system ingestors as a way of protecting the system from the entry of matter-energy that is inappropriate in size, frequency, quality, etc., for the units of the system. Clearly, this filtering process does not end with initial system entry; in most highly specialized systems there are two features that ensure that the matter-energy inputs are further and further filtered so that the highly specialized units have sufficiently specialized input, that is, within the narrow range of tolerance necessitated by the unit. The first of these two features is the distribution system which will not be discussed here but which may be thought of as a series of filtering devices. The second is the internal organization of the system so that units within it increase in specialization from the boundary to the center.

The American health care system, and the emergency medical subsystem in particular (unlike their British counterparts) are not characterized by this second feature. Not only is the U.S. emergency medical system an important entry point to the general health system as previously documented, but it is also a highly specialized unit to which the public has open and direct access. The nature of ingestors for the health system is thus of obvious importance and they may be characterized, compared, and evaluated in terms of the following criteria: 1) *Financial Accessibility:* This refers to the matter of how much initial entry at a given treatment site costs and the degree to which the patient personally will have to meet that charge prior to treatment. Although certain treatment sites are free (neighborhood health centers, industrial clinics, etc.), emergency rooms are reasonably financially accessible also because of current health insurance provisions as well as the legal difficulties of hospitals insisting on payment before treatment and the relative ease of avoiding payment altogether due to the very high accounting expenses of following up on small bills.

2) *Geographic Accessibility:* Numerical availability and spatial location are clearly vital characteristics of system ingestors. In general, there are obviously more private physician's offices than emergency rooms. But in many central city areas in the U.S. from which private physicians have relocated to the suburbs, emergency rooms may well represent geographically the most available entry point. The Chicago community area in which Cook County Hospital is located has 13 private physician offices to serve a population of over 70,000 individuals. In this context, it is hardly surprising that Cook County Hospital emergency rooms treat well over 1000 patients daily and the emergency rooms of other hospitals within the same community area a similar total number. It is in precisely these areas that hospital emergency rooms will have to bear the overwhelming burden of increased utilization.

3) *Temporal Accessibility:* For how long a period

during a day or a week are the entry points available as system ingestors? Physician's offices are open only a few hours a day and not on weekends. Nonhospital clinics are typically closed on weekends and in the evening. By contrast, hospital emergency rooms are open at all times and are so through legal and regulatory necessity rather than personal predilection. Ironically, emergency rooms are not only available more often to their clientele than other entry points are to their's but they also function as an alternative off-hours stand-by entry point for the clientele of all other ingestors. Thus, hospital and nonhospital clinics and private physicians will advise their patients to seek treatment during their own off-hours at the emergency department. As with financial accessibility, the temporal availability of all entry points except the emergency room is in large part within the autonomous discretion of the ingestor itself; for the emergency room, external rules are imposed through accreditation and licensing requirements as well as the constraining influence of civil case law defining the legal liability of hospitals.

4) *Clinical Selectivity:* How selective is each entry point? The growing trend toward specialization among physicians obviously implies that the physician's office as an entry point is becoming highly selective. The general decline of the general practitioner and the as yet low incidence of specialists in family practice underline this factor. In addition, the subspecialization of certain specialties (pediatrics, internal medicine, etc.) indicates that the quasi-generalized concern of many clinicians may disappear entirely. Hospital and nonhospital clinics as alternative entry points are similarly becoming highly selective. Admittedly, the selectivity may not be on the basis of clinical condition (although there is much of this in

the typical organization of hospital specialty and subspecialty clinics) but rather in terms of financial eligibility or geographic residence or program eligibility. In contrast, the hospital emergency department cannot be selective as to clinical condition. Further, the emergency room is typically denied (for reasons of legal liability) the filter mechanisms in the form of receptionists, nurses, answering services, and appointment schedules that allow entry points to deny or delay system entry without involving the physician himself. Although "triage" experiments have been attempted with mixed success, emergency rooms lack the counterpart of a receptionist who tells a potential patient that the doctor is taking no new patients, or does not deal with the reported symptom, or cannot see the patient until "three weeks from Thursday."

5) *Probability of Comprehensive Care:* Closely associated with the degree of clinical selectivity for system entry imposed by the several ingestors is the vital characteristic of how comprehensive the medical care is likely to be at and beyond each entry point. Is the concern only with the presenting symptom and the specific system involved, or is it likely to lead to comprehensive diagnosis and therapy for all the patient's symptoms and signs and even those of his family? Traditionally, of course, the general practitioner was thought of as providing comprehensive care *par excellence* while emergency room medical care was seen as inherently fragmented and episodic. Although probably such a distinction still exists, it is clear that the gap is narrowing. The specialization of physicians has substantially reduced the probability of comprehensive care for the patient who enters the health care system by means of a solo practitioner (though not for patients of multispecialty group practice). Similarly, it is clear that emergency departments at teaching

hospitals, through the in-house availability of specialists and the range of specialty clinics, can and do offer the prospect of comprehensive care as well as the technology that it requires.

6) *Probability of Continuous Care:* The criterion here is the differential probability associated with each entry point that the patient will receive care only from that source rather than being referred from treatment site to treatment site. Ironically, in a health system as specialized as the American one, the probability of comprehensive care bears an inverse association with the probability of continuous care in all settings except for the largest multispecialty clinics. Again, the emergency room has been regarded as inherently able to provide only episodic discontinuous care in contrast to the general practitioner providing more continuous care. But in practice the tendency of many emergency departments (again most likely those in teaching hospitals) to encourage return visits both for follow-up reasons (suture removal, cast checks, etc.) and in the event of symptom recurrence, as well as the apparent large-scale desire of the patients themselves to return for continuing primary care (often in the absence of private sources of care), has by accident and design made the hospital emergency room a source of continuous care for substantial segments of the population. Significantly, the emergency room may well be developing into the only widespread treatment setting where comprehensiveness of care is compatible with continuity of care outside of a handful of the larger hospital-based multispecialty group services.

7) *Professional and Technological Competence:* Related to the previous discussion of the increasing level of specialization of system units from the boundary to core is another important parameter of system entry

points: the quality of human and physical resources available directly at that point. Given the burgeoning growth and expense of technology available and necessary for contemporary diagnosis and therapy, and its resulting concentration in hospitals, hospital-based ingestors (emergency departments and clinics) in general have a higher order of technological competence than nonhospital ingestors. Indeed, a patient using the health system through a private physician's office may be subsequently referred to exactly the same resources that the patient entering the system through the emergency room had access to at his initial visit.

8) *Facilitation of System Flow:* In highly articulated and specialized systems, the presence of relatively few discrete entry points (as opposed to a situation, for example, where matter-energy can be absorbed by porous tissues continuously and ubiquitously across the boundary) is indication of the importance of an ingestor's ability to facilitate appropriate flow throughout the system. By "appropriate flow" is meant the ability of the entry point to process and return to the environment input that is beyond the tolerance levels of frequency, volume, and specialization of internal system units and to distribute to the internal units only that input which is sufficiently differentiated. This is of particular relevance for the health care system in view of the often (but mistakenly) made statement that it does not much matter at which ingestor a patient enters the system since he will eventually be referred to the clinically appropriate treatment site. This assumption, for example, underlies much of the public health screening programs which typically count their success and end their activity with the identification of positive cases rather than with ensuring that the positives receive appropriate and continu-

ing therapy. Judged in this light, solo practitioners (whether general practitioners or specialists) are probably low facilitators of system flow because of the organizational and financial disincentive involved while emergency departments are high facilitators in view of their hospital base and the insistence of many hospital staffs that emergency room patients be referred to them for continuing care.

9) *External Efficiency:* Highly specialized service systems operating with finite and externally allocated resources must clearly be concerned with the efficiency of entry points. In general, two types of efficiency may be delineated in terms of whether the ingestor activities are being evaluated in relation to the goals of the external environment or in relation to those of the internal system units. The external efficiency of system entry points, then, refers to such things as unit costs, utilization of physical and human resources per unit of time, and such general parameters as availability to the general population. The economics of scale and the high level of specialization generally indicate that external efficiency is high for emergency departments and large group practices and low for solo structures.

10) *Internal Efficiency:* In terms of the internal goals of the system and of its units (which may differ from the goals of the environment), entry points fulfill certain tasks such as filtering incoming matter-energy for subsequent rerouting to other units, and as a stand-by substitute for those units in the event of their nonavailability. In this sense, service systems differ from nonservice systems since the latter seek to maximize output and profit as a direct function of utilization. The more consumers a supermarket or cinema has, the greater the profit made by its system units. In contrast, service systems such as health, education,

and welfare do not generate internal resources in the same way and are much more dependent upon environmental resources and consequently on environmental dictates. As a result, service systems must maintain a balance between maximizing environmentally-determined input and minimizing input that is seen as inappropriate for the system units themselves. The hospital emergency department performs this balancing for the general health care system by functioning as a nonselective entry point while referring to other units appropriately filtered input. Similarly, it operates generally as an adaptive mechanism to stabilize the system in the face of potentially disruptive changes. Thus the trend of physician specialization combined with a reluctance to make house calls or to be available at night and weekends is a potentially disequilibrating trend that has not yet impaired the stability of the system. That it has not is entirely attributable to the adaptive function of the emergency room as a residual substitute treatment site. In this sense of performing necessary functions for other system units, emergency rooms as entry points exhibit a high level of internal efficiency and serve a function quite unlike their expected one.

Conclusions

The suggestion throughout this discussion has been that it is impossible to consider the present status of emergency medical services and their future development except by an evaluation of the key role played by them (and the hospital emergency department, in particular) in the wider health care system. The spectacular increase in visits to hospital emergency rooms over the last two decades is not attributable to any increase in clinical emergencies, nor do clinical emergencies account for most visits to this treatment site. Rather, the causal factors are to be found in the adaptive functions performed by the emergency room to enable the entire health care system to adjust to imbalances in other system units. All systems have adjustive mechanisms to regulate imbalance and ensure that they function smoothly. The changing role of the hospital emergency department can best be understood as an adaptive or homeostatic mechanism in the over-all health care system in much the same way as sweat glands operate in the human biologic system; that is, as a regulator or "sponge" which by changing its own behavior reduces imbalances or disequilibrating factors elsewhere in the system. The imbalances in the health care system include geographic maldistribution of physicians, the relative absence of a private health care system in many inner-city areas, the reluctance of physicians to make house calls and to be available at night or on weekends, the general shortage of primary care physicians, great financial barriers to utilization, and the concentration of specialized technical and human resources in hospitals. The relatively weak boundary maintenance processes of the emergency medical subsystem and the nonselective permeability of its entry points has created a situation where the hospital emergency room, through substantially increased utilization, allows the total system to adjust to these imbalances.

This adaptive function has several implications. First, by having this adaptation performed exclusively by one unit (rather than equally by all), any motivation for the units responsible for the imbalances to change is removed with the disequilibrating processes persisting and increasing until a system breakdown occurs. This is a distinct possibility and, indeed, may already have occurred in certain inner-city areas.

Even emergency rooms have finite resources and finite capacity and their ability to act as a sponge in "soaking" up the demand rejected elsewhere in the system is not limitless. The prospect of this systemic breakdown will be brought substantially closer by National Health Insurance if the removal of financial barriers is not preceded or accompanied by parallel structural changes in the system. Indeed, there are those who advocate National Health Insurance, in part, because of the reform possibilities of systemic collapse.

The second implication of the adaptive function of the emergency room is that those tasks for which it is pre-eminently specialized to undertake are being severely impeded. Specifically, the substantial and increasing number of nonurgent cases devolving on the emergency room because of this adaptive role detract from its ability to respond to clinical emergencies. Ironically, the volume of primary medical nonurgent care imposes its burden differentially so that those hospitals most specialized to provide trauma care are least called upon to provide it. Thus, in the Chicago area teaching hospitals see relatively fewer clinical emergencies than the smaller, less specialized hospitals without any teaching programs. This is, of course, because the larger teaching hospitals are primarily functioning as primary health care centers because of the emergency room's adaptive role. The net result is that the most specialized of hospital facilities in terms of medical resources are being forced into the least specialized in terms of the treatment needs of their emergency department patients.

The final implication of this matter is the most depressing. Since the changing role of the hospital emergency department is largely determined by imbalance elsewhere in the system, the direction and speed of these changes cannot be influenced endogenously by internal reform in the emergency medical subsystem. If one is sweating in response to excessive heat it is wiser to get into the shade rather than to directly block the pores of the skin. In the same way, changes elsewhere in the system must come before there can be any effective long-term solutions to the problems presently besetting hospital emergency rooms.

These wider changes clearly ought to take into account the interrelatedness of all system units and other insights available from social systems analysis. Hopefully, one of the insights will be the potentially wider role of the hospital emergency room and the considerable advantages it possesses as a health system entry point relative to other treatment sites. The argument of this paper is not that emergency rooms cannot and ought not provide primary health care. Rather, it is that they are compelled to provide this service by default and in the absence of coordinated planning. It is a burden carried unacknowledged and almost alone. Hospital emergency rooms have much potential in delivering comprehensive and skilled primary care if, and only if, this potential is planned and coordinated as part of wider structural reform that will reduce imbalance elsewhere in the health care system.

REFERENCES

1. Geoffrey Gibson, O.W. Anderson, and G. Bugbee, *Emergency Medical Services in the Chicago Area,* Center for Health Administration Studies, University of Chicago, 1970.
2. J. R. Kirkpatrick and L. J. Tabenhaus, "The Non-Urgent Patient on the Emergency Floor," *Medical Care,* 5:1, January-February, 1967, pp. 19-24.

3. Sidney S. Lee, J. A. Solon, and C. G. Sheps, "How New Patterns of Medical Care Affect the Emergency Unit," *Modern Hospital,* 94:5 May, 1960, pp. 97-101.
4. H.A. White and P. A. O'Connor, "Use of the Emergency Room in a Community Hospital," *Public Health Reports,* 85:2, February, 1970, pp. 163-168.
5. Marvin A. Lavenhar, R. S. Ratner, and E. R. Weinerman, "Social Class and Medical Care: Indices of Nonurgency in Use of Hospital Emergency Service," *Medical Care,* 6:5, September-October, 1968, pp. 368-380.
6. James G. Miller, "Living Systems: Basic Concepts," *Behavioral Science,* 10:3, July, 1965, pp. 193-237; and "Living Systems: Structure and Process," *Behavioral Science,* 10:4, October, 1965, pp. 337-379.

Part II

Patterns of Emergency Room Utilization

INTRODUCTION

Traditionally, the role of the emergency room has been to provide immediate treatment for acute illnesses or injuries. Within the last fifteen years, however, there have been dramatic changes in the nature and scope of treatment provided in hospital "emergency rooms." The extent of use has, of course, increased at an alarming rate; it is estimated that the number of emergency room visits in the United States doubled between 1960 and 1970. Perhaps even more important is their increased utilization, especially by the socially disadvantaged, as sources of treatment for nonemergent conditions. This growing trend has been the focus of much study, some authors even suggesting that the emergency room is becoming a "family physician" for the urban poor.

The evolution of the emergency room away from its traditional role is the focus of three articles in this section. In a study of the emergency rooms in four hospitals in New York City, Torrens and Yedvab (1970) found that "each served a different population in a different way, and that each fulfilled a quite different role for its patients and its community." The "Central Urban" hospitals' patients were more likely to be poor, less likely to present complaints of traumatic origin, and more likely to be seeking relief for flu, colds, or minor gastrointestinal problems. On the other hand, the "Suburban" hospital's patients were of higher social class, were more likely to have a private physician, and the majority were presenting traumatic complaints. Thus in the suburbs, the emergency room is still largely (though not exclusively) a trauma treatment center, while for the urban poor it provides the multiple services of a "family physician." The authors distinguish a third role: "substitute for the private physician and for the outpatient department during the off-hours when these services are not available." Of course, to a greater or lesser extent, every emergency room performs each of these roles, but Torrens and Yedvab feel the important point is that one can no longer speak "about 'the' emergency room, as if all emergency rooms were similar and a single model would suffice to describe them all."

Torrens and Yedvab's typology of emergency room roles is nicely complemented by a typology of emergency room utilizers developed by Alpert, Kosa, Haggerty, Robertson, and Heagarty (1969). Interviewing 4,320 families at Children's Hospital in Boston, Alpert, *et al.* found that the families could be divided into those with stable relationships to physicians, those with unstable relationships to physicians, those with stable hospital relationships, and those with unstable hospital relationships. This typology is based on the families' stated "usual" source of care, and the extent to which the "usual" is actually relied on. Not surprisingly, it was found that disadvantaged families (those on welfare, of low income, Negro, or with Spanish surnames) were most likely to rely on emergency rooms as their usual source of care. Those who indicated that they had a stable relationship with the hospital were also most likely to return to the emergency clinic for follow-up visits or to return with another child. Thus, large numbers of this emergency room's users were in fact utilizing it for on-going family health care.

The article by Lavenhar, Ratner, and Weinerman (1968) is an attempt to develop a more detailed understanding of which patients use emergency rooms for nonurgent conditions. Although it is clear from the two preceding articles that a lower socioeconomic group is associated with this pattern of use, Lavenhar, *et al.* were unable to demonstrate a relationship between social class and ratings of the urgency of the medical conditions of patients admitted to the Yale-New Haven Hospital's emergency room during a two-week period. Consequently, they examined the relationship of 17 demographic, socioeconomic, and medical care variables to patients' urgency status. The factor analyses suggested that "nonsocioeconomic variables interact differently within different social classes. This underscores the importance of evaluating the interaction of demographic, medical care and socioeconomic determinants in motivating individuals to seek help for nonacute medical conditions at an emergency facility."

The next group of articles are concerned with relationships between clinic staff and clinic patients, and the impact of these relationships on patient care. A common theme is that the medical competency of staff does not assure adequate medical care if unaccompanied by sensitivity to the individual needs, problems, and styles of patients.

Zola's article (1963) reports an interview study carried out in the outpatient departments of a large urban hospital. He found that the patient's ethnic background, the physician's specialty, and the spatial organization of the clinic had a significant impact on the effectiveness of the communication between physician and patient, and on the quality of care received. He presents three case studies which suggest that physicians' insensitivity to the emotional and social problems of patients can have serious medical implications.

This idea is given more rigorous study in Satin and Duhl's article (1972). Starting with the assumption that treatment "is a social encounter between patient and staff, couched in medical terminology and taking place in a medical setting but greatly influenced by the backgrounds and expectations of the participants," they examine the perceptions of physician, patient, and a psychiatrist-interviewer. Based on 257 interviews at the emergency room of an urban general hospital, they conclude that physicians generally fail to recognize social and environmental problems, or else translate them into medical categories. Patients whose problems were considered "psycho-social" by the psychiatrist-interviewer were less likely to receive follow-up help and less likely to receive psychiatric help in the emergency room than those so diagnosed by physicians.

Satin and Duhl generally adopt the perspective of the interviewer in examining the treatment encounter. An interesting contrast is provided by Solon, Sheps, Lee, and Jurkowitz (1958) who examine the staff's perspective on patients in outpatient departments. Interviewing staff physicians, visiting physicians, nurses, and social workers, they found general agreement that patients obtain outpatient services in a variety of use patterns. However, there were significant differences in attitudes toward patients between the nurses and physicians, on the one hand, and social workers on the other. The former expressed considerably more hostility towards patients' "shopping around" and overutilization of the clinics. The authors point out that "How people use a hospital outpatient department—for what basic purposes and with what specific patterns—must be in part influenced by the attitudes and behavior of the staff..."

Although the two groups of articles in this section appear to cover very different ground, they have in common an appeal for more individualized, differentiated approaches to the provision of care in the emergency room. They ask us to recognize that each emergency room serves a different population with different needs, and that each emergency room patient is an individual whose needs are emotional and social as well as physical.

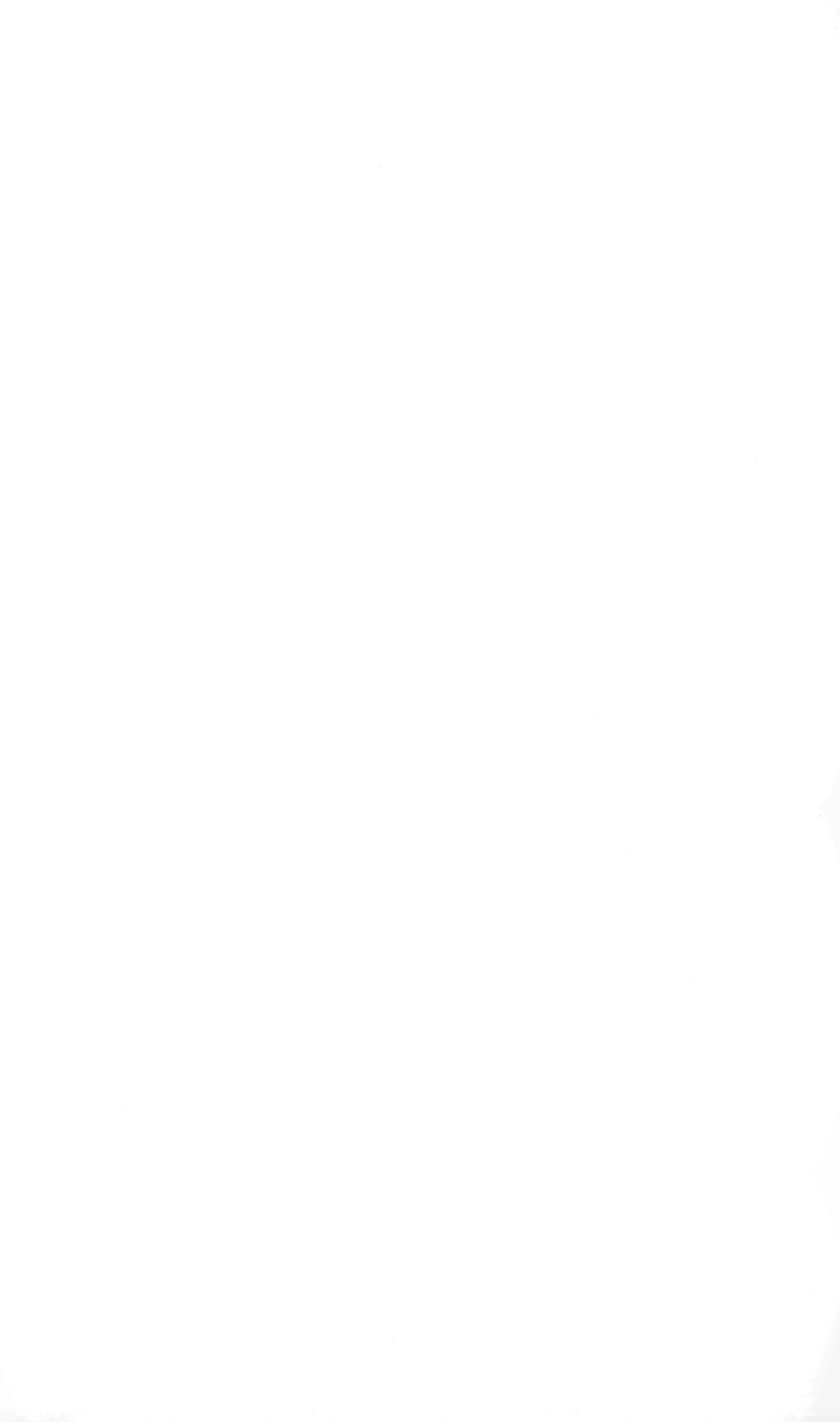

6. Variations Among Emergency Room Populations: A Comparison of Four Hospitals in New York City*

Paul R. Torrens, M.D., M.P.H.

Donna G. Yedvab, M.B.A.

In the years since the end of World War II, emergency rooms of hospitals across the country have experienced a rapid and marked increase in utilization. Emergency rooms which had previously cared for handfuls of patients, utilizing only small numbers of nurses and doctors, have each year been confronted with more and more patients who require greater allocations of space, staff, and funds.

Although the trend had been in progress for some time, the nation's attention was first drawn to this problem by the reports of Shortliffe in 1958 and Skudder, McCarroll, and Wade in 1961, which pointed out that the country's emergency rooms were experiencing a sharp rise in numbers of patients and that the percentage of patients using the emergency rooms for non-urgent reasons was increasing as well.[20, 23] Coincidentally, a report from the Nuffield Hospital Trust in England in 1960 revealed that the same trend was taking place there, even though the National Health

*Reprinted from *Medical Care,* January-February, 1970, Vol. VIII, No. 1.

Service supposedly guaranteed each individual a personal physician.[17]

In 1960 also, Lee, Solon, and Sheps carried out the first detailed analysis of an individual hospital's emergency room population at the Beth Israel Hospital in Boston.[14] This excellent study was followed in the next few years by similar studies of the emergency room populations of the Children's Medical Center, Boston,[4] Guy's Hospital, London,[7] Los Angeles County Hospital,[33] Yale-New Haven Hospital,[28,29,31] the emergency hospital and ambulance system of the city and county of San Francisco,[10] the Englewood (N.J.) Hospital,[22] the participating hospitals of the Michigan Blue Cross Plan,[26,27] the Vancouver General Hospital,[19] the New York Hospital,[18] the Hartford Hospital,[21] the Glasgow Royal Infirmary,[6] Boston City Hospital,[12] the Charleston County Hospital,[5] and Genessee Hospital, Rochester.[13] As the results of these various studies became available, a number of hospitals began to experiment with the organization of their emergency room services, either by instituting a "triage" system to expedite and improve patient care,[28,29] or by installing a full-time staff of private physicians whose professional efforts would be limited to the emergency room alone.[13]

As a result of all this effort, a considerable amount of information and experience has become available regarding the emergency rooms of the nation's hospitals. Most of the information, however, has been gathered in individual hospitals, as the result of work done in that hospital alone. With the exception of the Michigan Blue Cross Study,[26,27] there have been no studies involving emergency room populations of several hospitals. Since the purposes, the techniques, the study samples, and the definitions have varied so widely from study to study, it has been difficult to compare the information gathered in one emergency room with that gathered in another. Much useful information *has* been gathered, but meaningful cross-comparisons have not been possible.

In 1965, the Community Health Studies Unit of St. Luke's Hospital Center in New York launched a study of patients utilizing the emergency room facilities at four hospitals in New York City, in an attempt to determine the importance of urban hospital emergency rooms as a source of general medical care.[25] While the purpose of that study was to gather information about the emergency room as a medical care resource, it also provided a unique opportunity to compare four emergency room populations in some detail.

This report will concern itself with a comparison of these four emergency room populations and will include a discussion of the role of studies of this kind on emergency room planning and organization in the future.

METHOD

The study was carried out during an 18-month period from early 1964 to mid-1965. During the course of the study, a total of 1,113 patients was selected to participate according to a carefully-designed sampling system* and was interviewed by a team of specially-

*In preparation for the study, the research staff reviewed the emergency room records for each of the four hospitals to determine the distribution of patient-visits by hour of the day and day of the week at each hospital for the year prior to the study. Once the pattern was determined for each hospital, a sampling design was developed which distributed study interviews in direct proportion to this past pattern of patient visits.

trained, bilingual interviewers, as they waited to receive medical care in the emergency room. In the interview, extensive information was obtained about the patients themselves, their prior patterns of medical care, and their present medical problems. At the same time, information was gathered about the types and amounts of services provided to these patients by the emergency staff after the interview was completed.

The four hospitals involved in the study were located in four different sections of the city and represented a cross-section of all hospitals in New York City. They were not selected randomly for the study or as representatives of certain portions of the hospital population, but rather were originally included in the study because their administrative staffs expressed interest in taking part. In retrospect, it was realized that each of the hospitals represented a different geographic locale, had a different administrative organization, and served a different population, giving the study staff a unique opportunity for a widely-diversified look at New York City emergency room populations.

Hospital #1 was a 558-bed voluntary hospital located in midtown Manhattan, near the hotel-shopping-business center; among other things, it maintained a busy ambulance service as part of the New York City-wide ambulance system. Hospital #2 was a 713-bed voluntary hospital also located in Manhattan, but in a low-income residential area of apartment houses and tenements, somewhat removed from the midtown area; it did not operate an ambulance service. Hospital #3 was a 1363-bed municipal hospital located toward the periphery of the city, in a middle-income area of one, two, and three-family residential buildings; it operated an ambulance service that covered a wide geographic area which included several major highways. Hospital #4 was a 268-bed voluntary hospital located in a middle-upper income suburb at some distance from the heart of the city which was surrounded by relatively prosperous single-family homes. It also maintained an ambulance service which covered a rather wide geographic area, including three major expressways.

The 1,113 patient-interviews were distributed among the four hospitals in the following fashion:

	Interviews
"Central Urban" Hospital #1	356
"Central Urban" Hospital #2	380
"Peripheral Urban" Hospital #3	174
"Suburban" Hospital #4	203

The distribution of the interviews among the four hospitals, by hour of the day and day of the week, is given in Tables 1 and 2. This distribution directly parallels (and is drawn from) the patient-volume distribution of emergency room visits at the four hospitals during the year previous to the study, by reason of the original sampling design.

Table 1
Distribution of 1,113 Patient Interviews by Hour of the Day, by Hospital of Interview

Time of interview	'Central Urban' Hospital (#1)	'Central Urban' Hospital (#2)	'Peripheral Urban' Hospital (#3)	'Suburban' Hospital (#4)
8:00 a.m. to 4:00 p.m.	52%	53%	41%	46%
4:00 p.m. to midnight	38	38	41	47
Midnight to 8:00 a.m.	10	9	18	7
Not determined	0	0	0	0
Total patients interviewed	%100 #356	100 380	100 174	100 203

Table 2
Distribution of 1,113 Patient Interviews by Day of the Week, by Hospital of Interview

Day of interview	'Central Urban' Hospital (#1)	'Central Urban' Hospital (#2)	'Peripheral Urban' Hospital (#3)	'Suburban' Hospital (#4)
Monday	9%	14%	16%	15%
Tuesday	17	9	10	19
Wednesday	17	23	13	10
Thursday	18	20	31	15
Friday	19	17	13	16
Saturday	13	13	12	16
Sunday	7	4	5	9
	0	0	0	0
Total patients interviewed	%100	100	100	100
	#356	380	174	203

(In reviewing the emergency room experience of the four hospitals for the year prior to the study, preparatory to the development of a sampling design, it was noted that the four hospitals did not vary markedly in the hourly distribution of their emergency room patient-visits; all four hospitals saw approximately half of their emergency room patients between 8:00 a.m. and 4:00 p.m., approximately one-third between 4:00 p.m. and 12 midnight, and the remaining approximately 15 percent between midnight and 8:00 a.m. It was also noted that there was no marked difference among the hospitals with regards to the distribution of patient visits by day of the week and that all four hospitals had a slightly higher percentage of patient-visits during the middle of the week over what would normally be expected and a generally decreased number of visits on Sunday. All of these observations were reflected in the sampling design for the study.)

RESULTS

Descriptive Characteristics

Among the 1,113 patients interviewed in the four hospitals during the course of the study, 60 patients (5.4 percent) were under the age of one, 314 patients (28.2 percent) were aged 1 to 14, 530 patients (47.6 percent) were aged 15 to 44, 158 patients (14.2 percent) were aged 45 to 65, and 51 patients (4.6 percent) were aged 65 or over. There was surprising similarity among the patients in the four hospitals in this respect, with no marked difference being noted among the four populations. Also, there were approximately equal numbers of males and females in the study populations, with only slight variations being noted among the four hospitals.

All patients interviewed in the study were classified according to a social class index which gave increasingly higher ratings for people with greater income, more education, and more highly skilled occupa-

Table 3
Social Class Index for 1,113 Patients Interviewed, by Hospital of Interview

Social class index	'Central Urban' Hospital (#1)	'Central Urban' Hospital (#2)	'Peripheral Urban' Hospital (#3)	'Suburban' Hospital (#4)
3, 4, 5, 6	50%	63%	38%	8%
7, 8, 9, 10	35	26	44	48
11, 12, 13	12	8	9	38
Not determined	3	3	9	6
Total patients interviewed	%100 #356	100 380	100 174	100 203

tions.* As can be seen in Table 3, the population in the four hospitals varied widely in this regard, with the "central urban" hospitals #1 and #2 serving a population with predominantly low social class indices, with the "suburban" hospital #4 serving a population with predominantly high social class indices, and with the "peripheral urban" hospital #3 serving a population intermediate between the two extremes.

Approximately one-third of the 1,113 patients interviewed in the study were Negroes; however, the variation among hospitals was quite marked. The population at the "suburban" hospital #4 included no Negroes at all, the population at the "peripheral urban" hospital #3 (which was also the only municipal hospital in the study) contained almost two-thirds Negroes, and the "central urban" hospitals #1 and #2 contained 24.7 percent and 37.6 percent, respectively.

The same wide variation among the hospitals held true for the percentage of native-born Puerto Ricans in the four different interview populations, with the

*The Social Class Index was compiled from a rating scale based on a four-category occupational classification, a five-category educational-attainment classification, and a four-category income scale. In general, respondents who fall into social class indices 3, 4, 5, and 6 would have a yearly income of less than $5000, would not have completed high school, and would be involved in mostly unskilled occupations. Respondents in social class indices 7, 8, 9, and 10 would have incomes between $5000 and $7500, would have completed high school or a few years of college, and would have clerical, sales, or semi-skilled positions. Respondents in social class indices 11, 12, and 13 would have incomes of more than $7500 a year, would have completed college, and would be employed in managerial or professional occupations.

"central urban" hospitals #1 and #2 having 22.0 percent and 15.7 percent native-born Puerto Ricans, while the "peripheral urban" hospital #3 had only 0.6 percent and the "suburban" hospital #4 had none at all.

Financial Status and Health Insurance Coverage

Approximately one-quarter of the 1,113 patients interviewed were receiving financial assistance of some kind from some governmental agency, the greatest of which by far was a local welfare department. The percentage of people receiving assistance varied widely between the hospitals, as might be imagined, with only 1 percent of the patients at the "suburban" hospital #4 receiving welfare assistance, while 32 percent of the patients at the "central urban" hospital #2 fell into this category (Table 4).

Table 4
Governmental Financial Assistance Received by
the 1,113 Patients Interviewed, by Hospital of Interview

	'Central Urban' Hospital (#1)	'Central Urban' Hospital (#2)	'Peripheral Urban' Hospital (#3)	'Suburban' Hospital (#4)
None	73%	62%	75%	90%
Welfare (supplement)	3	6	3	0
Welfare (total)	13	25	8	1
Veterans Administration	0	1	1	1
Unemployment Insurance	1	1	3	0
Social Security	5	2	6	5
Pension	1	1	1	2
Workmen's Compensation	1	0	0	1
Other	0	1	2	0
Not determined	3	0	1	0
Total patients interviewed	%100 #356	100 380	100 174	100 203

144 Emergency Medical Services

A review of the various types of health insurance plans held by the 1,113 patients interviewed further served to underline the difference among the four hospital populations. In the two "central urban" hospitals #1 and #2 and in the "peripheral urban" hospital #3, approximately one-half to two-thirds of the population did not possess any type of private health insurance policy; by contrast, only 19 percent of the population interviewed at the "suburban" hospital #4 did not have any health insurance coverage (Table 5).

Present Medical Problem

With regard to the presenting complaint for which the 1,113 patients had come to the four emergency

Table 5
Types of Health Insurance Coverage for
the 1,113 Patients Interviewed, by Hospital of Interview

Insurance coverage	'Central Urban' Hospital (#1)	'Central Urban' Hospital (#2)	'Peripheral Urban' Hospital (#3)	'Suburban' Hospital (#4)
None	54%	60%	51%	19%
Blue Cross	10	8	3	15
Blue Cross-Blue Shield	16	13	14	35
Health Insurance Plan of New York (HIP)-Blue Cross	2	1	2	3
Group Health Insurance (GHI)-Blue Cross	1	1	3	2
Union Health Plan	9	10	18	9
Other	4	5	7	16
Not determined	4	2	2	1
Total patients interviewed	%100 #356	100 380	100 174	100 203

rooms seeking care, there was a wide disparity among the four hospitals in the study, as shown in Table 6. In the suburban hospital #4, 68 percent of the patients interviewed had come seeking treatment for trauma of some sort. In the "peripheral urban" hospital #3 and the "central urban" hospital #1, this figure was 25 percent and 36 percent respectively; in the "central urban" hospital #2, this figure was only 8 percent. By contrast, only 5 percent of the patients in "suburban" hospital #4 had come seeking relief for flu, cold or minor gastrointestinal problems, while this figure was 15 percent for the "peripheral urban" hospital #3, 25 percent for the "central urban" hospital #2, and 13 percent for the "central urban" hospital #1.

In keeping with the figures in Table 6, the length of time that the patient's complaint had been present be-

Table 6
Presenting Complaints for the 1,113 Patients Interviewed, by Hospital of Interview

Presenting complaint	'Central Urban' Hospital (#1)	'Central Urban' Hospital (#2)	'Peripheral Urban' Hospital (#3)	'Suburban' Hospital (#4)
Trauma	36%	8%	25%	68%
Flu, cold, or minor upper gastrointestinal complaint	13	25	15	5
Other G. I. complaint	2	3	3	1
Musculo-skeletal	8	12	5	4
Ear, nose, throat	5	13	8	3
Skin	7	8	9	3
OB-GYN	1	3	9	1
Cardiac	4	3	3	2
All others	24	25	23	13
Total patients interviewed	%100 #356	100 380	100 174	100 203

fore the patient sought emergency room care varied widely among the four patient populations.

As shown in Table 7, for the patients interviewed at the "suburban" hospital #4 (where traumatic problems had greatly predominated), the presenting complaint had been present for less than 12 hours; at the three other hospitals, by contrast, the presenting complaint had been present for less than 12 hours in only 24 percent of the patients interviewed at the "peripheral urban" hospital #3, in only 15 percent of the patients interviewed at "central urban" hospital #2, and in only 31 percent of the patients interviewed at "central urban" hospital #1. Indeed, in the patient population interviewed at these last three hospitals (1, 2, and 3), almost two-thirds of the patients had their presenting complaint for more than two days before seeking medical care in the emergency room, and in approximately 10 percent of them, the primary complaint had been present for six months or more.

Table 7
Time with Presenting Complaint for the 1,113 Patients Interviewed, by Hospital of Interview

Time with presenting complaint	'Central Urban' Hospital (#1)	'Central Urban' Hospital (#2)	'Peripheral Urban' Hospital (#3)	'Suburban' Hospital (#4)
0-11 hours	31%	15%	24%	68%
12-23 hours	7	8	9	11
24-47 hours	12	13	16	2
2-6 days	23	28	28	7
1-4 weeks	14	17	15	3
1-5 months	6	8	2	3
6 months or more	7	11	6	6
Total patients interviewed	%100 #356	100 380	100 174	100 203

Table 8
Previous Treatment of Presenting Complaint for the
1,113 Patients Interviewed, by Hospital of Interview

Previous treatment	'Central Urban' Hospital (#1)	'Central Urban' Hospital (#2)	'Peripheral Urban' Hospital (#3)	'Suburban' Hospital (#4)
None	57%	50%	26%	41%
Self	19	19	52	38
Private physician	5	7	0	10
Emergency room	6	11	5	1
Outpatient department	3	6	5	1
Other	10	7	3	9
Total patients interviewed	%100	100	100	100
	#356	380	174	203

Approximately half of all the 1,113 patients interviewed in the study had not attempted to obtain any medical treatment for their complaint nor had they attempted to treat themselves prior to coming to the emergency room for care. As shown in Table 8, the only significant differences among the hospital populations in this regard is that twice as many patients in the "suburban" hospital #4 and in the "peripheral urban" hospital #3 tried some form of self-treatment before seeking aid in the emergency room than did the patients in the "central urban" hospitals #1 and #2.

A review of the methods by which the 1,113 patients interviewed in the study were transported to the emergency room further serves to point up the differences between the four hospitals' population. As can be seen in Table 9, the majority of the patients at the "suburban" hospital #4 and the "peripheral urban" hospital #3 (85.7 percent and 51.2 percent, respectively) came to the emergency rooms of these hospitals by private automobile, while most of the patients at the "central ur-

148   Emergency Medical Services

ban" hospitals #2 and #1 (81.7 percent and 89.5 percent, respectively) either walked or came by some form of public transportation. These figures are doubly interesting, since they not only provide some added insight into the economic status of the patients, but also give some rough indices of the independent mobility of the patient population interviewed.

Care Provided in Emergency Room During Visit

Not only did the presenting complaints vary considerably from hospital to hospital, but, as might be expected, the manner in which each hospital handled these complaints differed considerably as well. For example, each hospital followed a pattern all its own in the use of x-ray and laboratory tests for its patients, a pattern that seemed to be directly related to the

Table 9
Means of Transportation to the Hospital for the 1,113 Patients Interviewed, by Hospital of Interview

Means of transportation	'Central Urban' Hospital (#1)	'Central Urban' Hospital (#2)	'Peripheral Urban' Hospital (#3)	'Suburban' Hospital (#4)
Ambulance	8%	0%	5%	6%
Police vehicle	0	0	1	0.5
No vehicle; patient walked to hospital	36	30	0.5	3
Subway	11	7	0.5	0
Bus	17	26	29	2.5
Taxi	18	28	10	1
Private car	8	8	52	86
Not determined	2	1	2	1
Total patients interviewed	%100 #356	100 380	100 174	100 203

Table 10
Laboratory Tests and X-ray Ordered by Physicians for the 1,113 Patients Interviewed, by Hospital of Interview

Laboratory tests and x-ray	'Central Urban' Hospital (#1)	'Central Urban' Hospital (#2)	'Peripheral Urban' Hospital (#3)	'Suburban' Hospital (#4)
None	60%	72%	75%	58%
At least one x-ray procedure	20	8	21	32
At least one laboratory test	7	14	4	7
At least one x-ray procedure and one laboratory test	1	1	0	3
Not determined	12	5	0	0
Total patients interviewed	%100	100	100	100
	#356	380	174	203

amount of trauma seen in that emergency room (Table 10). At the "suburban" hospital #4, where 68 percent of the presenting complaints were related to trauma, 35 percent of the patients received an x-ray of some sort; at "central urban" hospital #2, where only 8 percent of the presenting complaints were related to trauma, only 9 percent of the patients received an x-ray during the course of their medical care.

The hospitals differed considerably with respect to the number of medications prescribed for the patients interviewed. Table 11 shows that 92 percent of the patients interviewed at the "suburban" hospital #4 did not receive a prescription for any medication, while this figure for the other three hospitals ranged from 32 percent to 52 percent. It is also worth noting that approximately 10 percent of all the 1,113 patients interviewed during the course of this study received three or more prescriptions for medications at the time of their visit to the emergency room.

Possibly much of this variation in ordering laboratory tests and x-rays and in prescribing medications is related to the source of follow-up care which the patients were directed to obtain after their emergency room visit. As will be seen in Table 12, most of the patients (72 percent) at the "suburban" hospital #4 were referred to a private physician for follow-up care, while at the other three hospitals, most of the patients who required follow-up care were referred to a hospital outpatient clinic. (It should also be noted that the emergency rooms of municipal hospitals in New York City also serve as the "admitting office" for those hospitals. For that reason, the percentage of patients in the one municipal hospital in the study, "peripheral urban" hospital #3, who were admitted to the hospital after the emergency room visit, is probably falsely high when compared to the other three hospitals.)

As a further point of difference among the four hospitals included in the study, an attempt was made to determine who was billed for the cost of each patient's

Table 11
Prescriptions Issued for the 1,113 Patients Interviewed, by Hospital of Interview

Number of prescriptions issued	'Central Urban' Hospital (#1)	'Central Urban' Hospital (#2)	'Peripheral Urban' Hospital (#3)	'Suburban' Hospital (#4)
None	52%	33%	32%	92%
1	21	27	30	3
2	10	20	28	1
3	3	7	8	2
4 or more	1	7	1	0
Not determined	13	6	1	2
Total patients interviewed	%100	100	100	100
	#356	380	174	203

Table 12
Recommended Follow-up Care after the Emergency Room Visit for the 1,113 Patients Interviewed, by Hospital of Interview

Recommendation	'Central Urban' Hospital (#1)	'Central Urban' Hospital (#2)	'Peripheral Urban' Hospital (#3)	'Suburban' Hospital (#4)
No further care needed at this time	32%	31%	39%	4%
Private physician	4	1	5	72
Outpatient clinic	41	53	42	11
Emergency room	1	2	0	1
Transfer to another hospital	1	2	1	2
Admission to hospital	5	2	12	5
Other	5	3	1	1
Not determined	11	6	0	4
Total patients interviewed	%100 #356	100 380	100 174	100 203

emergency room visit (Table 13). Obviously, one hospital ("peripheral urban" hospital #3) was immediately excluded since it was a municipal hospital and as such did not bill anybody for the care they received in the emergency room.* At the "suburban" hospital #4, 65 percent of the bills were sent to third-party payers of some type and only 24 percent were billed directly to the individual patients. At the two "central urban" hospitals, two-thirds of the bills were presented to the individual patients themselves, and only a relatively

*Since the time this study was carried out, New York City has instituted a system of charges for patient care in the emergency rooms and outpatient clinics of all the municipal hospitals. At the time of the study, however, there was no attempt to charge patients for medical care received in the emergency rooms of municipal hospitals.

small number were sent to third-party payers. (At one of these hospitals, "central urban" hospital #2, all the third-party billing, 26 percent of the total, was sent to the welfare department and none to any other third parties.)

Medical Care During Year Prior to Interview

As the last point of difference among the four hospitals, an attempt was made to review each patient's pattern of medical care during the year prior to interview, in order to determine the relative importance of the emergency room as a source of general medical care. As one of the points covered, patients were asked to report the frequency with which they had used ambulatory medical services during the year prior to their emergency room visit and to describe the site of these services; as a check on the reliability of patient-

Table 13
Billing for the 1,113 Patients Interviewed by Hospital of Interview

Person or party to whom bill was directed	'Central Urban' Hospital (#1)	'Central Urban' Hospital (#2)	'Peripheral Urban' Hospital (#3)	'Suburban' Hospital (#4)
Patient	62%	68%	0%	24%
Blue Cross-Blue Shield	1	0	0	41
Group Health Insurance	0	0	0	1
Other insurance	0	0	0	14
Workmen's Compensation and Liability	8	0	0	7
Welfare Department	11	26	0	2
Other	1	2	100	2
Not determined	17	4	0	9
Total patients interviewed	%100 #356	100 380	100 174	100 203

Table 14
Most Frequently Utilized Sources of Ambulatory Medical Care during the Year Prior to Interview for the 1,113 Patients Interviewed, by Hospital of Interview

Most frequently utilized source of ambulatory medical care	'Central Urban' Hospital (#1)	'Central Urban' Hospital (#2)	'Peripheral Urban' Hospital (#3)	'Suburban' Hospital (#4)
No ambulatory medical care during the year prior to interview	44%	23%	22%	27%
Emergency room	15	16	8	4
Outpatient clinic	13	34	22	11
Private physician	25	15	40	57
Health department health station	2	7	6	0
Not determined	1	5	2	1
Total patients interviewed	%100	100	100	100
	#356	380	174	203

reporting, the records of the four hospitals included in the study were also reviewed and compared with the patient's reports of utilization of services at these hospitals. Table 14 shows the distribution for the most frequently utilized sources of ambulatory medical care during the year prior to interview.

Obviously, the use of patient-reports of prior utilization of ambulatory medical services has many dangers, as has been pointed out by several studies in recent years.[16,24] However, in an intensive study done on a small subsample of the patients interviewed in this study, it was found that there was only 3 percent under-reporting and 4 percent over-reporting of utilization of ambulatory medical services. This general result has since been duplicated by other workers in

New York City,[11] further reassuring us as to the general accuracy of the patient reports of prior utilization of ambulatory medical care.

DISCUSSION

In reviewing the studies of emergency room populations carried out since Lee's initial study in 1960, one is frequently presented with results which are conflicting or even contradictory. For example, the report from one hospital emphasizes that the greatest volume of patients come to its emergency room in the evenings and on the weekends,[5] while reports from other hospitals state that their busiest hours occur during the daylight hours of weekdays.[2,13] One set of reports points out that patients come to their emergency rooms seeking care for problems that are mostly related to trauma,[6,10,19,22] while another report states that trauma and related problems play a small role in its emergency room patient population.[18]

In the same vein, a report from a hospital in Boston states that its patients seemed to resemble the general population in Boston as a whole,[4] while one report from New Haven and another from Los Angeles state that their emergency room patient population is drawn heavily disproportionately from the lowest socioeconomic groups in the community.[32,33] One hospital reports from the Midwest that most of the patients surveyed had personal physicians available to them, and the reason they used the hospital emergency room was frequently tied up with their inability to reach him.[27] Another report from a hospital in the East states flatly that one of the main reasons its patients use the emergency room is that they are unable to obtain satisfactory private medical care.[31]

In terms of what should be done to improve emergency room staffing and organization, the published reports are equally confusing. A report from one large university hospital recommends the development of "triage" systems in the emergency room to help patients reach more appropriate sources of medical care [28, 29] while another report states that comprehensive health care services should be available in the emergency room itself.[33] Several reports stress the desirability of utilizing house staff and other physicians in training in the emergency room since it is potentially such a good learning experience for them,[30] while other reports encourage hospitals to consider the use of full-time staffs of attending physicians in the emergency room. [1, 3]

The reason for these apparently divergent findings and opinions becomes clear when viewed in the context of the study reported in this paper. In this four-hospital study, it was very apparent to the study staff that each of the emergency rooms included in the study were quite different from all others in the study, that each served a different population in a different way, and that each fulfilled a quite different role for its patients and its community.

The emergency rooms of the two "central urban" hospitals, for example, handled a population which was largely poor, uncovered by health insurance, and unaffiliated with other regular sources of medical care; in general, patients came to these facilities seeking medical care for nonemergency health problems and their follow-up care after the visit was to be provided by the hospital itself. In this respect, these two populations resembled the hospital populations described by Weinerman[28] and Wingert.[33]

By contrast, the emergency room at the "suburban" hospital served a population which was mainly middle/upper class, well-covered by health insurance, and regularly receiving medical care from some regular source other than the emergency room, usually a private physician in the community. In general, these patients came to this emergency room seeking care for genuine emergencies, usually related to trauma, and their follow-up care was to be provided by some source other than the hospital itself, usually a private physician. The "suburban" hospital's population resembled the population described in the Michigan Blue Cross study.[26, 27]

The position of the "peripheral urban" hospital and its population is difficult to define exactly, since it has characteristics of both the "central urban" hospitals and the "suburban" hospital. It resembles the "central urban" hospitals in that its population is composed largely of low and low-middle class minority group members with a low rate of health insurance coverage, whose emergency room problems were primarily nontraumatic and whose follow-up care would be provided primarily by the hospital outpatient department. On the other hand, it resembles the "suburban" hospital in that only a small percentage of the population are receiving financial assistance, most of the patients came to the hospital by private automobile, and much of their medical care during the year prior to this emergency room visit had been received in a private physician's office. This mixture of features is probably caused by its semisuburban (or "peripheral urban") location on the one hand (which would make it resemble the "suburban" hospital) and its "free" municipal hospital status on the other (which would make it attractive to the groups which are also drawn to the "central urban" hospitals). How the results from this "peripheral urban" hospital would compare with any other hospital reported in other studies would be hard to say, since it has many characteristics in common with other municipal hospitals in the country, yet has many features which are unlike most of these central-city institutions.

A review of the results of this four-hospital study, and of the other studies published in the past, suggests that emergency rooms in the United States now fulfill three general roles, any one of which may predominate and all of which may be present to some degree in any emergency room.

In the first role, the emergency room serves as the trauma-treatment center for the community, providing acute emergency care for problems related to trauma, accidents, and other serious, unpredicted events. In this role, the emergency room services a complete cross-section of the socioeconomic spectrum and works in close cooperation with the police and fire departments, ambulance services, and other community resources.

In its second role, the emergency room of many hospitals seems to be serving as substitute for the private physician and for the outpatient department during the off-hours when these services are not available or not appropriate to the particular patient's problem. While this role is historically newer than the first role for the emergency room and probably open to more debate, the figures from the Michigan Blue Cross study and from the present four-hospital study indicate that the hospital emergency room is becoming more and more of a partner both with the private physician in his practice and with the outpatient department.

In its third role, the emergency room of most of the central-city hospitals is serving as the "family physician" for the poor, particularly the minority group poor. In this role, the emergency room is seen as the place to go for all health problems, whether they are urgent or not; it is also seen as the logical entry point to the entire medical care system. In fulfilling this role, as opposed to the first two, the emergency room functions with relatively poor coordination and cooperation from other health or social resources in the community.

Unfortunately, most emergency rooms seem to have assumed these various roles without any conscious planning on anyone's part; rather the roles seem to have simply evolved in response to the patient's needs and are not the result of any carefully considered plan of action. Indeed, McCarroll and Skudder pointed out the discrepancy between what hospital administrators thought should happen in their emergency rooms and what was really going on. In their study, the majority of the administrators contacted stated that their emergency rooms were being primarily used for nonurgent problems, yet three-quarters of them felt that the emergency room services should be restricted to the treatment of emergencies only.[15]

What can be done about this situation? How can emergency room services be better planned in the future? First of all, it seems obvious that those responsible for planning the future of their emergency rooms should know what role the facility is actually fulfilling in its community right now. Is it primarily a trauma-treatment center for the whole area, is it an after-hours substitute for the private physician and the outpatient department, is it the "family physician" for the poor, or is it some combination of all three?

Once this factual information is available, the facility must be reviewed to see whether it is really organized to carry out its actual role in the most effective manner possible. If, for example, the emergency room is really the trauma-treatment center for the community, an attempt should be made to see whether it is equipped and staffed to really handle that function in the best manner possible. The administrator might consider joining his hospital with others in the area to establish a regional plan for the treatment of trauma, with one or two large centers taking on the responsibility presently dispersed between many smaller ones.

If the administrator discovers his emergency room spends a considerable amount of its time providing support for the private physician and the outpatient department in their off-hours, he may wish to review that situation and determine whether it should continue to do so. If it is determined that this is an appropriate use of the emergency room, he may then wish to build in systems for better communication and coordination of care between the emergency room and these two other providers of care.

The most difficult decision facing hospital administrators (and increasingly, the most frequent one) is what to do if he discovers that his emergency room is really serving as the "family physician" for the poor of the community. His choices (and the recommendations he has received in various articles in the professional literature) are endless, expensive, and frustrating. As one alternative, he can establish a screening or "triage" procedure to expedite the patients' progress out of the emergency room to more appropriate facilities for comprehensive medical care; to do this, however, he must be sure that these facilities exist and that they are as acceptable to the present emergency room patients as is the emergency room itself.

As a second alternative, he can try to improve his emergency room by the addition of new types of professional workers, such as public health nurses, social workers, psychiatrists, and other people whose skills are not regularly available to the emergency room staff and patients on a full-time basis. Although this by itself won't turn the emergency room into a good "family medical care" unit, it would certainly improve the quality of what is presently being done there.

The final alternative is to try to make his emergency room a center for comprehensive medical care, by completely revamping its organization, staff, equipment, and physical surroundings. While several authors have suggested this,[9,33] it seems unlikely that this will ever be possible or practical. Indeed, even if this were possible, it seems inadvisable to attempt it. If our society wants the poor (particularly the urban poor) to receive comprehensive medical care, it should stop fooling itself into thinking that the emergency room is the place to provide it and should start looking to other, more congenial settings.

A more promising solution is to develop alternative sources of comprehensive care which are equally accessible and attractive to the present emergency room population. Two obvious sites for this type of program would be the outpatient department of large hospitals or the new neighborhood health centers which are developing all over the country, if these two facilities could be organized to provide the kind of care the community requires. Once these are established and functioning smoothly, the emergency room could then become a point of initial contact and referral, much as Weinerman, Hilkovitz, and others have suggested.[8,32]

CONCLUSION

Very frequently, one reads in the medical care or hospital administration literature of "the emergency room" or "the emergency room crisis." The implication is that one emergency room is much the same as another and that a standard model will suffice in describing all facilities of this type. This is simply not so.

In the four-hospital study discussed in this report, it was very apparent that each of the emergency rooms was quite different from all the others, that each served a different population in a different way, and that each fulfilled quite a different role for its patients and its community.

The results of this study suggest that the role each emergency room assumes is shaped in a special way by the particular needs of the people of its area for medical care and by the willingness of the hospital facility to adapt to those needs, whatever they may happen to be. In general, emergency rooms in the United States now have three general roles, any one of which may predominate and all three of which may be present to some degree in every emergency room. These roles are: trauma-treatment center, private physician and outpatient department substitute in off-hours, and "family physician" for the urban poor.

In the past, the emergency room has been described as "the weakest link in the hospital chain."[21] While this criticism may be true in some ways, it should be reemphasized that the emergency room has proven to be one of the most useful, flexible, and productive areas of the modern hospital ... and deserves all the help and support it can get.

REFERENCES

1. Abbott, V. C.: Attending doctors staff emergency room. *Mod. Hosp.*, June, 1962.
2. Barry, R. M., Shortliffe, E. C., and Wetstone, H. J.: Case study predicts load variations patterns. *Hospitals*

34:34, 1960.
3. Beaven, W. E.: Medical staffing of emergency rooms: a trial of group practice. *Med. Ann. D. C.* 34:173, 1965.
4. Bergman, A., and Haggerty, R.: The emergency clinic. A study of its role in the teaching hospital. *Amer. J. Dis. Child.* 104:36-44, 1962.
5. Bradham, G. B.: An analysis of 2,418 emergency room admissions. *J. S. Carolina Med. Ass.* 61:127, 1965.
6. Browne, M. K.: An analysis of patients attending the casualty department. *Brit. J. Clin. Pract.* 17:325, 1963.
7. Fry, L.: Casualties and casuals. *Lancet* 1:163, 1960.
8. Hilkovitz, G.: The emergency room in the teaching hospital. *J. Med. Educ.* 41:724, 1966.
9. James, G.: Medical advances in the next ten years: the implications for the organization and economics of medicine. *Bull. N. Y. Acad. Med.* 41:14, 1965.
10. King, B. G., and Sox, E. D.: Emergency medical service system—an analysis of the workload. *Public Health Rep.* 82:995, 1967.
1. Kirchner, C., Lerner, R. C., and Clavery, O.: Reported use of medical care sources by low-income in-patients and out-patients. *Public Health Rep.* 84:107-117, 1969.
12. Kirkpatrick, J. R., and Taubenhaus, L. J.: Non-urgent patient on the emergency floor. *Medical Care* 5:19, 1967.
13. Kluge, D. N. et al: The expanding emergency dept. *JAMA* 191:801, 1965.
14. Lee, S., Solon, J., and Sheps, C.: How patterns of medical care affect the emergency unit. *Mod. Hosp.* 94:97, 1960.
15. McCarroll, J. M., and Skudder, P. A.: Conflicting concepts of function shown in national survey. *Hospitals* 34:35, 1960.
16. National Health Survey: *Health Interview Responses Compared with Medical Records.* U. S. Public Health Service, Washington, D. C. Series D, No. 5, p. 29, 1961.

17. Nuffield Provincial Hospitals Trust: *Casualty Services and Their Settings—A Study in Medical Care.* London, Oxford University Press, 1960.
18. Reed, J. I. et al.: Quantitative survey of New York hospital emergency room, 1965. *New York J. Med.* 67:1335, 1967.
19. Robinson, G. C., and Klonoff, H.: Hospital emergency services for children and adolescents: a one-year review at the Vancouver general hospital. *Canad. Med. Ass. J.* 96:1304, 1967.
20. Shortliffe, E. C., Hamilton, T. S., and Naroian, E. H.: The emergency room and the changing pattern of medical care. *New Eng. J. Med.* 258:20, 1958.
21. Shortliffe, E. C.: Emergency rooms—weakest link in hospital care? *Hospitals* 34:32, 1960.
22. Sklar, H. S.: Acute problems of suburban adolescents. A survey of emergency room visits. *Clin. Pediat.* 7:220, 1968.
23. Skudder, P. A., McCarroll, J. R., and Wade, P. A.: Hospital emergency facilities and services, a survey. *Bull. Amer. Coll. Surg.* 46:44, 1961.
24. Solon, J., Sheps, C., Lee, S., and Barbano, J.: Patterns of medical care: validity of interview information on use of hospital clinics. *J. Health Hum. Behav.* 3:29, 1962.
25. Torrens, P. R., and Yedvab, D. G.: *Impact of Emergency Services Upon Patterns of Ambulatory Care.* (photo-offset) Division of Medical Care Administration, U. S. Public Health Service, April, 1969.
26. Vaughn, H. E., Jr.: *Hospital Emergency Room Utilization Study,* Michigan Blue Cross Association, Research and Statistical Division, October, 1965.
27. ———: Why Patients use Hospital Emergency Departments? *Hospitals* 40:59-62, 1966.
28. Weinerman, E. R., and Edwards, T.: Triage systems show promise in management of emergency depart-

ment load. *Hospitals* 38:55, 1964.
29. Weinerman, E. R.: Effects of medical "triage" in hospital emergency service. *Pub. Health Rep.* 80:389, 1965.
30. ———: Out-patient clinic services in the teaching hospital. *New Eng. J. Med.* 272:947, 1965.
31. ———: Determinants of use of hospital emergency service. *Amer. J. Pub. Health* 56:1037, 1966.
32. ———: Innovation in ambulatory services. *J. Med. Educ.* 41:712, 1966.
33. Wingert, W. A.: The demographical and ecological characteristics of a large urban pediatrics outpatient population and implications for improving pediatrics care. *Amer. J. Pub. Health* 58:859, 1968.

7. The Types of Families That Use an Emergency Clinic*

Joel J. Alpert, M.D.

John Kosa, Ph.D.

Robert J. Haggerty, M.D.

Leon Robertson, Ph.D.

Margaret C. Heagarty, M.D.

Utilization of hospital emergency clinics is increasing constantly. At the Children's Hospital Medical Center, for example, use of the emergency clinic has grown in ten years from 4,500 visits per year (1957) to more than 50,000 visits per year in 1967. The lack of available physicians in the community, the increase in insurance coverage for hospital emergency room visits, the constant availability of the emergency service, and the use of the emergency service by the physician are suggested explanations for this increased use.[4] Not all families, however, use the emergency clinic for the same reasons or with the same degree of consistency. Some use it for true emergencies, others as a source of ongoing care. This differential utilization has been associated with economic status, with high-income families said to use the emergency

*Reprinted from *Medical Care,* January-February, 1969, Vol. VII, No. 2.

clinic for true emergencies while low-income families use it as a source of ongoing care.[5]

The emergency clinic offers an important, technically competent service to the low-income population. This same service, however, is indicted as part of a system of health care which is described as episodic and fragmented. As a result, the low-income families that use emergency clinics have been selected as the target population to reap the benefits of new comprehensive care programs. Sigmond has suggested that when such comprehensive alternatives are provided, families will turn away from the emergency facility.[2]

This study reports a detailed examination of the users of one hospital's emergency clinic. It is an attempt to differentiate users of the clinic, to describe different types, i.e., to develop a typology of the users of this medical facility, to distinguish their social characteristics, and to suggest possible uses for such a typology.

METHOD

The data were collected at the Medical Emergency Clinic of the Children's Hospital Medical Center as part of a longitudinal study of health care. This clinic, like so many emergency services, fulfills many functions. It is used as a place of referral by many physicians, as an emergency facility by families unable to reach their usual physicians, and as a regular community clinic by low-income families living in the neighborhood. Surgical emergencies are not handled in this clinic, but are seen in a special surgical emergency clinic.

For a six-month period in 1964, the parent accompanying each child seen with a new illness was interviewed. If the family returned during the interview period with this child or another child in the family with a new complaint, identifying data were obtained but the family was entered only once for the statistical analysis. Respondents were interviewed between 9:00 a.m. and 9:00 p.m., when approximately 92 percent of the clinic patients are seen. A previous study of this clinic suggested that those patients seen in the 9:00 p.m. to 9:00 a.m. hours are not significantly different from the daytime users.[1]

The parent, usually the mother, was given a questionnaire by a trained lay interviewer. The questionnaire contained two questions which related to utilization of the clinic and the reason for the visit. The parent was asked: "Do you have a doctor who usually looks after the children when they are ill?" (yes or no) and "How did you happen to come to the clinic for this visit?" The second question could be answered (1) "referred by a private physician," (2) "couldn't get my doctor," (3) "people recommended the clinic," (4) "because of a previous visit," (5) "the clinic is the best place to take the children," and (6) "the hospital is my doctor." Some respondents gave multiple reasons. The questions were asked to establish whether the family had established a relationship with a particular physician whom they usually consulted when the children needed medical attention, and the degree to which the respondent relied on this physician.

TYPOLOGY

The combination of answers to the two questions yielded four types of utilizers of the Children's Hospital: The family that had a stable relationship with a physician (stable—M.D. relationship); the family that had an unstable relationship with a physician (unstable—M.D. relationship); the family that had a stable relationship with the hospital (stable-hospital relationship); the family that had an unstable relationship with the hospital (unstable-hospital relationship) (Fig.1).

Families who, by this definition, had stable relationships with physicians were those who first answered that they had established relationships with particular physicians and indicated that they came to the emergency clinic because they were referred by or could not contact them. Families defined as having unstable relationships with physicians were those who, although claiming to have physicians they usually consulted, came to the clinic without contacting them for such reasons as "people recommended it," "previous visits," "the clinic is the best place," or "the hospital is my doctor."

Families defined as having stable relationships with the Children's Hospital did not have established relationships with physicians and came to the clinic because "the clinic is the best place" or "the hospital is my doctor." The last group, those who had unstable relationships with the hospital, were those who had no usual physicians and came to the clinic because of previous visits or because people recommended the clinic; because they were referred by physicians; or because they couldn't reach a physician, having previously indicated that they did not customarily consult a particular physician.

Three hypothetical situations were presented to every third respondent, to assess what the families perceived as normal behavior with respect to typical needs for medical care. Each respondent was asked which source of care he would select in each situation: (1) The need for care for acute illness. "Your child has

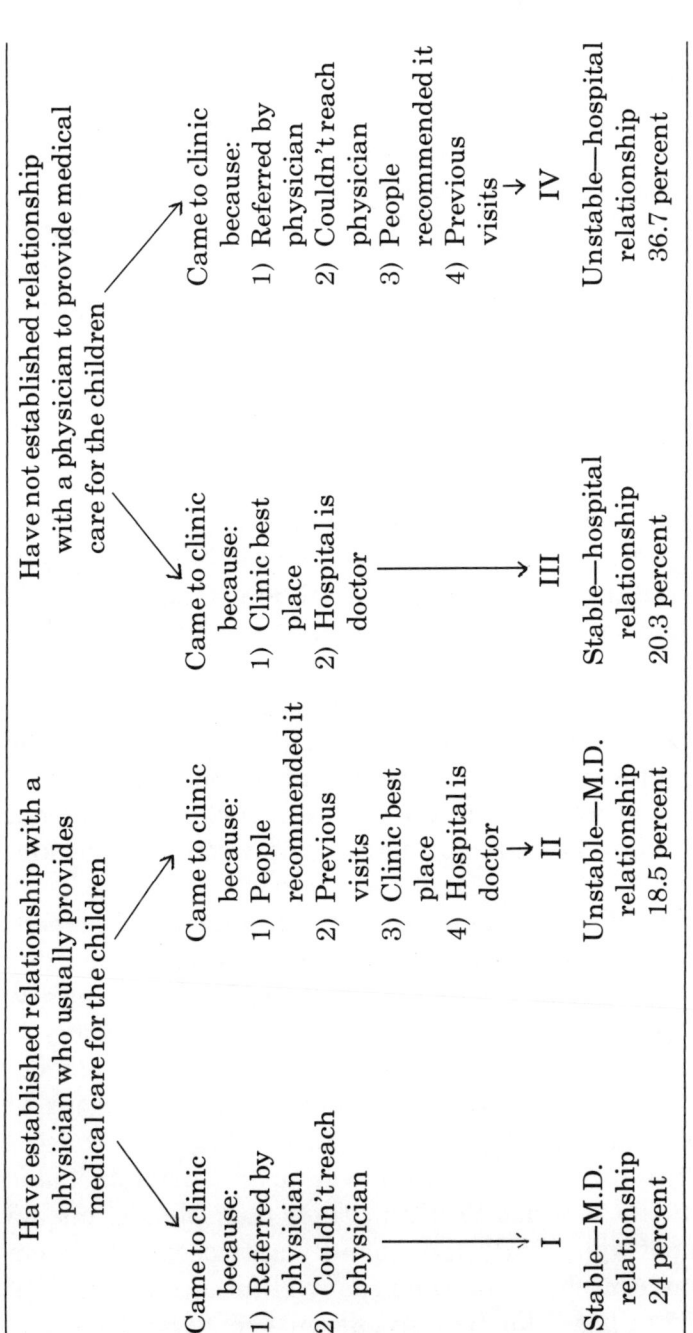

Figure 1. The four types of utilizers (N = 4,320).

a temperature of 104 degrees. Where would you go?" (2) The need for preventive services. "Your child needs a booster shot. Where would you go?" (3) The need for care for chronic illness. "Your child has an illness such as diabetes. Where would you go?" In each case, the respondent was given a choice between his physician and an institution (i.e., hospital or well-baby clinic).

RESULTS

Four thousand, three hundred and twenty families were interviewed. A random check of the register sheet of the clinic indicated that 96 percent of eligible respondents were interviewed. These families made 5,600 visits during the time period.

Sixty-one percent of the families were Catholic, 31 percent Protestant, 3.2 percent Jewish. Seventy-one percent were white and 26 percent Negro. Only 1.8 percent had annual incomes above $10,000; 7.8 percent less than $3,000, 40 percent between $4,500 and $7,500.

As the data presented in Table 1 indicate, 42 percent of the sampled families had physicians whom they usually consulted when the children were ill. Eighty-five percent of the families with incomes in excess of $10,000 had physicians who usually provided medical care for the children, compared with 16 percent of those on welfare.

Reasons for coming to the clinic are shown in Table 2. Of the families that had their own physicians, 43 percent apparently did not attempt to contact them before coming to the emergency clinic. Almost half of the families who had bypassed their usual doctors had made previous visits to the emergency clinic, one-third claimed that the clinic and not the doctor was the best source of care for the children, and a small proportion went so far as to claim that the Children's Hospital was their doctor.

As defined, 24 percent of the families had stable-M.D. relationships, 18.5 percent an unstable-M.D. relationship, 20.3 percent stable-hospital relationships, 36.7 percent unstable-hospital relationships.

Not surprisingly, the four types of utilizers had conspicuously different background characteristics (Table 3). Disadvantaged families, that is, those on welfare, of low income, Negro, or with Spanish surnames, were most likely to be in the unstable-hospital group. The percentage of disadvantaged families was lowest in the stable-M.D. group and highest in the unstable-hospital families. Disadvantaged families made up more than half of the unstable-hospital families. Families who lived more than three miles from the hospital were most likely to be in the stable-M.D.

Table 1
Families That Have Their Own Doctors

	No. of families	*Families that have particular physicians who usually provide medical care for the children (percent)*
All families	4,320	42
Income		
On welfare	621	16
Less than $3,000	333	24
$3,000-$4,500	1,369	38
$4,500-$6,000	1,009	55
$6,000-$7,500	452	62
$7,500-$10,000	191	63
More than $10,000	75	85

Table 2
Reasons for Coming to the Emergency Clinic

How did you happen to come to the clinic for this visit?	Families that have established relationships with physicians who usually provide medical care for the children (N = 1,829) (Percent)	Families that do not have physicians who usually provide medical care for the children (N = 2,431) (Percent)
Referred by a private physician	49	2
Couldn't get my doctor	8	*
People recommended it	18	21
Because of a previous visit	23	46
The clinic is the best place to take children	14	24
The hospital is my doctor	1	15

* Less than half of one percent.
Percentages add up to more than 100 because some respondents listed multiple reasons.

Table 3
Selected Characteristics of Four Types

Percentage Distribution of Families

	Stable-M.D.	Unstable-M.D.	Stable-Hospital	Unstable-Hospital	Total
On Welfare (609)	2	14	25	59	100
Income under $4,500 (2,300)	14	16	23	47	100
Negro (1,127)	7	9	30	54	100
Spanish (145)	15	9	20	56	100
Families with no hospital insurance	19	22	46	44	100

Table 4
Medically-related Behavior of the Four Types of Clinic Utilizers

	Stable-M.D. (N=1,037) (Percent)	Unstable-M.D. (N=785) (Percent)	Stable-hospital (N=862) (Percent)	Unstable-hospital (N=1,558) (Percent)
Family came back for one repeat visit	8	11	20	18
Family came back for two or more repeat visits	2	3	9	7
Family came back for repeat visit with the same child	6	9	16	14
Family came back for repeat visit with another child	4	5	13	10

Table 5
Preferences for Medical Facilities of the Four Types of Clinic Utilizers*

	Stable-M.D. (389) (Percent)	Unstable-M.D. (284) (Percent)	Stable-hospital (286) (Percent)	Unstable-hospital (454) (Percent)
Your child has a temperature of 104 degrees; where would you go?				
Hospital	11	15	46	40
Private doctor	82	76	48	52
Where would you go to get shots for the baby?				
Well-baby clinic	28	36	82	71
Private doctor	67	60	16	25
Your child has a chronic illness, where would you go?				
Hospital	49	55	74	59
Private doctor	45	40	23	34

*Questions asked every third interviewee only ($N = 1{,}413$). Percentages do not add up to 100 percent because minor category answers are not listed.

group (37 percent) and least likely to be in the stable-hospital group (12 percent). Families who relied on the hospital, compared with those who relied on physicians, were less likely to have hospital insurance (45 percent vs. 20 percent), but this finding has less importance since the advent of Medicaid.

Stable-hospital families were most likely to come back for repeat visits in the six-month study period and most likely to come back for multiple repeat visits (Table 4); they were also most likely to bring other children. Stable-M.D. families showed the opposite behavior and were least likely to come back for repeat visits, while the two other types fell between.

The hypothetical situations presented to the families described different medical needs, yet the answers showed great consistency. In each situation (Table 5) the stable-hospital families, compared with the other categories, were most likely to select a hospital or clinic and least likely to select private physicians; the stable-M.D. families were least likely to select a hospital and most likely to select private doctors.

DISCUSSION

Patients who use medical resources in a way that can be described as haphazard, irrational, and detrimental to continuity of care are not exclusively clinic patients. Private practitioners can give many examples of patients who use one physician or hospital for one symptom and another physician or hospital for another symptom. Solon has differentiated, for example, between a patient's central source of care, which he says he usually goes to, and his volume source of care, the source he goes to most often.[3] As suggested by Torrens,[4] families using emergency clinics at different hospitals are not all of the same type and use the hospital for different reasons. In his study, the central urban hospital functioned as a general clinic, while the private suburban hospital was used principally for genuine emergencies and when the patients could not locate their private physicians. It is possible that such differences in use and users exist within each hospital.

We reasoned that the typology could explain the complex pattern of utilization by considering the interplay of the user's "usual pattern" of medical care and the degree to which the "usual" was relied on. The rationale for the proposed typology was based on the recognition that many patients claim a usual source of care and can name a personal physician to whom they turn for needed care, but in fact do not rely completely on this usual source. There were two types of families who said they had their own doctors. The first relied on the physician except for referrals and emergencies, and the second relied on the doctor only occasionally. A similar typology was hypothesized among the families who did not have their own doctors. Those who said "the hospital is the best place" or "the hospital is my doctor" might very well have more stable relationships with the hospital than those who came because they were referred or it was recommended.

The three hypothetical medical situations added another dimension to the typology. The first situation referred to high fever, an anxiety-provoking, acute illness requiring urgent action. Here the families with stable-M.D. and unstable-M.D. relationships predominantly claimed to consult private physicians, while half of the "hospital" families said they would seek the services of private doctors rather than relying on the hospital.

The second situation referred to immunizations as a routine preventive measure. Here the pattern of fragmented curative and preventive service appeared most clearly. While most of the families who had relationships with particular physicians would go to them, the "hospital" families apparently would tend to use the well-baby clinic. Those families with stable relationships, whether with the hospital or with the doctor, were more consistent in their claimed utilization. For example, more families with stable-hospital relationships said they would use a well-baby clinic and more families with stable-M.D. relationships would use the doctor, compared with their "unstable" counterparts. This was also true of the "acute-illness" vignette.

Although this pattern persisted in the responses to the third example, a chronic illness, for the first time as many as half of the families with either stable-M.D. or unstable-M.D. relationships would take their children to the hospital. The hospital is seen as the place to go for long-term or complicated problems.

The degree of reliance on any medical facility, that is, the stability of the relationship, appears to correlate with advantaged status. Patients who have stable relationships with one medical service, be it doctor or hospital, are socially more advantaged when compared with those who have unstable relationships with the same medical services.

The proposed typology permits classification of the population using an emergency clinic. Such an approach is a reminder that "clinic patients" are not all the same. Each family that uses an emergency clinic does so for complex reasons and motivations associated with, for example, medicine-taking or appointment-keeping. A simple questionnaire administered in any emergency clinic might help decide who the patients are and how the clinic services are being used. Furthermore, it might be easier to change the utilization pattern of one type of patient compared with another type. Is it possible that Medicare and Medicaid will enable those families who until now have relied mainly on hospital clinics to rely on private physicians, assuming such physicians are available? Perhaps the private practitioner can learn something about the way his patients use his services by such an instrument. Could a public clinic, by offering a comprehensive care program, change the relationships of certain families from unstable to stable? Is it possible to predict, by screening families based on this typology, what the responses of the families to the offer of a comprehensive care program will be? It is known that not all families respond equally when an offer of comprehensive care is made,[6] and further study might lead eventually to ways of changing health care patterns if more were known about motivation for seeking medical care.

SUMMARY

Four thousand, three hundred and twenty families were surveyed in an emergency clinic over a six-month period to determine whether they had established relationships with particular private physicians to provide medical care for their children. The reasons for the clinic visits were determined. A typology of users of the emergency clinic was developed which examined the relationship between the usual source of care and degree of reliance on this source. Twenty-four percent of the families studied had stable relationships with physicians and 36 percent had unstable relationships with the hospital. Those who had unstable relationships with the hospital were most likely to be disadvantaged families. It is possible to screen emergency clinic patients with such a typology.

REFERENCES

1. Bergman, A.B., and Haggerty, R. J.: The emergency clinic. *Amer. J. Dis. Child.* 104:36, 1962.
2. Sigmond, R. M.: Areawide planning for emergency services. *J.A.M.A.* 200:308, 1967.
3. Solon, J.: Patterns of medical care: Sociocultural variations among a hospital's outpatients. *A.J.P.H.* 56:884, 1966.
4. Torrens, P. R., and Yedvab, D. G.: Outpatient care. *Hospital Topics* December, 1966, p. 71.
5. Weinerman, E. R., Ratner, R. S., Robbins, R., and Lavenhar, M. A.: Yale studies in ambulatory medical care: Determinants of use of hospital emergency services. *A.J.P.H.* 56:1036, 1966.
6. White, M., Alpert, J., and Kosa, J.: Hard to reach families in a comprehensive care program. *J.A.M.A.* 201:801, 1967.

8. Social Class and Medical Care: Indices of Nonurgency in Use of Hospital Emergency Services*

Marvin A. Lavenhar, M.P.H.

Robert S. Ratner, M.A.

E. Richard Weinerman, M.D., M.P.H.

In the past few decades, the volume of patient visits to hospital emergency services has increased substantially. Much of the increment has been attributed to the use of emergency facilities for a wide variety of nonurgent conditions.[8]

In an attempt to reverse this trend in the Emergency Service of the Yale-New Haven Hospital, an initial screening procedure (medical triage) was instituted in 1963. This screening technique entailed brief medical evaluation of all incoming patients to determine the type and priority of services needed and to provide appropriate referral. Despite the implementation of the medical triage program, a high proportion of patients with nonurgent conditions continued to present themselves at the emergency facility.[9]

*Reprinted from *Medical Care,* September-October 1968, Vol. VI, No. 5.

In order to explain this persistent trend, a detailed study was made of the characteristics of emergency service patients according to the urgency of their conditions.[10] One of the perplexing findings of that investigation was the inability of an occupation-education index of social class to differentiate between patients with urgent and nonurgent conditions in the emergency service setting. The present study was undertaken in an effort to explain this apparent lack of association with social class, and to develop more appropriate indices for the prediction of use of a hospital emergency service for nonurgent conditions.

SUMMARY OF PREVIOUS RESEARCH

Study Population

The original study population consisted of 2,028 patients who visited the Yale-New Haven Hospital Emergency Service during the two-week period from July 9 through July 22, 1964. Descriptive data for each patient visit were collected from the Emergency Service record. In addition, more detailed information about socioeconomic and medical care variables was obtained through personal interviews of a 20 percent subsample (402) of these patients. The sampling and interview procedures used have been described.[10] The present report pertains to the subsample population only.

Definitions of Urgency Classifications

During the study period, the resident physician on duty evaluated and rated the presenting condition of each patient as emergent, urgent, or nonurgent according to the following definitions:

Emergent: condition requires immediate medical attention; time delay is harmful to patient; disorder is acute and potentially threatening to life or function.
Urgent: condition requires medical attention within the period of a few hours; there is possible danger to the patient if medically unattended; disorder is acute but not necessarily severe.
Nonurgent: condition does not require the resources of an emergency service; referral for routine medical care may or may not be needed; disorder is nonacute or minor in severity.

Since relatively few of the presenting conditions were classified as emergent, for purposes of analysis the emergent ratings were combined with those in the urgent category to provide a contrast with the group of patients with nonurgent conditions. Only the latter group was considered inappropriate for treatment at a hospital emergency facility.

Socioeconomic Status and Medical Care Patterns

A strong relationship between an individual's social class position and his utilization of medical care services, particularly for treatment of mental illness, has been reported.[1,5,6] Moreover, two previous studies focusing on hospital emergency services found evidence of a direct association between low socioeconomic status and nonurgent presenting conditions.[2,4] A possible weakness in these latter studies, however, was the assumption that all individuals residing in the same geographical area belonged to the same social class.

In the previous analysis of the patient population of this emergency service, the authors wished to test the hypothesis that patients in deprived socioeconomic circumstances were more likely than others to use the emergency service for nonurgent conditions. The Hollingshead Two-factor Index, based on the occupation and educational level of the head of the household weighted by a ratio of 7:4, was selected as the most appropriate and convenient measure of social-class position.[1] The relevance of this index to analysis of medical care utilization had already been demonstrated.[1,5,6] Since the index value was determined for each patient separately, it was deemed to be a more sensitive indicator than a general measure based on geographical location.

The anticipated positive relationship between low socioeconomic status and nonurgency was not confirmed, however. It was reflected only indirectly by a significant association between social class and use of a private physician as the usual source of medical care. This factor of relationship with private medical care associated positively with the urgency of presenting conditions in the Emergency Service. However, as is clearly demonstrated in Table 1, the Two-factor Index as a direct measure of social-class position was itself not significantly associated with urgency rating in this patient population.

An examination of the characteristics of the study population provides some leads to explain the inapplicability of the Two-factor Index in this setting.

Table 1
Urgency Rating by Social Class

Social class	Urgent	Nonurgent	Total	Percent nonurgent
I-III	29	47	76	61.8
IV	62	82	144	57.0
V	70	105	175	60.0
Total	161	234	395	59.2

$X_{2df}^2 = .58$. $.80 > P > .70$.

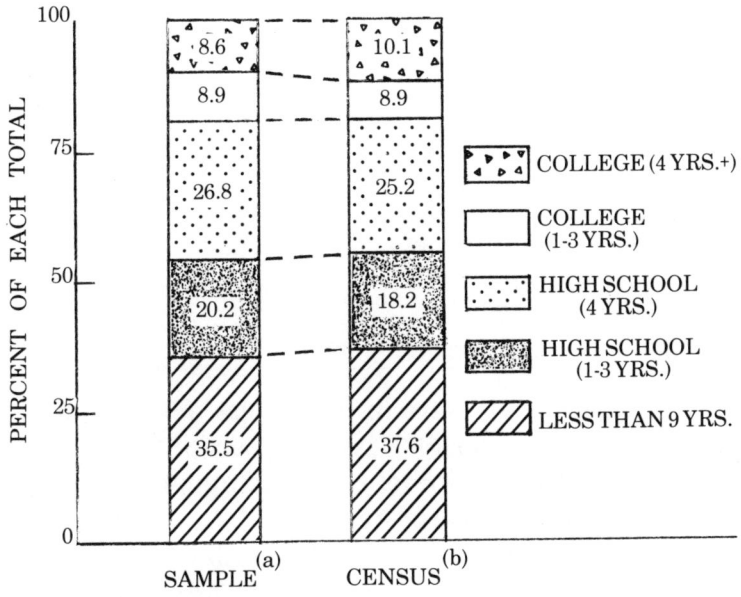

(a) Refers to head of family.
(b) Includes all persons 25 years and older.
Fig. 1. Percentage distribution by educational status, interviewed subsample and New Haven area.

When compared with the general New Haven population, the Yale-New Haven Hospital Emergency Service patient sample included a larger proportion of unmarried individuals, minority group members, inner-city residents, and low-social-class members. On the other hand, despite their predominantly "lower-class" profile, the levels of education attained by the patient population were closely comparable to those of the New Haven population (Fig. 1).

Further indications of the atypical composition of the study population are shown in Tables 2, 3, and 4. The association between social class and family income was noticeably weak (Table 2). An unusually large proportion (22 percent) of patients in the highest

Table 2
Social Class by Income Level

Income level	Class I-III	Class IV	Class V	Total	Percent Class I-III	Percent Class V
$0-4,999	17	68	132	217	8	61
$5,000-7,499	17	49	28	94	18	30
$7,500 and over	42	22	12	76	55	16
Total	76	139	172	387	20	44

social classes (I-III) were in the lowest income classification (less than $5,000). Neither occupational level nor educational attainment, the components of the Two-factor Index, were significantly related to urgency status (Tables 3 and 4). This inability to demonstrate a strong relationship between any one of the socioeconomic variables examined and the urgency status of patients precludes the applicability of the Two-factor Index or any other "all-purpose" social-class index in this medical care setting. Instead, it emphasizes the need to develop a new, more specific index which takes into consideration the complex interrelationship between relevant socioeconomic, demographic, and medical care variables.

Table 3
Urgency Rating by Occupational Level

Occupational Level	Urgent	Non-urgent	Total	Percent Non-urgent
1-3	32	41	73	56
4-6	87	130	217	60
7	46	64	110	58
Total	165	235	400	59

$X^2_{2df} = .34 \quad .90 > P > .80.$

PRESENT INVESTIGATION

Research Objectives

The specific aims of this research were:
1. To demonstrate methods of developing indices relevant to the specific circumstances of medical care situations.
2. To derive appropriate predictive indices of use of the Yale-New Haven Hospital Emergency Service for non-urgent conditions.
3. To assess the relative importances of various demographic, socioeconomic and medical care variables in influencing the use of emergency facilities for nonurgent medical problems.
4. To elucidate the observed incongruence between a two-factor index of social position and the "urgency" status of a sample of Emergency Service patients.

Methodology

Preliminary analyses of the study data indicated that the use of the Emergency Service for nonurgent conditions was influenced by a complex of interrelated variables, most of which were qualitative.

Table 4
Urgency Rating by Educational Level

Educational Level	Urgent	Non-urgent	Total	Percent Non-urgent
1-2	14	22	36	61
3-4	59	84	143	59
5-6	67	95	162	59
7	21	34	55	62
Total	161	235	396	59

$X_{3df}^2 = .24.$ $.99 > P > .95.$

Therefore, a method of multivariate statistical analysis, applicable to qualitative variables, was employed; the gross results were presented in the previous report.[10] Since the population available for analysis was relatively small, only a handful of variables could be taken into consideration at any one time. Therefore, this procedure yielded little information beyond that provided by the univariate analyses.

For the present research, it was decided to employ multivariate statistical techniques that would allow exploration of the complex interrelationships among several variables in both the overall sample population and in selected subgroups. The two techniques applied to the study data were the principal-axis method of factor analysis (with varimax rotation) and multiple linear regression analysis. Although it was recognized that these methods are not specifically applicable to qualitative data and could not provide definitive results, it was nevertheless assumed that they could provide some additional knowledge about the interrelationship of the variables known to be associated with "urgency" status. Mathematical computations required for these techniques were executed by the IBM 7094 computer at the Yale Computer Center.

Factor analysis. The method of factor analysis, frequently used in studies utilizing socioeconomic status to predict and/or evaluate health status,[3] provides a means of reducing a large number of correlated variables to a smaller matrix of uncorrelated factors. The varimax rotation procedure often assists in clarifying the interpretation by reducing the total number of prominent variables within each factor.

Findings of the previous research were used to select 17 variables which were expected to be related indirectly or directly to urgency status. These variables were categorized and assigned discrete values (Table

5), with higher values indicating closer relationships to nonurgency. After excluding all records for which information about any one of the 17 variables was

Table 5
Factor Analysis Research Variables

Variables	Categories and Scale Score
Day of week	Mon.-Fri. (1); Sat.-Sun. (0)
Time of visit	8 a.m.-10 p.m. (1); 10 p.m.-8 a.m. (0)
Census tract	Core city (1); outer city (0)
Sex	Male (1); female (0)
Age (years)	1-14 (4); 15-24 (3); 25-54 (2); 55 plus (1)
Marital status	Never married, separated, divorced (1); married, widowed (0)
Ethnicity	Negro, Puerto Rican (1); white (0)
Years at current address	Not a New Haven resident, less than six months (2); six months-two years (1); more than two years (0)
Usual source of medical care	Emergency service (2); outpatient clinics (1); private physician (0)
Has regular private physician	No (1); yes (0)
Emergency service visits in past year	Over 6 (3); 3-6 (2); 1-2 (1); none (0)
Medical help sought before coming to the Emergency Service	No (1); yes (0)
Source of referral to the Emergency Service	Self (2); lay (1); medical (0)
Family income level	Under $2500 (5); $2500-5000 (4); $5000-7500 (3); $7500-10,000 (2); Over $10,000 (1)
Occupational level	(1-7)
Educational level	(1-7)
Social class	(1-5)

lacking, a total of 378 patient records was available for analysis.

The factor analysis procedure was applied to the study data in two stages. Initially, six analyses were performed, one for each of two urgency categories within each of three social-class strata. It was anticipated that this primary approach would assist in providing further explanation of the unsuitability of the Two-factor Index of Social Position as an indicator of urgency status. The second stage of this analysis was intended to explore the interdependence of variables within each urgency classification. Therefore, social class subdivisions were eliminated and factor structures were developed and compared for the entire urgent and nonurgent populations.

Multiple regression analysis. In an effort to develop a more suitable predictive index, multiple linear regression analysis was applied to the study data. Regression analysis provides an estimate of the proportion of "criterion variance" that can be accounted for by the complete system of predictor variables or by portions of that system. It was anticipated, therefore, that this procedure would assist in identifying those variables that are most appropriate for determining an individual's likelihood of using the Emergency Service for nonurgent reasons (criterion variable). In addition, application of this technique results in an equation for predicting the unknown criterion of a new subject from his known set of predictor scores.

Since most of the variables available for analysis could not be measured on a conventional numerical scale, all of the simple and "interaction" variables selected were first dichotomized (Table 6). For each of these variables, patients with the characteristic listed were assigned a score of 1 for that variable; otherwise, a score of 0 applied. To obtain determinate estimates,

Table 6
Multiple Regression Analysis Research Variables

Simple Predictor Variables	T ratio	Interaction Variables	T ratio
1. Weekday visit	0.2	24. (1) × (2)	-0.1
2. Daytime visit	-0.1	25. (1) × (3)	-0.6
3. Core-city resident	1.0	26. (2) × (3)	0.5
4. Male	-1.1	27. (2) × (4)	1.3
5. Age under 15	-3.4*	28. (3) × (6)	0.1
6. Age 55 or over	-2.0*	29. (3) × (9)	-0.0
7. Unmarried	1.5	30. (3) × (20)	-1.8
8. Minority group	-0.5	31. (4) × (8)	0.5
9. Short residential tenure	-0.1	32. (7) × (8)	0.3
10. High occupation	-1.0	33. (7) × (18)	-0.9
11. Low occupation	-1.1	34. (8) × (9)	0.7
12. High education	-1.0	35. (8) × (18)	-1.2
13. Low education	-0.2	36. (8) × (20)	0.4
14. Self referral	1.1	37. (9) × (14)	0.7
15. Medical referral	-1.2	38. (9) × (18)	-0.6
16. Usual source, M.D.	2.5*	39. (11) × (20)	0.5
17. Usual source E.S.	1.8	40. (12) × (14)	0.9
18. No private M.D.	0.5	41. (12) × (20)	-1.3
19. Frequent use of E.S.	0.4	42. (13) × (20)	0.1
20. Low income	1.3	43. (14) × (20)	-1.6
21. High income	-1.5	44. (3) × (8)	0.2
22. Social class I-III	0.4	45. (18) × (20)	2.4*
23. Social class V	1.3	46. (21) × (22)	-1.6
		47. (20) × (23)	-0.3
		48. (3) × (23)	-0.6
		49. (18) × (23)	-1.2
		50. (18) × (22)	1.2

Criterion variable: Nonurgent medical condition

*Significant at the 95 percent level of confidence.

one category of each variable was eliminated. That is, only one alternative was retained for dichotomous variables, and two alternatives were retained for trichotomous variables. With the variables transformed in this manner, the method of regression analysis of dummy variables described by Suits[7] was applied, utilizing 23 simple and 27 interaction predictor variables for each of 378 subjects. The significance of the multiple-correlation coefficient and of the contribution of each predictor variable was tested.

Predictor variables that did not contribute significantly were eliminated from subsequent analyses. This resulted in two final multiple linear regression equations, each of which could be utilized as an index of nonurgent use of the Emergency Service. Since both the predictor variables and the criterion variable could take the values of 0 or 1, the regression equations yielded estimates of the criterion which were bounded by 0 and 1 and which could be interpreted as probabilities associated with nonurgency.

Findings

Results of factor analyses. Since the results of the factor analyses are extensive, only the highlights of the findings will be presented, with emphasis upon factors which were easily interpretable after rotation and upon those which focused attention on contrasting subgroups of the urgent and nonurgent categories within each social stratum.

Factor I of the urgent group describes an outer-city population which usually resorted to private medical care but came to the Emergency Service during working hours in times of acute medical urgency. Factor I of the nonurgent category depicts a low-income professional group (perhaps advanced students and/or their families) which was unable to afford or lacked motivation to seek private medical care. This group did not seek medical help before coming to the Emergency Service, but considered the emergency facility to be its primary source of medical care.

Thus, surprisingly enough, when social class was determined exclusively by occupational and educational attainment, distinct differences in medical care patterns were observed even within the top three social classes. These differences apparently were related

Social Classes I-III

	Urgent	Nonurgent
Number of factors examined:	5	6
Cumulative variation explained:	72 percent	74 percent
Factors compared:	I	I
Variation explained by each:	18 percent	19 percent
Variables (factor loadings):	Time of visit (.77) Census tract (-.72) Usual source of care (-.52) Regular M.D. (-.74)	Marital status (-.51) Usual source of care (.79) Regular M.D. (.80) Family income (.74) Medical help sought (.51)

to income and convenience factors which influenced the recourse to emergency facilities under conditions of medical nonurgency. The large number of advanced students and their families that were based at the hospital or in close proximity to the medical center probably accounted for the liberal use of the Emergency Service facilities by class I-III persons. Presumably this group did not interpret reliance upon the Emergency Service as having "lower-class" connotations, either because they, as transients, were not motivated to establish stable medical care patterns, or because they were aware of the wide range of medical services which were conveniently accessible to them.

Within social class IV, patients with urgent medical conditions fell into two major categories as represented by Factors V and VI. One subgroup sought other medical help before being referred to the Emergency Service. The other main subgroup comprised a low-income, working-age population which generally did not rely on the emergency facility but did go directly to it in times of urgent medical need.

For the population whose members presented themselves with nonurgent conditions, Factor III delineates a group of patients who utilized the emergency facility as a primary source of care on weekends. Factor IV focuses upon a non-working-age population whose members came to the Emergency Service primarily during the convenient daytime hours.

Attempts to seek medical help before coming to the Emergency Service seemed to reflect the true urgency of the medical problem for the Social Class IV patients. Age also appeared to be a significant determinant of nonurgent use, suggesting that class IV persons in the more vulnerable young/old age groups tended to make use of the Emergency Service for regular and preventive health care. In contrast, class IV persons in the working-age groups generally first applied to other available medical resources, such as employment clinics and private physicians, but resorted directly to the emergency facility on weekends when other medical sources were not readily accessible.

Social Class IV

	Urgent	Nonurgent
Number of factors examined:	7	6
Cumulative variation explained:	76 percent	67 percent
Factors compared:	V; VI	III; IV
Variation explained by each:	12 percent; 18 percent	12 percent; 10 percent
Variables (factor loadings):	*Factor V* Medical help sought (-.88) Source of referral (-.72) *Factor VI* Age (.77) E.S. visits (-.57) Income (-.45)	*Factor III* Medical help sought (.72) Source of referral (.59) Day of of week (-.71) *Factor IV* Age (-.75) Time of visit (.67)

Class V persons presenting with acute medical conditions were represented by two prominent groups. Factor I describes a minority group population which has relied heavily on the emergency facility in times

Social Class V

	Urgent	Nonurgent
Number of factors examined:	6	6
Cumulative variation explained:	70 percent	66 percent
Factors compared:	I; II	II; III
Variation explained by each:	14 percent; 13 percent	11 percent; 11 percent
Variables (factor loadings):	*Factor I* Ethnicity (.73) E.S. visits (.73) Usual source (.69) *Factor II* Age group (.74) Years at current address (.84) Private M.D. (.56)	*Factor III* Ethnicity (-.71) Census tract (-.78) *Factor II* Age group (-.64) Marital status (.72) Family income (.55)

of medical need. Factor II delineates a residentially unstable working-age population with no regular private medical care.

The class V persons with nonurgent conditions were represented by one group of white, outer-city residents (Factor III), and by a combined young/old low-family-income segment of the population (Factor II).

Even within the lowest social class, differences in age composition and in ethnicity appeared to influence the recourse to emergency facilities. Persons in the young/old age groupings tended to utilize the Emergency Service as an all-purpose clinic. Ethnic differences were not quite as pronounced but seemed to be correlated with other variables in influencing the use of the emergency facility.

The factor analyses of the entire "urgent" sample and of the total "nonurgent" sample, over all social classes, showed the effects of socioeconomic variables on the utilization of the emergency facility. Factor I of the nonurgent group and Factor II of the urgent segment comprised socioeconomic variables exclusively and accounted for the most variability in their respective groups. However, they still accounted for less than 20 percent of the within-group variability. Age-group distribution appeared to be the only other variable which contributed alone to medical urgency.

The inability of any one factor to account for more than 20 percent of the within-group variability in any one of the eight factor analyses cited further explains the unsuitability of the Two-factor Social Class Index in predicting the nonurgent use of the Emergency Service. The factor analyses strongly suggest that non-socioeconomic variables interact differently within different social classes. This underscores the importance of evaluating the interaction of demographic, medical care, and socioeconomic determinants in motivating individuals to seek help for nonacute medical conditions at an emergency facility.

Results of the multiple regression analyses. The significance of the contribution of each predictor variable was tested by means of T-ratios. Results are pre-

Social Classes I-V

	Urgent	Nonurgent
Number of factors examined:	6	6
Cumulative variation explained:	65 percent	63 percent
Factors compared:	II; V	I; III
Variation explained by each:	17 percent; 7 percent	19 percent; 9 percent
Variables (factor loadings):	*Factor II*	*Factor I*
	Educational level (-.82)	Family income (.70)
	Occupational level (-.89)	Educational level (.85)
	Social class (-.95)	Occupational level (.89)
	Factor V	Social class (.95)
	Age group (.73)	*Factor III*
	Family income (-.67)	Age group (-.47)
		Time of visit (.49)

Table 7
T-ratios of Variables Selected from
Preliminary Multiple Regression Analysis

Variables	T-ratios
1. Age under 15	-3.38
2. Age 55 or over	-3.11
3. Unmarried	1.53
4. Self-referral	2.64
5. Usual source (Emergency Service)	.23
6. No regular private physician	.16
7. Low income	.54
8. Low social class	-.60
9. Low income x no regular private physician	1.20

sented in Table 6. Among the simple predictor variables, only *age* and *usual source of medical care* contributed significantly. The fact that only one of the 27 interaction variables was found to be statistically significant was surprising, indicating the possibility that the variables for the most part exerted independent effects.

After examination of the T-ratios and the intercorrelations between variables, it was decided to retain nine of the original predictor variables and to fit a regression analysis to this subset. The variables retained and their corresponding T-ratios are shown in Table 7. Once again the prominent variables are *age* and *usual sources of medical care*—overshadowing the effects of such influences as *low income or low social class* as far as prediction of nonurgency is concerned.

For practical purposes, it was considered desirable to perform two final regression analyses, each providing a predictive equation which would yield an index of nonurgency, and each derived from different subsets of the nine selected predictor variables.

An "Emergency Service Index" was then derived from the five variables listed in Table 8, including two medical care variables that were ascertainable only from direct questioning of the patient at the emergency facility. The two age variables were most important in predicting urgency status. The interaction variable *(low income x no regular private physician)* and *type of referral* also contributed significantly. Although *marital status* was not a statistically significant variable, it was uncorrelated with the other variables and exerted an influence which approached significance throughout the regression analyses. The Emergency Service Index suggests that an unmarried individual aged 15-54 who is in the low-income bracket, has no regular private physician relationship, and is self-referred to the Emergency Service is most likely to attend for nonurgent medical reasons.

The variables of *age, marital status,* and *family income* were used to develop a *"Demographic Index."* These variables are readily ascertainable from many sources and are generally available without recourse

Table 8
Emergency Service Index*

Variable	(No.)	T-ratio	Regression Coefficient
Age under 15	(1)	-3.44	-.22
Age 55 or over	(2)	-3.17	-.26
Unmarried	(3)	1.62	.10
Self-referral	(4)	2.78	.14
Low income x no regular private physician	(9)	2.96	.15

*Multiple correlation coefficient = 0.32; F ratio = 8.67; intercept = 0.51.

Regression equation: $P = .51 - .22X_1 - .26X_2 + .10X_3 + .14X_4 + .15X_9$.

Table 9
Demographic Index*

Variable	(No.)	T-ratio	Regression Coefficient
Age less than 15 years	(1)	-3.41	-.22
Age 55 years or more	(2)	-3.96	-.33
Unmarried	(3)	1.33	.08
Low income	(7)	2.28	.12

*Multiple correlation coefficient = 0.27; F ratio = 7.47; intercept = 0.59.

Regression equation: $P = 0.59 - 0.22X_1 - 0.33X_2 + 0.08X_3 + 0.12X_7$.

to personal interviews. From Table 9 it is apparent that the age-group variables dominate the Demographic Index, which characterizes a patient who uses the Emergency Service for nonurgent medical conditions as being unmarried, aged 15-54, and in the lowest income category.

In regression analysis the square of the multiple correlation coefficient provides an estimate of the proportion of criterion variance that can be accounted for by the predictor variables and thereby yields an indication of the predictive efficiency of the regression equation. In this respect, the two final regression equations are somewhat disappointing, in that each explained less than 10 percent of the criterion variance. However, it should be recognized that when a binary criterion is used in regression analysis the multiple correlation coefficient is probably underestimated.

Another means of examining the "goodness of fit" of the regression model is to cross-tabulate the regression estimates of the criterion against the observed distribution of urgency status. The probability of nonurgency was estimated for each of the 378 sample members and with each of the two final regression models. The probability estimates were divided into three categories (under 0.50, 0.50-0.69, and 0.70 or more) and the corresponding observed distribution of the sample population by urgency status was determined. Results are shown in Tables 10 and 11. In both indexes, the proportion of nonurgent patients rises significantly with increasing probability of nonurgency. The predictive ability of the Demographic Index (Table 11) was comparable to that of the Emergency Service Index (Table 10) in the higher probability range, but not quite as good in the range under 0.50.

The regression indexes of nonurgency can be used as a guide to identify, for health education purposes, that subgroup of the Emergency Service patient population which has been inclined to use the emergency facility for nonurgent medical needs. For example, when applying the Emergency Service Index to the study population, patients who were assigned probability scores on nonurgency exceeding 0.70 represented 24 percent of the total sample, 31 percent of the nonurgent population, and only 14 percent of the urgent patient visits. Similarly, utilizing the Demographic Index and focusing on 31 percent of the total

Table 10
Emergency Service Index: Observed versus Predicted Urgency Distribution

Prob. (Nonurgent)	Urgent	Non-urgent	Total	Percent Nonurgent
0.00-0.49	44	21	65	32.3
0.50-0.69	88	134	222	60.4
0.70-0.99	21	70	91	76.9
Total	153	225	378	59.5

$X_{2df}^2 = 31.48$. $P < .001$.

Table 11
Demographic Index: Observed versus Predicted
Urgency Distribution

Prob. (Nonurgent)	Urgent	Non-urgent	Total	Percent Nonurgent
0.00-0.49	53	39	92	42.4
0.50-0.69	72	96	168	57.1
0.70-0.99	28	90	118	76.3
Total	153	225	378	59.5

$X^2_{2df} = 25.35.$ $P < .001.$

patients with probabilities greater than 0.70 yields 40 percent of the nonurgent visits and 18 percent of the urgent visits in the population under study.

Although the regression models do not provide an exceptionally good fit to the observed urgency distribution, a comparison of the fit of the regression models in Tables 10 and 11 with that of the Social Class Index in Table 1 easily demonstrates the superiority of the regression models in this medical care environment.

DISCUSSION

The Two-factor Index of Social Class Position, based on a weighted average of occupational and educational attainment scores, has proven to be an effective means of explaining medical care utilization patterns in various medical care settings. The inability to demonstrate a direct relationship between this index of social class and the urgency of the presenting medical condition in the specific Emergency Service population under review was, apparently, due to the atypical socioeconomic characteristics observed in this particular group of patients. Specifically, social-class position was found not to be highly associated with family income in this population. Moreover, factor analyses revealed that, within each social class, intervening variables such as age, income, ethnicity, and usual medical care patterns exerted varying influences on the utilization of the Emergency Service. The findings account for the unsuitability of the Two-factor Index, or any other "all-purpose" social index, for discriminating between urgent and nonurgent medical conditions at the Yale-New Haven Emergency Service.

The multiple linear regression technique was used to develop a more appropriate index for this medical care setting. The two measures derived, the Emergency Service Index, based on a weighted average of five demographic and medical care variables, and the Demographic Index, developed from a weighted average of four demographic variables, each provided a closer fit to the observed distribution of urgency status than did the Two-factor Index of Social Position.

Both regression models emphasize the importance of a patient's age in discriminating between urgent and nonurgent use of the Emergency Service. Patients aged 15-54 were the prime users of the emergency facility for nonurgent-conditions. The factor models, however, indicate that certain young and old segments of the patient population, particularly in the lower socioeconomic groups, utilized the Emergency Service routinely as an all-purpose clinic. Therefore, in addition to age distribution, other intervening factors such as *marital status, family income,* and *usual medical care patterns* are required to assist in discriminating between urgent and nonurgent use of the Emergency Service.

Despite the pertinence of the above findings, caution must be exercised in interpreting the results of regression analysis when a binary criterion is used. Although the tests of significance utilized are generally quite robust, the real test of the goodness of fit is still the accuracy of prediction when the regression equation or index is applied to independent observations. Since the amount of data collected in this study was not adequate for subdivision for testing purposes, tests of validity should be applied on new data from a similar population.

Although the indexes derived are more appropriate than the simple index of social class, it is apparent that further study of the determinants of use of the Emergency Service is indicated.

SUMMARY

The interrelationships among selected demographic, socioeconomic, and medical care variables were examined in a random subsample of 402 of 2028 consecutive patients at the Emergency Service of the Yale-New Haven Hospital.

The lack of association between an occupation—education index of social class and the use of the emergency station for nonurgent conditions has been examined and explained, to some extent, by the application of factor analysis to the study data.

The method of multiple regression analysis has been proposed as a means of developing indexes more relevant to the specific medical care setting. This technique was applied to derive two new indexes of use of the Emergency Service.

The relative importance of various demographic, socioeconomic, and medical care variables in influencing the recourse to the emergency facility for nonurgent medical problems has been evaluated. The need for additional motivational analysis has been emphasized.

REFERENCES

1. Hollingshead, A. B., and Redlich, F. C.: Social Class and Mental Illness. New York, John Wiley, 1958.
2. Kwass, S. K.: Social Class Differences in Emergency Room Attendance. Student thesis, Yale University, 1958 (unpublished).
3. Lebowitz, M.D., and Malcolm, J. C.: Socio-economic analysis of the Alameda County Health Department jurisdiction. *A.J.P.H.* 54: 1876, 1964.
4. Lee, S. S., Solon, J. A., and Sheps, C. G.: How new patterns of medical care affect the emergency unit. *Mod. Hosp.* 94:97, 1960.
5. Myers, J. K., and Roberts, B. H.: Family and Class Dynamics in Mental Illness. New York, John Wiley, 1959.
6. Myers, J. K., Bean, L. L., and Pepper, M. P.: Social class and psychiatric disorders: A ten-year follow-up. *J. Health Hum. Behav.* 6:74, 1965.
7. Suits, D. B.: Use of dummy variables in regression equations. *J.A.S.A.* 52:548, 1957.
8. Weinerman, E. R., and Edwards, H. R.: Yale studies in ambulatory medical care: I. Changing patterns in hospital emergency service. *Hospitals* 38:55, 1964.
9. Weinerman, E. R., Rutzen, S. R., and Pearson, D. A.: Yale studies in ambulatory medical care: II. Effects of medical triage in hospital emergency service. *Public Health Rep.* 80:389, 1965.
10. Weinerman, E. R., Ratner, R. S., Robbins, A., and Lavenhar, M. A.: Yale studies in ambulatory medical care: V. Determinants of use of hospital emergency services. *A.J.P.H.* 56:1037, 1966.

9. Problems of Communication, Diagnosis, and Patient Care: The Interplay of Patient, Physician and Clinic Organization*

Irving Kenneth Zola, Ph.D.

As every beginning medical student learns, history taking is a major diagnostic tool. Such interviewing requires a great deal of skill and understanding, and when there are reasons for reticence and fear, such as in an initial medical visit, even greater demands are placed on the doctor and the patient in their attempt to communicate with one another.[1,2] The nature of this communication, moreover, is determined by a number of nonmedical factors, three of which will be delineated in this paper: the patient's ethnic background, the physician's medical specialty-orientation, and the clinic's spatial design and organization. An attempt will be made to demonstrate how each of these may operate to prevent or limit communication between patient and doctor and thus affect ultimate diagnosis and treatment.

*Reprinted from *Journal of Medical Education*, October 1963, Vol. 38, No. 10.

THE PATIENT'S ETHNIC BACKGROUND

A number of studies have noted that both the diagnosis and treatment which psychiatric patients received were related to their social class[3-6]. There has, however, been little speculation about the effect of social background on the diagnosis and treatment of medical patients and their physical disorders.[7] During a study on the decisions of lower-class Italians, Irish, and Anglo-Saxons to seek aid at the Medical, Eye, and Ear, Nose and Throat (ENT) Clinics of a large urban hospital, proportionately more Italians were found to be labeled "psychiatric problems" by their physicians. This was despite the fact that there was no evidence that psychosocial problems were more frequent among them. On three general ratings of such problems* there were no statistically significant differences between the ethnic groups and thus no objective reason to expect the greater frequency of "psychiatric diagnosis" in one group over another.

Such differences in diagnosis might, however, be related to how the patients presented themselves and thus how they were perceived and ultimately diag-

*In obtaining a measure of the amount and nature of psychosocial problems in the study population, all the patients were rated on three categories: (1) Note was made of the spontaneous mention by the patient of being "very nervous," or of "nerves" being one of his greatest problems. (2) Note was made of the spontaneous mention of very pressing and difficult vocational, personal, or interpersonal situations (e.g., in the process of getting a divorce, having to care for a mentally ill husband or child, hating present work and life etc.). (3) A clinical psychologist rated the patient's interview responses as to the "presence of obvious psychological problems interfering with adequate functioning."

nosed and treated. In the larger study, basic differences were found between the Italians and the Irish (the Anglo-Saxons occupied a middle position but more often resembled the Irish) in the way they presented their chief complaints and illnesses and in the specific circumstances surrounding the decision to come to a doctor. The over-all study is reported elsewhere,[8,9] but some specific findings on the Italians are pertinent: they tended to show diffuse reactions to being sick; they reported more symptoms and stated more often that the symptoms made them irritable and difficult to get along with; and, in describing the specific circumstances bringing them to a doctor they more often felt that their symptoms interfered with social and personal relations, or mentioned the presence of an interpersonal crisis. In another study of Italians, Zborowski[10] felt that their "uninhibited display of reactions" to pain and their overinvolvement with symptoms would tend to provoke distrust in the doctors treating them. Since the Italians in our sample might also be perceived as "overacting," we speculated that this might have influenced the high number of psychiatric diagnoses.

The hypothesis that the patient's social background (i.e., ethnicity) and thus the way he presented himself influenced his diagnosis was tested by examining a group of cases where no medical basis for the symptoms had been found. It was felt that in these cases the operation of nonmedical factors would be most clear. So that we might err on the side of conservatism, a number of diagnoses which did little more than describe the patient's symptoms were excluded. (For example, "vitreous opacities" referred to the fact that the patient saw spots in front of his eyes, while "tinnitus" meant he heard hums, rings, buzzing, etc. It is interesting to note, however, that these "descriptive" diagnoses were attributed primarily to the Anglo-Saxon and Irish patients.) Because the number of males which fit these criteria was too small for statistical comparisons, the hypothesis was only tested on a subsample of women: ten Italians, thirteen Irish, and six Anglo-Saxons.

When the previously mentioned ratings of psychosocial problems were applied to the above three groups, no statistically significant differences were found. Each of these three groups were then further subdivided by the implied etiology of their symptoms. The first category, "psychogenesis implied," were patients with one of three diagnoses: tension headache, functional complaint (e.g., functional pain in the left arm) and emotional disorder (e.g., anxiety, depressed, neurotic, etc.). The second category consisted of patients where no explicit psychogenesis was implied. It included only those women in whose cases the physician had explicitly stated there was "no pathology" and a few cases of asthenopia (meaning tired eyes). Table 1 shows how the doctors diagnosed patients where no organic basis for their complaints had been found. It is worth noting that the two "psychogenesis" cases of the Anglo-Saxons had the most obvious psychopathology in the entire sample of two hundred. One of these presented herself as being "mentally ill" and had been referred by the local Mental Health Association. The second entered the interview reeling and unsteady, accompanied by the distinct aroma of liquor and was subsequently diagnosed by her physician as "alcoholic."

In short, when no medical disease was found, the Italians were diagnosed as having a psychological problem while the Anglo-Saxons and Irish were not. Since psychosocial problems were equally present in all groups, there was no reason to expect one of the

TABLE 1

PHYSICIAN DIAGNOSES OF FEMALE PATIENTS WITH NO ORGANIC BASIS FOR SYMPTOMS

	Italian	Irish	Anglo-Saxon
Psychogenesis Implied	11	2	2
No psychogenesis Implied	1	9	4
Total	12	11	6

Italian vs. Irish, X^2 equals 10.60 (corrected for continuity), $P < .01$

three ethnic groups to have more diagnoses in the "psychogenesis implied" category. Thus one can only conclude that the patient's ethnic background, which influenced the way she presented herself and her complaint, may have inordinately and inappropriately influenced the diagnosis by the examining physician.

THE PHYSICIAN'S SPECIALTY-ORIENTATION

The forces which affect the doctor-patient communication stem from attributes of the doctor as well as the patient. What the patient tells the doctor is influenced, for example, by what cues and interests he perceives and thus what he thinks the doctor wants to hear. What the doctor wants to hear is, in turn, the product of his own background, training, and specialty-orientation.

When attention was focused on the doctor's recognition of patient concerns directly related to his symptoms and his decision to seek aid, evidence was found of a barrier in doctor-patient communication. Our material indicated that not only were there many instances where such concerns were not considered but that recognition, or lack of recognition, of these concerns was more marked at one clinic than another. While more patients with psychosocial problems appeared in the Medical Clinic population, proportionately fewer were acknowledged at either the Eye or the ENT Clinics. (Incidentally, the tendency toward giving the Italians, rather than the Anglo-Saxons or Irish, diagnoses which implied a psychogenic basis was most evident at the Eye Clinic, least at the Medical, with the ENT intermediate.) Thus, a person, regardless of the nature of his presenting complaint, had the best chance of his personal and psychosocial problems being recognized if he was first seen by a doctor in the Medical Clinic, and the worst chance if seen by a doctor in the Eye Clinic. This seemed to imply that there was a differential tendency on the part of specialty-orientations to be aware of the present personal concerns of the patient.

Unfortunately, no objective statistical material was collected on what transpired between the patient and his doctor. The research situation, however, often permitted the author to speak with both the doctor and the patient after the latter was seen. By systematic record review, it was also possible to check the nature of his treatment (including mention of reassurance, guidance, etc.) and his medical progress. From this information and from the more systematically collected interview data, it was possible to create a fairly complete picture of the patient's concerns, both medical and otherwise, surrounding his decision to seek aid. The following cases are illustrative of instances where the psychosocial concerns of the patient were not recognized.

No Organic Pathology

Mary B. was twenty-three, married, and in her seventh month of pregnancy with her first child. She felt she was nearsighted and that it had been too long since her last check-up (i.e., three years). In recent months she had suffered from headaches in and around her eyes and some dizziness. On examination, the doctor found "no visible problem" and told her to return PRN. Since she was pregnant he explained to the author that he did not think it necessary to check her glasses since the prescription would only change once she had delivered. "I told her to return then if she was still bothered by them (i.e., headaches). Her vision was 20/20 with glasses." Why then did this patient come in with such minor problems? The research interview revealed that she was extremely embarrassed about her appearance and felt that this was affecting all her relationships. About three months ago, she broke her glasses (they were presently taped together), but "we didn't have the money with my husband out on strike." "The other day my cousin was over at the house and I was talking about being ashamed of the glasses and how I look 'cause we were going to a wedding." When asked about the general effect of her symptoms (i.e., headache, etc.) she responded, "Well I might have stayed home when I could have gone out . . . or go to bed rather than go out . . . I couldn't go to a movie or anything like that (the way I looked) . . . and so my husband had to go with his brothers." Again and again, she somewhat defensively told how much her husband was against her coming to this clinic but she felt that she could not wait any longer and so went against his wishes.

In understanding this case, it is irrelevant whether the embarrassment and her anxiety stem really from the taped and broken glasses or is related more to her pregnancy; the point is that she has come to the doctor. While he has examined her calling card (i.e., the symptoms) and quite correctly dismissed her ocular symptoms as minor and inconsequential, he did not recognize her more pressing concerns. Knowledge of these might have led to their discussion, a prescription for a new pair of eyeglass frames, or a referral elsewhere. The patient, however, returned empty-handed and discouraged to a husband who told her not to come here in the first place.

Minor Organic Pathology

Carol C. was a forty-five-year-old, single bookkeeper. Within the past year, her mother died and shortly thereafter her relatives began insisting that she move in with them, quit her job, work in their variety store and nurse their mother. With her vacation approaching, they have stepped up their efforts to persuade her to try this arrangement. Although she had a number of minor aches and pains, her chief complaint was a small cyst on her eyelid (Diagnosis: Fibroma). She feared that it might be growing or could lead to something more serious and so felt that it should be checked now (the second day of her vacation) before it was too late. It was only in a somewhat mumbled response to the question of what she expected or would like the doctor to do that she made a connection between the stress she was undergoing with her family and her present insistence on taking care of the cyst. From a list of possible outcomes to her examination, she chose, "Maybe a hospital(ization) . . . Rest would be all right . . . (and then in a barely audible tone) just so they (family) would stop bothering me." The examining physician acceded to her request for removal of the fibroma and referred her to the out-patient operating room. The cyst, however, was only her calling-card and its removal only temporarily alleviated her difficult and threatening interpersonal situation. Her subsequent pattern of medical care bore this out.

Within two weeks after recovery from the operation, she returned to the Eye Clinic still claiming that something was wrong with her eyes. She was sent to Refraction but the tests revealed that glasses were unnecessary. Four months later, she returned again to the Eye Clinic, this time presenting headaches in and around her eyes as the chief complaint. Once again she was examined by an opthalmologist and once again she was refracted. This time, the doctor noted in the record, "Headaches not thought to be on an ocular basis." He did, however, prescribe Collyrium 26 and told her to see her local medical doctor for a more complete examination. (According to her replies in the research interview, she did not really have one.) Seven months later, she appeared at the Emergency Ward with "terrific headaches." She was examined by the attending physicians and given a skull series. The final report states there was no pathology, "though possibly increased intracranial pressure." Several weeks later, she turned to still another avenue of help and asked for an appointment at the Medical Clinic. Here again she presented chiefly the complaint of headaches but this time accompanied by a great deal of bloating and belching. After a series of tests, there appeared in the record the first documented awareness of an underlying psychogenic problem. The final diagnosis was functional headache and epigastric distress. In the course of the last two years, this woman has presented herself at the clinics of the hospital on five separate occasions, involving some ten visits, with as many doctors and technicians and countless tests and examinations.

Major Organic Pathology

Paul W. was thirty-nine, married, a college graduate and presently between assignments as a waiter. A week prior to this visit, his face had become chapped when he had gone for a long walk on a windy, rainy day. He applied cold cream and almost immediately his face began to swell. At about the same time, he noticed a loss of vision in his right eye but he decided to wait awhile before doing anything. As he put it, "I like to feel self-sufficient." When asked when he considered himself sick enough to go to a doctor, he replied, "I don't know ... something obviously calling for medical aid, like appendicitis ... I feel most people go too frequently, magnify their symptoms out of proportion ... If they had greater knowledge of self and physical functions, they wouldn't go as often ... I only go when I can't help myself." As an example, he cited a recent incident. "Last summer I cut my foot and allowed it to become poisoned . . . it became pretty bad . . . When the glands in my groin started to swell and pain, it was time to see a doctor . . . and that was the first time in years." When asked what made him come now, he replied, "Every man has a dream . . . and this (symptoms) affected mine. You see, I do some writing and that's why we follow the resorts. In between jobs I'm able to do this (writing), but if my eyes go, I couldn't drive to the resorts . . . My worry reached a peak last night. It was the first time that it (symptoms) became so prominent that it affected my continuity, my ability to concentrate and do my work." The physician, however, did not recognize his concern about self-reliance and independence that was reflected both in his general pattern of medical care and in his delay in seeking help for his current visual problem. Instead he told him that it was necessary to come back for further tests. Paul W. took the appointment slips and never returned. The probably major diagnosis of optic neuritis or multiple sclerosis only emphasizes the implications of this break in treatment.

While it is expected that there would be instances where the patient's psychosocial concerns would go unnoticed, two conclusions may nevertheless be drawn. (a) Lack of recognition was in large part due to the doctor's orientation and communication (or lack thereof) with his patient; and (b) this lack of attention was more frequent among the practitioners of one specialty rather than another (Eye and ENT vs. Medical). Perhaps the clinician cannot be concerned with the patient's psychosocial problems in their global and general dimensions. It nevertheless seems apparent from these cases that he must at least be concerned with those problems which pertain to the patient's presenting complaint and his decision to seek aid. If he does not recognize these concerns, the examining physician may lose an opportunity to treat his patients effectively.

THE CLINIC'S SPATIAL DESIGN AND ORGANIZATION OF WORK

While the organization and physical structure of a clinic is often thought to be determined by the nature of the disorders, the number of patients, and the most efficient mode of treatment, this very structure can also contribute to the dilemma of the physician in attempting to deal with the patient's "problems."

The clinics, for example, differed in physical structure. At the time of this study, each patient in the Medical Clinic was led by his doctor into a private examination room; in most instances, a room not visible to the other patients. In the ENT Clinic, only a curtain and a partition (open at the top) closed out the world of the doctor-patient from the world of the "waiting." The other patients were relatively near, sitting on benches only a yard or two away. The Eye Clinic, both in the screening room and the clinic proper, was the most open of all. No doors, screen, or walls—only six feet of space separated the patient being seen from those who were waiting. In many instances, he may be within "touching distance" of the patient being examined next to him.

An innovation at the Medical Clinic indicates that the physical setting of a clinic has more to do with a basic philosophy of patient care than with the limitations set by the disease under treatment. Though the medical examination rooms insured physical privacy (an enclosed room), the new chief felt that they did not insure psychological privacy and so had the walls extended to the ceilings. He felt that it was essential to better medical treatment to facilitate communication between the doctor and the patient and that by insuring complete privacy, he was removing one of the barriers.

The flow of patients and thus the demands on a doctor determine, in part, the amount of time he can spend with each individual. In the Medical Clinic, a modified block appointment system was in operation and limited numbers of patients are assigned to the staff. On the other hand, in both the ENT and the Eye Clinics, a sizeable proportion of patients were seen without appointment (Eye more than ENT). The majority of these "walk-in" patients were not strictly emergency cases, a fact well known to the staff.

Another organizational feature is worthy of mention which was, however, peculiar to the Eye Clinic—the utilization of paramedical personnel. The pattern of this use was especially crucial in the case of the patient who came in for such complaints as headaches, blurriness of vision, or difficulty in reading or seeing objects and whose final diagnosis indicates that "nothing is physically wrong." Initially, they were seen in the screening room or in the clinic proper. Upon examination, no ocular disease was detected. The doctor, however, felt that their eyes should be tested more thoroughly or that their glasses should be checked and so referred them to the Refraction Clinic. There they were seen by an optometrist and told that there was nothing wrong with their vision (20/20) or that there was no necessity to change the prescription of their glasses. Unless the patients requested it (they rarely if ever did), they were not referred back to their examining physician but sent along, still with their headache, their blurriness, their difficulty in seeing. The last person to see these patients was an optometrist who, by training and organizational role in this clinic, functioned primarily as a technician and thus was perhaps the one least likely to be in a position to help them, as well as the one least likely to be asked by these patients for further help.

Thus the utilization of paramedical personnel, the flow of patients, and the use of physical space served to make the Medical Clinic most suited to the recognition of the patient's psychosocial concerns and the Eye Clinic least well suited. More importantly, these features illustrate how the differing spatial structure and organization of the clinics implicitly supported the differing orientations of their physicians.

DISCUSSION

Originally, clinics began as dispensaries to screen patients for hospital admission and therefore were not conceived as treatment centers themselves.[11] The increasing number of chronically ill patients and the nature of their medical problems make it evident, however, that more and more patients will be treated in out-patient facilities. In one sense, then, this paper is an extension of previous studies,[12-15] which have called attention to the presence and importance of psychosocial problems in out-patient or ambulatory populations.

The major observations of this study suggest that the recognition of and attention to such problems are influenced by an interplay of several nonmedical factors: the patient's ethnic group membership as shown in the way he presents himself and communicates to the doctor; the examining physician's specialty-orientation as it is reflected in his tendency to overlook the patient's psychosocial concerns; and the clinic's spatial design and organization which can be either a stimulant or a barrier to communication. Particularly in cases where the medical condition is not clear-cut, these factors will influence the diagnosis and treatment which a patient receives.

None of these factors are immutable. The physical and spatial structure can be changed to assure more communication. Organizational changes are also possible. For example, in the special instance of the Eye Clinic, refractions might routinely precede the regular examination or some arrangement might be devised whereby patients are referred back to the examining physician, especially when nothing organic is found to account for his symptoms. All clinics could, without sacrificing emergency coverage, regulate the intake and flow of patients and thus allow more time for physician-patient contact. If an individual's condition goes untreated and therefore worsens or becomes more difficult to manage, or if, though untreated, he continues to seek a solution through different avenues, the total costs in time and money would certainly outweigh the costs of an extended or more thorough initial visit.

Physical and organizational changes are, however, only part of the story. Regardless of the degree of privacy, the patient may be unwilling to talk. Findings of the larger study[8] indicated that patients differed in the way they presented themselves to the doctor. It may also be inferred that they differed in what they thought relevant to their illness and what they deemed necessary to tell the doctor. In that paper, it was demonstrated that, in reality, patients of all three ethnic groups studied had major psychosocial problems and concerns which either caused or exacerbated their conditions or interfered with effective treatment. Yet, in part because of the way the patient initially presented his complaint (which differed by ethnic groups), the recognition of such problems was confined inordinately to one ethnic group. Thus greater attention must be given to the fact that illness or disease is not a purely physical and isolated problem but arises, is perceived, and treated within a social context and this, in turn, will affect the nature of all communication about it.

Doctor-patient communication is, however, a two-way street and evidence has been presented showing that physicians themselves were often unwilling to listen to or probe the patient. Moreover, it seems evident that the doctor's clinical training is at least partly responsible for his difficulty in recognizing and treating such problems and that the training for some specialties prepares one less well than does others. This last observation assumes greater importance as we realize that with the increasing sophistication of the lay population (as well as the increasing specialization of medical personnel) more and more people go directly to specialists or are referred to him at their own request.[16] While the specialist is necessarily concerned with the treatment of a specific organ or disease, the dilemma arises over what his responsibility is to the patient. In an ever-growing number of cases, there simply is no "family doctor"[17] to whom he can return the patient who has pressing psychosocial problems.

CONCLUSION

The question now becomes, should all medical practitioners be capable of recognizing and treating the psychosocial concerns and complaints of the patient. Some feel that this should be the task of other professionals or the task of a special group of medical specialists. To emphasize this point, Churchill[18] cited the following example:

"... a conscientious doctor responded to the call (re: a sick child) but found that the real reason for the vomiting and pain was an angry dispute between the child's parents. After a long day he (the doctor) has to stay until long past midnight in an effort to straighten matters out. An experienced visiting nurse or trained social worker or even the wise neighbor next door might have handled this situation."

While it is problematical to speculate who could best have helped these parents, it is completely unreasonable to expect that any professional or semiprofessional other than the physician would have been called in under any circumstances where the immediate problem was a child's vomiting and pain. A similar situation often confronts the specialist. With increasing sophistication and regardless of the "true" or underlying concerns of the patient or the etiology of his specific condition, patients with visual symptoms are more likely to consult an eye specialist, with a nasal condition, an ENT man, with a limb or back ailment, an orthopedist, etc. This has led men like Balint,[19] Magraw (observations on general practice,[20] and Yudkin (observations on pediatric practice,[21] to claim that psychosocial concerns and problems are part of most illnesses and that attention to them is integral to the effective practice of any medical specialty. Thus, while we cannot expect all specialties to be equally interested in the global and general concerns of the patient, we should expect the physician to be aware of those concerns which affect the patient's presenting complaint, his decision to come, and his subsequent willingness to continue in treatment.

If, as Coleman contends, the emotional distance and the barrier to patient-doctor communication:

". . . is not a necessary or inevitable result, nor the price the physician must pay for calling—it's merely the price he pays for the neglect of this aspect of his training..."[22]

then it is within the realm of medical education that a solution will have to be found. Certainly there is ample evidence, both in this paper and in other investigations, that the vast majority of patients are reticent, anxious, and even fearful of consulting a doctor. In other words, there is probably a general tendency toward delay. Cognizant of this phenomenon, physicians in general, regardless of the seriousness of the patient's presenting complaint, could acknowledge this anxiety and attempt to reinforce his openness as well as the very fact of his coming at all. There is too little awareness of the two-sidedness of the doctor-patient relationship.

"The roles of the doctor and patient are complementary, and it would be most unusual if ideas in role behavior held by patients were not interlocked with and reinforced by expectations of patients which are held by doctors."[23]

Perhaps the major step toward such awareness is the not-so-simple realization that the doctor can block or reject the patient's communication by his very reaction, or lack of reaction, to the patient's concerns and that this will have profound effects on how much he can help and treat his medical condition.

While the comments in this paper have relevance for the handling of all disorders, they seem to have particular relevance in the treatment and management of chronic illness. With the overwhelming majority of such disorders there is at present no instant cure, no miracle drug, no medical surgical procedure and yet there are continual requests and demands for help and support made by the patient. Treatment has become a question of controlling, maintaining, and rehabilitating—processes in which the patients themselves play the major role. With awareness of himself as well as of the patient, the doctor would be in a position to more intelligently intervene and support the patient's own efforts to cope with his disorder.

REFERENCES

1. Kahn, R. L., and Cannell, C. F. *The Dynamics of Interviewing.* New York: Wiley, 1957.
2. Magraw, R. M., and Dulit, E. P. The Patient's Presenting Complaint—Signpost or Goal? *Univ. Minn. Med. Bull.,* 29:329-340, 1958.
3. Hollingshead, A. B., and Redlich, F. C. *Social Class and Mental Illness.* New York: Wiley, 1958.
4. Kahn, R. L., Pollack, M., and Fink, M. Social Factors in Selection of Therapy in a Voluntary Hospital. *J. Hillside Hospital,* 6:216-218, 1957.
5. Kahn, R. L., Pollack, M., and Fink, M. Socio-psychologic Aspects of Psychiatric Treatment in a Voluntary Mental Hospital. *A.M.A. Arch. Gen. Psychiat.,* 1:565-574, 1959.
6. Siegel, N. H., Pollack, M., Kahn, R. L., and Fink, M. Social Class, Diagnosis, and Treatment in Three Psychiatric Hospitals. Paper Presented at the Annual Meeting of the American Sociological Association, St. Louis, Missouri, August, 1961.
7. Ruesch, J., Jacobson, A., and Loeb, M. B. Acculturation and Illness. *Psych. Monog.,* 62: 292, 1948.
8. Zola, I. K. Socio-cultural Factors in the Seeking of Medical Aid. Unpublished Ph. D. Thesis, Harvard University, 1962.
9. Zola, I. K. Socio-cultural Factors in the Seeking of Medical Aid: A Progress Report. *Transcultural Psychiatric Research,* 14:62-65, 1963.
10. Zborowski, M. Cultural Components in Response to Pain. *Patients, Physicians, and Illness.* E. G. Jaco, Editor. Glencoe, Illinois: Free Press, 1958. Pp. 256-268.
11. Washburn, F. A. The Out-patient Department and Emergency Ward, in *The Massachusetts General Hospital,* Boston: Houghton Mifflin, 1939. Pp. 199-236. 199-236.
12. Grobin, W. Personal Experience in the Practice of Internal Medicine. *Canad. Med. Ass. J.,* 79:259-265, 1958.

13. Mannucio, M., Friedman, S. M., Kaufman, M. R. Survey of Patients Who Have Been Attending Non-Psychiatric Outpatient Department Services for Ten Years or Longer. *J. Mt. Sinai Hosp.,* 18:32-52, 1961.
14. Shepherd, M., Fisher, M., Stein, L., and Kessel, W. N. N. Psychiatric Morbidity in an Urban Group Practice. *Proc. Roy. Soc. Med.,* 52:269, 1959.
15. Tyler, S. H. On the Nature of Private Practice and the Need for Psychotherapy. *Amer. Practit.,* 1:1303-1308, 1950.
16. Williams, T. F., White, K. L., Andrews, L. P., Diamond, E., Greenberg, B. G., Hamrick, A. A., and Hunter, E. A. Patient Referral to University Clinic. Patterns in Rural State. *Amer. J. Public Health,* 50:1493-1507, 1960.
17. Geiger, H. J. The Choice and Use of Physicians by Families: Physician Quality and Family Choice. Paper presented at the American Sociological Association Meetings, Washington, D.C., August 29-September 2, 1962.
18. Churchill, E. D. Medical Wants and Needs in Mature and Developing Nations. *Medical Times,* November, 1961.
19. Balint, M. *The Doctor, The Patient, and His Illness,* London: P. Homan, 1957.
20. Magraw, R. M. Psychosomatic Medicine and the Diagnostic Process. *Postgrad. Med.,* 25:639-645, 1959.
21. Yudkin, S. Six Children with Coughs, The Second Diagnosis. *Lancet,* 2:561-563, 1961.
22. Coleman, J. V. Mental Health, Patient Care and Medical Practice. *Integration of Mental Health Concepts with the Human Relations Professions.* 132 pp. Proceedings of a Lecture Series Sponsored by the Bank Street College of Education as a Memorial to Ruth Kotinsky, 1962. Pp. 30-42.
23. Apple, D. How Laymen Define Illness. *J. Health Hum. Beh.,* 1:219-225, 1960.

10. Help?: The Hospital Emergency Unit as Community Physician*

David George Satin, M.D.

Frederick J. Duhl, M.D.

In this report, we attempt to make two significant contributions to the understanding of the general hospital emergency unit (EU). First, comprehensive descriptive data on the patient's experience in the EU are provided. It is our thesis that interpretation of problems is influenced by the background of the evaluator; therefore, we report in detail the incidence of problems brought as interpreted by patient, attending physician ("physician"), and research psychiatrist ("interviewer") and contrast these points of view. We also report the proportions of patients taking various paths to the EU from the time of attempts to get help elsewhere to the time of admission. The administrative and medical responses of the EU are documented, as well as the dispositions made.

Second, we analyze the relationship between type of problem brought by the patient on the one hand and the paths taken to the EU and the service received on

*Reprinted from *Medical Care,* May-June 1972, Vol. X, No. 3.

the other, again contrasting the experience of groups as defined by patient, physician, and interviewer.

The increased prevalence of chronic disease, the development of techniques of ambulatory care, and the increased respectability of certain human disorders have changed the hospital outpatient service fundamentally in the past 25 years so that "its clearcut original function has evolved into a complex web of manifest and latent functions. ..."[23] A recent study of health insurance utilization indicated that EU visits accounted for 85 percent of the outpatient department use rate of 142 per 1000 people insured.[18] It was estimated that the number of EU visits nationwide doubled over the decade 1960-1970.

In trying to understand the function of the EU in the life of the community, we soon find the assumption of an objective exchange of symptoms for treatment inadequate. It is our thesis that what takes place is a social encounter between patient and staff, couched in medical terminology and taking place in a medical setting but greatly influenced by the backgrounds and expectations of the participants. Sir Aubrey Lewis has said: "the concept of health needs to be clarified: and we realize that it is hardly to be defined without reference to the material and the social environment within which each individual lives. ..."[7] The designation of "disease" depends upon the normal state of the individual, the reportability of changes, the language of description, the total functioning of the organism, and social environmental moulding. Parsons has extensively described the social role and deviance control implications of illness and its sanction by medical authorities.[11] The social and cultural factors influencing the search for professional attention have also been explored.[25,27]

The criteria and significant variables of a successful outcome to this encounter (i.e., "good patient care") are only gradually being identified. In one study, patients expected help with the presenting problem, but their judgment that a doctor was good depended much more upon his competence, interpersonal relations, and kindness.[17] On the other side of the encounter, it has been shown that there is a variable perception and acceptance by medical staff of patient needs and patterns of resource use, and physicians are often more intolerant and narrower than other medical professionals.[23] The interplay of these various factors determines the success of the mutual search for a satisfactory formulation of problems and a working relationship,[2] and the nature and accuracy of diagnosis and fulfillment of need.[26]

Although some ignore these considerations,[9,15] thoughtful administrative planning for the EU has pointed up the need for accurate data on input and outcome.[5,8,11] Scattered reports are available on factors influencing application to the EU, ranging from the assumption that it is a matter of simple convenience[22] to explorations of selective cultural,[25] social,[24] medical resource availability,[13,18] and disability perception[1] factors. Likewise, a few fairly comprehensive studies of the processing of patients within the EU[6,18] have been complemented by more selective reports on variations in volume of intake,[3] treatment agent,[12] and urgency of problem and diagnosis.[10,13]

The comprehensive data presented here on patient flow in the EU and the extent to which the needs of the participants are met by this facility are important both as a critique of current EU functioning and as source material for future planning for the health of the community.

METHOD

The research techniques used in this difficult research situation and our experience with them have been reported in detail elsewhere.[21] In brief, the setting was the EU of an urban general hospital. Patients were initially interviewed by clerks, and then seen by experienced triage physicians for simple treatment or referral to one of the wide variety of medical specialists (including psychiatrists and psychiatric social workers) available in the EU.

A total of 257 applicants to the EU for help with health problems were selected randomly.* Each was interviewed by one of three research psychiatrists as soon as possible after the applicant's arrival. While a wide range of theoretical and experience backgrounds was represented among these psychiatrists, a pretest in which each of a series of patients was interviewed by multiple psychiatrists revealed an extremely close agreement as to the presence and degree of psychosocial problems.

The interview schedule included both open-ended and limited-choice questions about background (demographic, socio-economic, and agency use), previous handling of the problems brought to the EU, and the nature of these problems. On the basis of this interview, the interviewer then recorded his diagnostic conclusions as to the presence, nature, and severity of the patient's problems. Since the interviewer did not do physical examinations or laboratory tests and was not an expert in physical illnesses, he relied heavily

*Details of patient background are reported elsewhere.[21]

on the treating physician's judgment in estimating physical problems. He was, however, the most skilled in eliciting evidence of psychiatric and social problems and most sensitive to their presence. Therefore, the interviewer's diagnosis of specific problems is reported only in regard to psychosocial problems, and his judgment is the criterion for the presence of such problems. His evaluation of the gross categories of patient problems is also reported.

After the patient was discharged from the EU his medical records were reviewed with respect to the administrative classification given him, the clinical specialties which treated him, the diagnoses made, and the disposition arranged. These raw data were then categorized. The patient's complaints were reviewed to determine the system involved: if some physical aspect of the body, it was labelled "physical"; if emotions, behavior, or a psychophysiologic reaction, it was labelled "psychiatric"; if relationships with specific other individuals or function in general social roles (e.g., work, finances), it was labelled "social." The specificity with which complaints were identified, their severity and duration, and the total number of complaints were also categorized. Similar categorization was done for the physician's diagnoses.

Impressionistic clinical judgments, including patient complaints, physician diagnoses, and interviewer diagnoses, are key variables in this study. There are no "objective" judges of "true" problems in a setting where all evaluators are parties to a social negotiation or represent biased viewpoints. However, we feel that it is justified and valuable to document carefully these clinical events and interactions which are so important to medical care delivery, and to analyze them and test the significance of the relationships found.

Table 1
Patterns of Patient Problems by Evaluator*

Problem	Evaluator		
	Patient (percent)	Physician (percent)	Interviewer (percent)
Physical only	83.2	84.1	25.2
Physical & psychosocial	4.9	6.7	60.9
Psychosocial only	12.0	9.2	13.9

Patient vs. physician: x^2 p < .001; Cramér's V = .346
Patient vs. interviewer: x^2 p < .001; Cramér's V = .249
Physician vs. interviewer: x^2 p < .001; Cramér's V = .279

*All problems identified by patient, physician, and interviewer were reviewed for this analysis.

RESULTS

Problems Brought

Table 1 shows the proportions of the major problem patterns.* It is clear that patient and physician agree more closely, seeing only physical problems in the great majority of patients, and mixed physical and psychosocial problems rarely.† The interviewer saw almost the same proportion of purely psychosocial problems, but many more psychosocial problems associated with the physical problems.

*A much more detailed analysis of the relationship between evaluations by patient, physician, and interviewer is reported in another report on prevalence of psychosocial problems and their relationship to other variables.[20]

†Cramér's V coefficient is a measure of degree of association between variables in a tabular analysis.[4] Its limits are 0 and 1 for all size tables, and thus is used here so that degree of association can be compared across tables of differing sizes.

When psychiatric and social problems were distinguished, there was most marked discrepancy in finding social problems. While 8.9 percent of patients voiced social complaints, only one such diagnosis was ever made by a physician. In contrast, interviewers found that 37.2 percent of patients had social problems.

Table 2 compares more specific problems identified by the patient and physician.* Agreement is 66.8 percent over-all. Physicians make 30.8 percent diagnoses of traumatic injury, compared to 23.4 percent for patients. Nonlocalized complaints (such as a fall) made by patients are given the whole range of physical and psychiatric diagnoses by the physician. Conversely, neurologic illness, a rather subtle diagnosis, is made almost twice as often by physicians, as often on the basis of psychiatric as neurologic complaints.

Major disagreements lie in the psychosocial area. Most glaringly, physicians make *no* first diagnoses of social problems (and only one such diagnosis ever); they diagnose about one-third of patients' social complaints as psychiatric and the rest musculoskeletal or EENT. The physicians' almost 50 percent higher psychiatric diagnoses come mainly from patient internal organ complaints. Problems of the surrounding physical world (train accidents, house fires, etc.) were presented by 7.7 percent of patients and never diagnosed by physicians.

The physician made more specific diagnoses than the patient in 48.6 percent of the cases, while the patient was more specific in only 7.9 percent; there was agreement in 43.6 percent.

*More detail on the type, severity, specificity, and recency of problems brought to the EU and the patient's general manner of presentation is given elsewhere.[21]

There was agreement between patient and physician on the severity of the problem in 61.6 percent of the cases; the physician estimated a more severe problem in 21.5 percent, and the patient in 16.9 percent (Table 3). Agreement between patient and interviewer was 56.6 percent, the interviewer making a more severe diagnosis in 27.8 percent of the cases, and the patient in only 15.5 percent.

Patients tend to see a very small proportion of problems as chronic, while physicians and interviewers saw a relatively small proportion as acute (Table 4).

Table 2
Specific Groupings of Problems by Evaluator*

	Evaluator	
Problem	Patient (percent)	Physician (percent)
Physical (total)	85.8	87.0
musculoskeletal	17.3	21.3
skin	16.9	16.6
pulmonary	11.6	9.2
gastrointestinal	7.6	10.0
eye, ear, nose, throat (EENT)	6.2	6.3
cardiovascular	4.5	4.2
urogenital	4.5	5.4
neurologic	3.6	6.3
miscellaneous	4.4	4.6
total body	9.3	2.9
Psychiatric	8.4	13.0
Social	5.8	0.0

*Only first problems identified by the patient and physician were considered in this analysis. This limitation was necessary for simplification of analysis and presentation. It is not unreasonable to assume that the evaluations are comparable, since, in the majority of cases, only one problem was identified, and in other cases the first problem identified is likely to have been the one considered most important.

Table 3
Severity of Problem by Evaluator*

Severity	Evaluator		
	Patient (percent)	Physician (percent)	Interviewer (percent)
Mild	31.2	31.5	19.6
Moderate	56.1	48.1	60.4
Severe	12.7	20.3	20.0

Patient vs. physician: x^2 p $<$ .001; Cramér's V = .394
Patient vs. interviewer: x^2 p $<$ .001; Cramér's V = .269
Physician vs. interviewer: x^2 p $<$ .001; Cramér's V = .455

*Only the first problems identified were considered, as in Table 2.

The patient also voices the smallest total number of complaints, reporting only one in 80.8 percent of the cases and three or more in 9.0 percent. The physician increases by one-third the proportion of cases in which more than one problem is identified (one problem = 69.1 percent; three or more = 10.6 percent), and the interviewer identified three or more in over half the cases (one problem = 21.1 percent; three or more =

Table 4
Duration of Problem by Evaluator*

Duration	Evaluator		
	Patient (percent)	Physician (percent)	Interviewer (percent)
Acute (less than 2 wks.)	72.2	64.4	38.5
Subacute (2-12 wks.)	15.9	5.9	2.7
Chronic (13+ wks.)	11.9	29.7	58.9

Patient vs. physician: x^2 p $<$ .001; Cramér's V = .268
Patient vs. interviewer: x^2 p $<$ .001; Cramér's V = .204
Physician vs. interviewer: x^2 p $<$ .001; Cramér's V = .376

*Only the first problems identified were considered, as in Table 2.

51.7 percent). All evaluators found that patients with physical problems were more likely to have only one problem. Patients and interviewers found that a higher proportion of patients with psychosocial problems had multiple problems; interviewers found this true especially among those with social problems.

Pathways to the Emergency Unit

An attempt to get help before coming to the EU was made by 53.4 percent of the patients. A medical resource was approached by 78.0 percent of these (about half trying a private doctor and one-third another unit in the study hospital), other professionals (including police and social agencies) by 4.3 percent, and nonprofessionals or self-help by 17.7 percent. Treatment was received by 20.3 percent of the total sample, and advice, support, or simple referral by 33.1 percent.

Patients came mainly from the surrounding area (83.1 percent from within five miles). Of the total sample, 36.7 percent were self-referred; medical authorities referred 30.7 percent, nonprofessionals (e.g., work associates and friends) 25.4 percent, and nonmedical professionals (often police and fire rescue squad) 7.3 percent. This hospital was chosen by 39.3 percent because they had been treated there in the past or were currently receiving treatment there. A forced choice was made by 35.1 percent (it was closest in an emergency, had special facilities not elsewhere available, or were directly referred), 23.3 percent because of its general reputation, and 16.3 percent because of convenience.*

Patients arrived at the EU alone in 30.0 percent of the cases, while 65.2 percent were accompanied by

*Total percentage is over 100 as more than one reason was given by some patients.

nonprofessionals and 4.4 percent by nonmedical professionals. In only one case did a medical professional bring a patient to the hospital. A study of EU records indicated that the peak time of arrival was between 4 and 7 PM, when 25.3 percent of the patients appeared. There was a rather even distribution over most of the rest of the day: 19.5 percent 8-11 AM, 19.1 percent noon-3 PM, and 17.9 percent 8-11 PM. The early hours of the morning saw a large drop-off: 11.3 percent midnight-3 AM, and 7.0 percent 4-7 AM.

Patients with physical complaints are significantly more frequently self-referred than medically referred, and only rarely referred by other professionals (Table 5). Self-referral and medical referral are equally important in those with psychiatric complaints, though other professionals are more involved here than with physical complaints. Most of those with social complaints are referred by other professionals and nonprofessionals. The physician and interviewer find diagnostic groups randomly distributed among referral sources.

Table 5
Source of Referral by Patient Complaint*

	Complaint		
Source of Referral	Physical (percent)	Psychiatric (percent)	Social (percent)
Self	40.2	33.3	8.3
Nonprofessional	20.1	16.7	25.0
Medical	31.2	33.3	16.7
Other professional	8.5	16.7	50.0
$x^2 \, p < .001$			

*Only the first problem identified was considered, as in Table 2. When separate analyses were done considering all complaints similar results were obtained, with statistical significance reached for physical ($x^2 \, p < .05$) and social ($x^2 \, p < .001$) complaints.

Other steps on the pathway to the EU were not significantly related to diagnosis, although a few interesting trends exist. A larger proportion of patients presenting psychiatric complaints have received treatment prior to EU admission than those assigned psychiatric diagnoses by physician or interviewer (28.0 percent vs. 16-19 percent). Also, patients with psychiatric complaints are less likely to come to the EU between midnight and 7 AM than those who receive psychiatric diagnoses (8 percent vs. 15-20 percent). The peak admission period for those with psychiatric complaints and those with psychiatric diagnoses appears to be 4-7 PM, thus puncturing the myth that such unreasonable people are largely responsible for inconvenient night calls.

Emergency Unit Response

Both administrative personnel and medical evaluators determine whether the patient is given full administrative documentation ("booked," i.e., accepted as a full patient evaluation and service contact), only listed in the daily log sheet ("logged," i.e., noted for legal purposes, but not considered a full patient service contact), or not documented ("not logged," i.e., not considered a patient at all, but an inappropriate or superficial inquirer). Of our sample, 87.6 percent were booked, 9.7 percent logged only, and 2.7 percent not logged.

The great majority, 89.3 percent, were cared for by the hospital house staff, while 6.3 percent were treated in the EU by private physicians; the remaining 4.4 percent were treated under a special arrangement for industrial accident cases. The distribution of clinical specialties among the attending physicians* was 24.9 percent general surgery, 22.8 percent internal medicine, 11.2 percent pediatrics, 10.3 percent psychiatry, 7.7 percent surgical subspecialties (e.g., urology, orthopedics), 3.9 percent neurology and neurosurgery, and 2.1 percent dentistry. Fully 24.5 percent were seen only by the triage physician. Clearly, he does much more than preliminary evaluation and assignment for more definitive management, often providing a quick definitive evaluation and treatment.

Referral to an outpatient clinic for further treatment was the disposition for 37.9 percent of the sample; 23.4 percent were admitted as in-patients, 16.1 percent were asked to return to the EU (although this facility is not intended for continued treatment), and 7.7 percent referred to private physicians. None was referred to a social agency. In addition, 12.1 percent were discharged with no follow-up plans, and 2.8 percent left before disposition plans were made. In terms of immediacy of continued treatment, 23.0 percent were admitted directly to follow-up resources, 48.4 percent were given appointments in the future, and 13.7 percent were to go only if necessary; no follow-up treatment plans were made for the remaining 14.9 percent.

Only the interviewer finds a significant bias in administrative classification of problem groups (Table 6). Almost one-fifth of those he diagnoses as having psychiatric problems are not accorded full patient status, and almost 5 percent are not recognized at all.† In contrast, the physician is least aware of bias in this regard, though he decides the legitimacy of the request for help: Cramér's V for first problem vs. book-

†Another paper deals in more detail with patients bringing psychosocial problems.[20]

*Percentages add up to more than 100 since about 7 percent of patients were seen by more than one clinical specialty.

Table 6
Administrative Status by Interviewer Diagnosis*

Status	Diagnosis		
	Physical (percent)	Psychiatric (percent)	Social (percent)
Booked	95.2	81.2	100.0
Logged	4.8	14.1	0.0
Not logged	0.0	4.7	0.0
x^2 p $<$ .004			

*Only the first problem identified was considered, as in Table 2.

ing status = .183 for interviewer, .111 for patient, and .084 for physician.

While diagnostic groups are referred to appropriate clinical specialties for care in the main, our data indicate that the association between the interviewer's diagnoses and treating clinical specialties is weakest, and patients he diagnoses as having social problems are *randomly* assigned (Table 7).* All evaluators agree that physical problems are cared for almost equally by medical and surgical specialists, though the triage physician cares for a quarter of the cases. Patients with psychiatric and social complaints and those given these diagnoses by the physician are cared for mainly by the psychiatric staff, though internists may see a sizable minority. In contrast, only

*Tables 7 and 8 are presented in this form for ease of comparison between problem groups and evaluators. Each row represents a tabular analysis of first attending clinical service vs. the presence of a particular problem type as identified by a specific evaluator. Only that part of the table relating to patients who *did* have that type of problem is presented, along with statistical tests on the table as a whole.

TABLE
Attending Clinical Service by Problem Group by Evaluator*

Problem	Service				$x^2 p$	Cramér's V
	Triage only (percent)	Medicine† (percent)	Surgery‡ (percent)	Psychiatry (percent)		
Physical						
patient	26.8	33.5	37.4	2.2	<.001	.673
physician	24.1	36.0	37.9	2.0	<.001	.744
interviewer	24.5	35.6	35.6	4.3	<.001	.450
Psychiatric						
patient	4.0	16.0	12.0	68.0	<.001	.733
physician	16.2	24.3	5.4	54.1	<.001	.714
interviewer	30.1	23.5	31.6	14.7	<.001	.344
Social						
patient	0.0	38.9	16.7	44.4	<.001	.389
physician§	0.0	0.0	0.0	100.0		
interviewer	22.0	31.7	37.8	8.5	ns	.081

*Only the first attending service was considered for simplicity of analysis and presentation. Since 93 percent of patients were seen by only one service, this simplification is not likely to have distorted the findings. All problems identified were considered in this analysis.
†Includes internal medicine + medical subspecialties (e.g., cardiology) + pediatrics + neurology/neurosurgery.
‡Includes general surgery + surgical subspecialties (e.g., orthopedics) + dentistry.
§Statistical tests are invalid as only one case is included.

10.3 percent of patients diagnosed by the interviewer as having psychosocial problems are seen by psychiatric staff; the great majority are cared for by nonpsychiatric staff (especially surgeons).

Patients diagnosed by the interviewer as having psychosocial problems again are found to receive less thorough help in disposition from the EU (Table 8). A considerably larger proportion of those he diagnoses as having psychiatric problems are referred to the EU or given no follow-up referral than of those so diagnosed by other evaluators. An even higher proportion of those the interviewer diagnoses as having social problems are given no follow-up referral.

In contrast, 92.0 percent of patients with psychiatric complaints are referred to treatment resources. Social complaints bring no such therapeutic response, however.

DISCUSSION

A review of the data gives strong support to the impression that, for a large proportion of the applicants to the EU, this facility functions much like a community physician.* Over 80 percent live nearby and choose the EU for reasons related to medical treatment (from their own past experience, recommendation, or reputation). For half it is the first resource applied to, and three-quarters have not previously been treated. A majority come at a convenient time during the day rather than randomly, and are referred by friends, relatives, or themselves. One-quarter were treated by the triage physician only, and for one-quar-

*The incidence of recent life stresses in this population, and their relationship to the problems brought is reported elsewhere.[19]

Table 8
Locus of Disposition by Problem Group by Evaluator*

Problem	Disposition					$x^2 p$	Cramér's V
	Out-patient (percent)	In-patient (percent)	Private physician (percent)	EU (percent)	No Follow-up† (percent)		
Physical							
patient	37.5	24.0	6.2	17.2	15.1	ns	.145
physician	37.2	24.7	6.5	17.7	14.0	ns	.192
interviewer	38.5	25.1	4.6	16.4	15.4	ns	.195
Psychiatric							
patient	48.0	40.0	4.0	0.0	8.0	<.059	.204
physician	42.1	34.2	10.5	2.6	10.5	ns	.181
interviewer	37.7	19.9	6.8	18.5	17.1	ns	.136
Social							
patient	45.0	25.0	10.0	10.0	10.0	ns	.077
physician‡	100.0	0.0	0.0	0.0	0.0		
interviewer	39.8	27.7	6.0	7.2	19.3	<.057	.201

*All problems identified were considered in this analysis.
†Includes patients sent home with no referral to follow-up resources and those who left the EU before disposition plans were made.
‡Statistical tests are invalid as only one case was given a social diagnosis.

ter no referrals for treatment elsewhere were made. This, coupled with the 14 percent who were told to get further treatment only if they felt the need, adds up to a picture strongly reminiscent of the busy family practitioner's office. The limited involvement of alternative medical resources before or after the EU contact is striking; only 31 percent were referred to the EU by medical authorities, only one person was brought by a medical professional, only 6 percent were treated in the EU by private physicians, and only 8 percent were referred back to such doctors after discharge.

Our thesis that the backgrounds and attitudes of the patient, physician, and interviewer influence their perceptions of applicant needs in the EU is supported by the sharp contrasts in their evaluations of the presenting problems. The patient, as a layman, concentrates on the presenting symptoms, thus reporting fewer, more recent, and less severe problems in vaguer terms. The physician and interviewer, as health professionals, tend to search for relevant history and less overt additional needs, thus reporting more, more chronic, and more severe problems. However, in terms of type of problem recognized, the evaluators group themselves differently. The patient and interviewer are more willing to recognize the broad range of problems, including psychiatric and social problems. In contrast, the physician is significantly unlikely to refer social and environmental problems to the EU and almost completely overlooks them in the EU. Either he is insensitive to such problems or feels that these are not legitimate needs for the EU to deal with, and must translate such complaints into the more orthodox medical categories of physical and psychiatric illness (thus accounting for some of the excess of physician psychiatric diagnoses over patient psychiatric complaints). Thus, as both a medical professional and one who is sensitive to psychosocial problems (which are likely to be chronic), the interviewer stands out in terms of the number, chronicity, and severity of problems and the frequency of psychiatric and social problems he diagnoses. It is interesting that almost all of these additional psychosocial problems he finds in conjunction with physical problems, and thus represent a more complex view of the applicant's problems rather than a complete disagreement with the other evaluators as to the applicant's needs.

The data on the relationship between the perception of applicant needs and the response received from the EU indicate that the overt psychiatric complaints of the patient get relevant attention so long as they are not social in nature. Such applicants, as a group, were more likely to have received treatment prior to coming to the EU than the group given psychiatric diagnoses by professionals. Likewise, they were more likely to see a psychiatrist in the EU itself. In contrast, almost 20 percent of those the interviewer diagnosed as having psychiatric problems were not "booked" as fully legitimate patients. This seems related to the attending physician's failure to recognize psychiatric problems, since he does not recognize an administrative classification bias in relation to diagnosis. Thus, patients with psychiatric problems may be turned away as having no important treatment needs. In fact, such applicants are often recorded as having needed "advice only," a much less respected status than those who received medical or surgical treatment.

Psychosocial problems were identified in about 17 percent of the sample by the patient himself, in 16 percent by the physician, and in 75 percent by the interviewer. Yet only about 10 percent were ever seen by the psychiatric service in the EU (about 15 percent of those found by the interviewer to have psychiatric problems and 9 percent of those he found to have social problems). Even in disposition, almost one-third of those with interviewer-judged psychiatric problems and one-quarter of those with social problems were not referred for regular treatment, and not one patient in our sample was referred to a social agency.

The traditional view of the hospital's role was relatively simple: "It has long been assumed that good patient care is provided in good hospitals; that is, if a hospital is well managed and staffed by competent physicians, nurses and other personnel, its patients must be receiving optimal care...."[17] But in the modern hospital, the differing needs, expectations, and prejudices of the parties to this social-professional encounter result in a complex interaction in terms of the very definition and perception of the problems being dealt with as well as the services rendered. The medical professions have long struggled to incorporate the emotional and social needs of their clients into their physical health perspectives. The sometimes uneasy accommodation reached has turned awkward again in the emergency unit, where psychiatric and, even more, social needs are only reluctantly recognized and dealt with and are often swept under the rug of more comfortably traditional physical diagnoses and treatment.

People with life problems turn to professional helping agencies when their own coping capacities or other environmental resources prove inadequate, or when this is the culturally sanctioned course of action. It is inappropriate to expect them to make fine distinctions as to the diagnostic categorizations of their problems or the admissions criteria or interest biases of professional agencies. Attempts at training them in this respect are not generally useful, since lay health care consumers cannot be expected to understand or be interested in these technicalities. People experience problems as urgent in some degree, and it is the responsibility of the professional planners and deliverers of helping services to see that adequate responses are available to those in need. Another report on the EU[21] supports findings in other medical facilities that this is the community expectation despite all educational and administrative efforts otherwise.

In this perspective, the hospital EU is an especially accessible and acceptable helping resource, since there are a minimum of administrative and even physical barriers to reaching it, and it carries the aura of special expertise of the hospital. It should, therefore, be prepared to act as a major crisis intervention and screening agency for the broad range of problems brought to it. This requires official acknowledgment of this repsonsibility and transmission of this attitude to the staff, since, in the EU studied, the availability of psychiatric staff by no means insured that psychosocial problems would be recognized and responded to. Staffing and facilities should be broadened to fulfill this function rather than being adequate only to the surgical emergency, with haphazard and inhospitable housing of other services. In addition to a broadened definition of their responsibilities, the staff needs to recognize that patients bring multiple, intertwined complexes of problems, and that the first one identified does not exhaust the staff's therapeutic responsibility.

There is also a need for nonpsychiatric staff training in the recognition of psychosocial problems which are most often overlooked now, and in techniques of dealing with such patients at least in a preliminary way. While psychiatric consultation and referral resources should be readily available, it is wrong to think that all awareness of and dealing with psychosocial problems can be left to them, such as by having a separate psychiatric triage physician. Our findings indicate that significant psychosocial problems often appear in conjunction with physical problems and may be expressed only secondary to the physical complaints. Therefore, those dealing with the physical problems must be the first to recognize and deal with the psychosocial problems. Also, there is a fear of acknowledging psychiatric problems and a stigma attached to seeking professional help with psychosocial problems. For these reasons, people often seek out physical health professionals for help, and may refuse to deal with psychosocial health professionals.

Finally, the EU must be seen as part of the broad range of health and welfare helping resources in the community. The paucity of more personal, "family practitioner" types of medical resources in the community (such as individual physicians, local group medical practices, or comprehensive community health centers) has been cited as a factor contributing to the increased use of EU's, along with the inefficiency and high cost of private medical care. Increased availability of such resources might reduce the demand for EU services to some extent, but some people will always find the available, high-status, and prompt intervention-oriented EU most appropriate to their needs, and the EU must be prepared to respond. Recognizing the broad range of community needs presented to it, it must have close and effective communications and referral relationships with a broad range of other units in a network of helping resources. In this way problems, once identified and responded to in a preliminary way, can receive follow-through help by the most effective helping agents, whether these be surgical, psychiatric, marital counseling, financial assistance, or other. In order to avoid the fragmentation of therapeutic relationships which notoriously leads to poor treatment results and patients dropping out of treatment, the staff in the EU should not specialize in this transient type of care, but be there only part-time while following through in other settings on the care of clients first contacted in the EU.

As has been mentioned, a generally responsive EU is so readily accessible to the community for help with a broad range of problems that it is very close to providing a general view of population needs defined as being "health problems." As such, it provides an extraordinary opportunity to evaluate and monitor community health needs, and a laboratory for the study of health care practices and the development of more effective ones. In these ways, medical practices can be adapted to the community's health needs, rather than attempting to adjust service requests to traditional institutional practice.

REFERENCES

1. Apple, D.: How laymen define illness. *J. Health Hum. Behav.* 1:219, 1960.
2. Balint, M.: The Doctor, His Patient and the Illness. New York, International Universities Press, 1957.
3. Barry, R., Shortliffe, E., and Wetstone, H.: Hospital emergency departments: case study predicts load variation patterns. *Hospitals* 34:34, 1960.
4. Blalock, H.: Social Statistics. New York, McGraw-Hill, 1960.
5. Lee, S., Solon, J., and Sheps, C.: A hospital emergency unit's function in medical care. Paper read before the Medical Care Section of the American Public Health Association, Atlantic City, N. J., October, 1959.
6. Lee, S., Solon, J., and Sheps, C.: How new patterns of medical care affect the emergency unit. *Mod. Hosp.*

94:97, 1960.
7. Lewis, A.: Health as a social concept. *Br. J. Sociol.* 4:109, 1953.
8. Lowden, J.: The casualty department. *Lancet* 1:955, 1956.
9. Manegold, R., and Silver, M: An overview of emergency medical care services. *JAMA* 200:300, 1967.
10. McCarroll, J., and Skudder, P.: Hospital emergency departments: conflicting concepts of function shown in a national survey. *Hospitals* 34:35, 1960.
11. Medical World News: What's wrong with hospitals? *Medical World News* 8:41, 1967.
12. Mendelson, J.: Emergency ward statistics at the Massachusetts General Hospital. Informal study, 1957.
13. Mestitz, P.: a series of 1817 patients seen in a casualty department. *Br. Med. J.* 2:1108, 1957.
14. Muller, J., Chafetz, M., and Blaine, H.: Acute psychiatric services in the general hospital: III statistical survey. *Am. J. Psychiat.* 124:46, 1967.
15. National Academy of Sciences/National Research Council: Recommendations for improving emergency medical services. *JAMA* 200:304, 1967.
16. Parsons, T.: Definitions of health and illness in the light of American values and social structure. *In* Patients, Physicians and Illness, E. Jaco, Ed. Glencoe, Ill., The Free Press, 1958; p. 165.
17. Reader, G., Pratt, L., and Mudd, M.: What patients expect from their doctors. *Mod. Hosp.* 89:88, 1957.
18. Research and Statistical Division: Hospital emergency room utilization study. Michigan Blue Cross, 1965.
19. Satin, D.: (Help): Life stresses and psychosocial problems in the hospital emergency unit. *Soc. Psychiat.*, 1972.
20. ———: Help!: Prevalence and disposition of psychosocial problems in the hospital emergency unit. *Soc. Psychiat.* 6:105, 1971.
21. ———:"Help": The hospital emergency unit patient and his presenting picture. In press.

22. Sigmond, R.: Areawide planning for emergency services. *JAMA* 200:308, 1967.
23. Solon, J., Sheps, C., Lee, S., and Jurkowitz, M.: Staff perceptions of patients' use of a hospital outpatient department. *J. Med. Educ.* 33:10, 1958.
24. Stoeckle, J., Zola, I., and Davidson, G.: On going to see the doctor: the contributions of the patient to the decision to seek medical aid; a selective review. *J. Chron. Dis.* 16:975, 1963.
25. Zola, I.: Illness behavior of the working class: implications and recommendations. *In* Blue Collar World: Studies of the American Worker, A. Shostak and W. Gomberg, Eds. Englewood Cliffs, N.J., Prentice-Hall, 1964; p. 350.
26. ———: Needed problems of research. Paper presented to the National Tuberculosis Association Conference on Medical Sociology and Disease Control, 1964.
27. Zola, I., and Spivak, M.: Psychosocial and cultural factors in seeing a doctor. Unpublished paper, 1963.

11. Staff Perceptions of Patients' Use of a Hospital Outpatient Department*

Jerry Solon, Ph.D.

Cecil G. Sheps, M.D.

Sidney S. Lee, M.D.

Maeda Jurkowitz

THE PROBLEM

Medical progress has magnified the importance of care for the ambulant patient. At the same time, its conquest of so many communicable diseases has enlarged the impact of the chronic diseases. The problem of meeting the needs of ambulatory patients, and particularly of those who are chronically ill, inevitably involves the organized framework of health services available through hospital outpatient departments.

The outpatient department has responded to social and technological changes in a manner characteristic of social institutions. Its clear-cut original function has evolved into a complex web of manifest and latent

*Reprinted from *Journal of Medical Education*, Jan. 1958, Vol. 33, No. 1.

functions. Whether the resultant role of the outpatient department is rational in terms of meeting current needs is laid open to question. The Beth Israel Hospital, of Boston, sharing a growing concern about the role of OPD's, recently embarked on a study to determine how its outpatients are currently using the hospital's clinics within their total patterns of medical care.

As a preliminary to interviewing patients about their use of the clinics and other sources of medical care, the research group interviewed staff members of the Outpatient Department. The staff's accumulated experience was sought as a means of anticipating patients' use-patterns, so that a sensitive interviewing schedule could be constructed for use with the patients. A wealth of information emerged from these discussions with the staff, and it is presently being used in planning interviews with patients.

Review of the staff interview material has meanwhile led the research investigators to be increasingly impressed with its significance beyond its immediate application to the interviews with patients. Staff perceptions of patients and their use-patterns may be seen as constituting an attitudinal climate which confronts patients who seek clinic services. However much they may be based on mere impressions, or even on misconceptions, the staff's beliefs and attitudes may assume an objective reality for the patient in the reception which he meets. Bigley suggests that "One of the reasons why a patient sometimes wanders from one institution to another is the unfriendly or unprofessional attitude of some member of the staff, who, though otherwise entirely proficient, defeats the chief aim of the clinic."[2] The converse of this is fully as much to be suggested. Where staff members are understanding and receptive toward the patient and he senses a climate of social warmth, he is likely to be influenced to seek his medical care there.

The staff's perceptions may thus themselves be a partial determinant of how and where patients seek their medical care. While this hypothesis is not amenable to testing with presently available data, study of the interview material for what it reveals of staff perceptions of patients and their use-patterns offers some useful background and understanding.

THE SETTING

The Beth Israel Hospital in Boston is a voluntary, medium-sized general hospital with an extensive teaching and research program. It has an outpatient department which, with 33 general and specialty clinics, is typical of the teaching hospital in a large metropolitan area. The OPD serves people who are referred or choose to come to it for medical care and are judged to be medically indigent. These patients, in turn, may serve as teaching material for medical students. While patients are subject to an admission procedure which determines their financial eligibility, there are no fixed income limits, eligibility being based on the individual's medical and economic situation. A standard charge is made for each clinic visit, but the fee is scaled down or cancelled in accordance with the individual's ability to pay.

The physical layout of this outpatient department is fairly typical of such institutions: large, open waiting halls with examining rooms around the periphery. There is, however, considerably less crowding, confusion, and hubbub than in most outpatient departments, since an organized appointment system for patients' visits is in operation.[4]

The clinics are staffed by unpaid physicians, who are in private practice, and by house staff. The former serve in the clinic in exchange for privileges of admitting private patients to the hospital and of otherwise using hospital facilities. Nurses and social workers, and most other ancillary professional and clerical personnel, are employed by the hospital on a salaried basis.

SCOPE AND METHOD

Information was gathered during the first half of 1957 through interviews with nurses, social workers, and physicians (Table 1). All the nurses who staffed the outpatient clinics are represented and those members of the social service department particularly involved in the outpatient department. Physicians included in the study represent approximately the number who staff the clinics on a typical day. The actual selection of physicians for inclusion was arranged by concentrating on the staff of six of the OPD clinics, encompassing the general clinics in medicine and surgery and four specialty clinics.

Professional staff members of the hospital's Medical Care Studies Unit conducted all interviews. The interviews were structured, but permitted open-end discussion at all points. The resultant data therefore represent the responses of the entire group on uniformly queried points, plus additional volunteered information from varying numbers of the staff.

The interview material was analyzed initially for its substantive information on patients' patterns of clinic use which were perceived by the staff. The character of responses among the several staff groups then led, in addition, to formulation of the following hypothe-

Table 1

Number of Respondents By Clinic

	Medical	Surgical	Diabetic	Gastro-intestinal	Eye	Genito-urinary	
Physicians (total)	17	6	5	6	10	8	52
Visiting	14	5	5	5	10	6	45
House staff	3	1	—	1	—	2	7
Nurses							10
Social workers							10
TOTAL							72

sis: Differences among staff members in their perceptions of clinic patients and their use-patterns are associated with the staff member's professional identification and his role in the institutional structure.

Qualifications. The findings which bear on this hypothesis do not presume to delve deeply, since they are culled from material which was fashioned primarily for the substantive data on use-patterns. The quantitative data presented are subject to wide chance variations, based as they are on a small population. They are employed in their literal form to impart the general understanding and insight which they suggest to the investigators.

While the results, of course, represent the Beth Israel Hospital, and the usual cautions about observing their possibly limited applicability are in order, there is no obvious reason to believe that this hospital is sharply atypical in regard to the subject matter under study.

FINDINGS

Variety of use-patterns. The hospital offers the services of the outpatient clinics to those who cannot afford to purchase medical care privately. How individuals avail themselves of these services is subject to many variations. The discussions with staff members of the outpatient department at Beth Israel Hospital have brought into relief four basic types of use-patterns (Chart 1). Staff observe patients using the hospital's clinics (a) for their central, principal source of medical care, (b) only for conditions calling for specialists' services, (c) for care related only to episodes requiring hospitalization, or (d) for follow-up of emergency conditions only. There is no sharp division of opinion among the staff regarding the existence of these four types of use. Only a few staff members felt that patients do not use the OPD in one or another of these ways. (A larger number did not know in order to judge one way or the other.)

These four basic use-patterns, together with other less prominent patterns, are manifested and elaborated in an almost endless variety of specific uses, according to the respondents. Patients may use the hospital clinics as their sole source of medical care, except for calling in a private general practitioner for home visits in acute illness. Some may use the hospital and nothing else, employing the emergency ward in acute situations. Some receive their general care privately, but turn to the OPD for specialty care. Some pass through the OPD to check on what their private physician has told them. Conversely, some are regular clin-

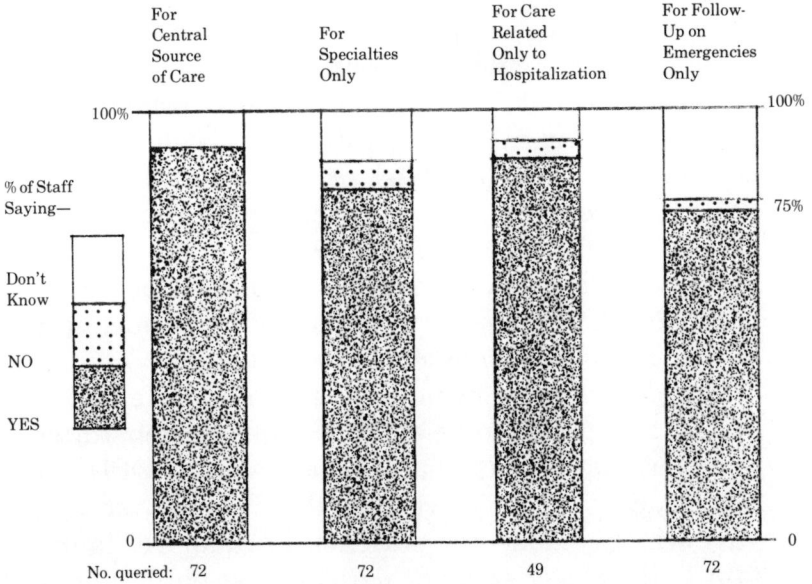

Chart 1. Patients' basic types of use of OPD
Staff's opinions as to whether some patients use OPD:

ic patients, but may consult a physician privately to verify what they've been told in the clinic. Some use a variety of OPD's in different hospitals, in ways which are either complementary, overlapping, or entirely duplicating. Some shift from private to clinic care when something "major" develops, as when surgery and hospitilization become involved. However, apparently more frequently, others reverse this shift and seek private care when surgery is indicated.

There are some who are not regular clinic patients at all, but have a brief clinic episode as an aftermath of an emergent condition which had precipitated them into the emergency ward. Then there are some whose brief brush with the clinics is in connection with getting some special diagnostic procedures performed, while they are under the private doctor's continuing management. These special-purpose contacts sometimes lengthen into continued management in the OPD. Some private patients are deliberately shunted over to the OPD when a physician exhausts his tolerance of a troublesome, demanding patient, or when a patient can no longer pay for private care.

Some people are said to use the OPD primarily to stock up on their favorite medications at low, or no, cost; others, to help establish or maintain their status as welfare recipients. Still others are said to come to OPD as a means of gaining access to the hospital ward for a "rest." And to many who are socially isolated, the OPD is a place to get away from loneliness, to meet friends, to have *something* to do.

This enumeration by no means exhausts the variety of uses suggested by the staff. It amply demonstrates, however, that both the basic function of the OPD and the specific way in which the OPD is employed may vary widely among the patients. Particularly important to the larger study of patients' use-patterns now under way is the fact that any one of the four basic use-patterns mentioned above leaves room for additional sources of care to be tapped by the patient. The patient may be using private doctors, or other hospitals, in addition to using Beth Israel Hospital.

Differences in Staff Perceptions. While virtually all the staff recognize the existence of the broad use-patterns noted earlier, differences appear among staff groups in their perceptions and attitudes concerning specific types of uses and practices. These differences reveal the diverse perspectives from which staff members view the OPD, and can be related to differential experiences, role prescriptions, and identifications.

Chart 2. Obtaining all care from Beth Israel Hospital

Distribution of staff, by their opinions as to
proportion of patients obtaining all care at BIH

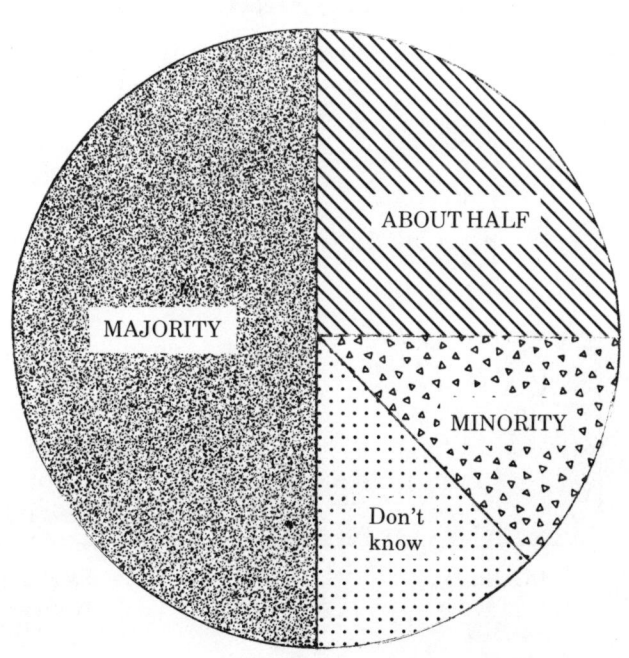

When the staff members were asked how many of the outpatients they believe to be getting *all* their medical care from Beth Israel Hospital, exactly half expressed the belief that a *majority* of the patients use only the one source for their care (Chart 2). However, the views of the visiting physicians on this question appear substantially different from those of the other staff members (Chart 3). Fewer visiting men than other staff members believed that a majority of the outpatients are receiving all their care at the one source. The opinion that merely a *minority* of the clinic patients obtain their care solely from Beth Israel Hospital is held only by visiting physicians (one-fifth of them are of this view). None of the house physicians, nurses, or social workers perceives this type of user (that is, those who get all their care at Beth Israel) to constitute anything less than half of the total

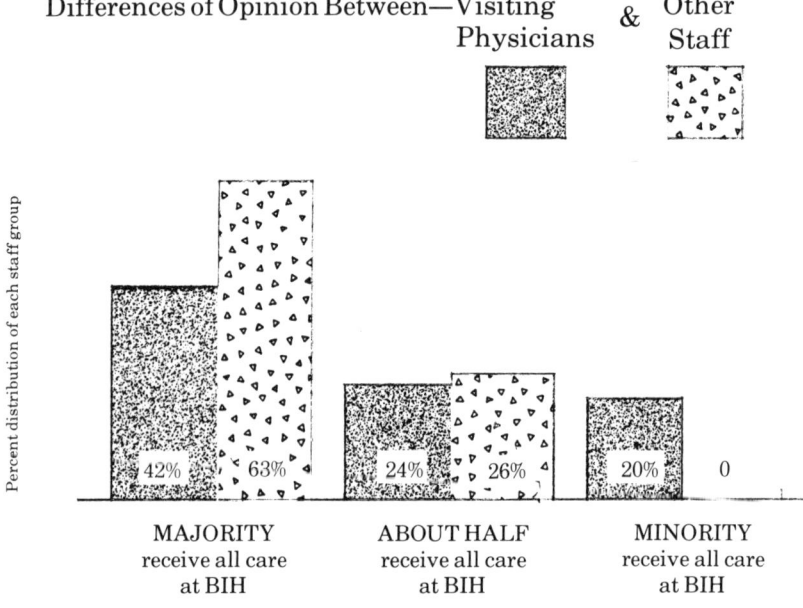

Chart 3. Use of Beth Israel Hospital for all care: Differences of Opinion Between—Visiting Physicians & Other Staff

patient group. The visiting physician is perhaps more likely, on purely experiential grounds, to have in mind doctors' referring private patients to the OPD for some occasional, special services. This interpretation is supported in part by the responses on the subject of referrals from private physicians to the OPD. The purpose of such referrals was often said to be the performance of diagnostic procedures, with the patient remaining under the continuing management of his private physician. Referral for such diagnostic work was noted by a larger proportion of the visiting physicians (69 percent) than of the rest of the staff (48 percent).

The visiting physician is, of course, not rooted in the institution as are the other staff members. His focal role is in his private practice, whereas the others—house physicians, nurses, and social workers—are performing their professional roles as full-time staff within the hospital. The differences of perspective which flow from this are undoubtedly not merely at the level of objective observations, but probably have a large attitudinal element as well. This attitudinal element is of course shaped by many forces besides identification with the OPD. Professional-group membership certainly enters into this strongly, and perhaps more strongly than the extent of identification with the hospital.

Attitudinal differences among staff groups break through in relation to the practice of "shopping around." This refers to patients' going to different places for care of the same condition. The staff's reactions to this practice were sought in terms of their general attitude (Chart 4). Slightly more than one-half of the total group evidenced general acceptance or understanding of patients' shopping, while 38 percent had an over-all critical attitude toward the practice. Social workers are sharply distinguished from the others, identifying strongly with the patient: only 20 percent expressed general opposition to the practice, while 80 percent were accepting and understanding of patients' engaging in "shopping around."

Whatever the general attitude toward patients' shopping, some disadvantageous features of the practice were almost always mentioned by the staff (Chart 5). Some of the staff (24 percent) placed their criticism on the type of patient who would engage in "shopping around" for medical care. Some of the same or others were critical because of the waste of community resources (22 percent), because they felt the experience of shopping was not good for the patient psychologically (38 percent), or because the patient's medical care suffered thereby (78 percent). Again, the social workers are distinctively oriented: they expressed *no* criticism of the type of patient; and, whereas only one-third of other staff members were troubled by possible psychological effects of the shopping experience on the patient, seven of the ten social workers expressed this type of concern.

Chart 4. General Attitude of staff toward "shopping around"

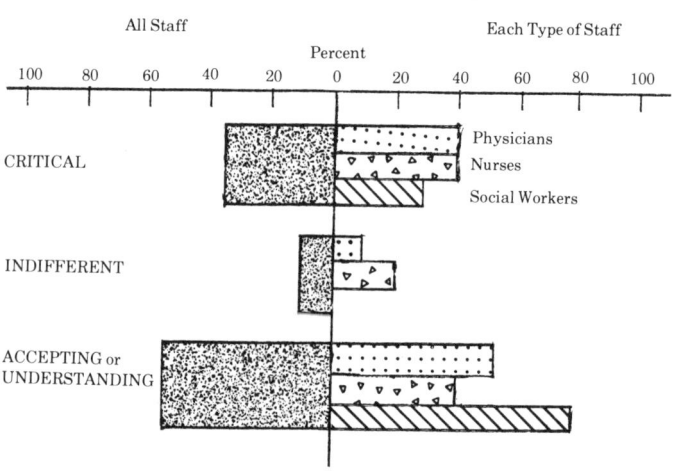

The nurses, interestingly, are aligned quite similarly to the physicians, in terms of both their general attitudes and specific criticisms (cf. Chart 4 on general attitude toward shopping). They expressed direct criticism of the shopping type of patient almost as frequently, relatively, as did the physicians. Significantly, observation in other institutions prompted Burling and his associates to comment that "A conflict in attitudes toward outpatients which permeates the entire clinical staff is most obvious in the nurse. On the one hand she feels compassion for the underprivileged, and on the other hand a scorn for the weak and unsuccessful person which is reinforced by the widespread assumption in this country that poverty indicates moral turpitude. There is a persistent undercurrent of aggression against charity patients which is rarely allowed direct release...."[3] The present study does not

Chart 5. Specific criticisms of "shopping around."

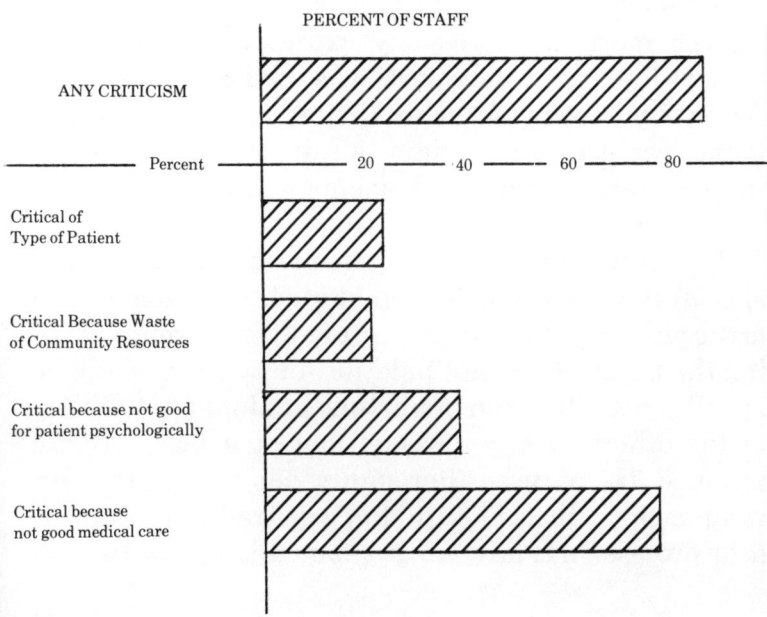

permit nearly as strong a conclusion, since a sympathetic, understanding approach appears to predominate among the group studied. However, the evidence gives support to recognition of some ambivalence.

It is interesting to note that, although the subject of shopping arouses considerable and sometimes heated comment, about 80 percent of the staff regard it to be a practice of only a small number of patients. Only one out of every ten among the staff believe that *many* patients "shop around."

The staff's personal reactions to patients' shopping were directly solicited in the course of interviewing. No such reactions were solicited, however, in connection with asking whether patients make excessive use of the clinics. Four out of every five queried on this point responded that, to a greater or lesser extent, patients do visit the clinics more frequently than is medically necessary. One-third of these respondents were moved, in addition, to express some criticism of this alleged overutilization. Significantly, all but one of the explicit objectors were physicians.

Even more spontaneously expressed, although in only 11 instances, to be sure, was the belief that if patients "had to pay" for what they received, they would make less use of the clinic. Again, in all but one of these instances, it was physicians who made this type of observation.

The visiting physician may be recognized as having special impulses which prompt such expressions. He is the only one of the several professional groups staffing the OPD who is not paid for his service. While he spends only a fraction of his time against the full time of the others, it is time taken out of a busy private practice. He may be thoroughly adapted to this arrangement, which has the force of tradition and certain professional advantages; but this equilibrium is threatened when, in his view, patients are occupying his valuable, contributed time needlessly.

It is the physician, again, who feels abused when he regards the OPD as sometimes "stealing" patients from private practitioners. Patients do at times, and under various sets of circumstances, shift from private care to clinic care. This happens ordinarily when a patient is no longer able to pay for private care, and is referred to, or seeks out, the OPD. However, when other reasons prompt a private patient to become a clinic-user, the label "patient-stealing" is applied. Although the survey did not explicitly seek the information, one-fourth of the respondents mentioned that "stealing" occurs. Most of these, as would be expected, were visiting physicians.

Social workers, on the other hand, more frequently refer to a practice known as "unloading." This term is used to describe a private physician's referral of a patient to the OPD when the patient's funds have been exhausted or his neurotic demands have become too much to handle. These problems would naturally tend to bear in on the attention of the social worker, whose role revolves around the patient in relation to his personal and social problems.

The financial factor, it may be noted, threads through much of the interview material. This is quite understandable inasmuch as medical indigency is the basis of eligibility for OPD services. It is further understandable in that the operation of this eligibility criterion appears to be under some question: fully two-thirds of the staff, in discussing the composition of the OPD patient population, expressed the belief that some of the people who use the OPD could afford to receive this care privately (Chart 6). Among the visiting physicians, three-fourths made such statements, and in most cases accompanied their remarks with criticism of such patients. Among the rest of the staff, one-half observed this financial discrepancy, but only a small number of these expressed open criticism. Those who did were nurses; social workers offered no criticism.

The perceptions which the staff has of patients in social and intellectual terms must have a profound influence on relationships with the patients. In the course of describing the clinic population, some of the staff noted that the patients are generally of limited education and intelligence. In characteristically patterned form, this was mentioned by one-fifth of the physicians, one-tenth of the nurses, and none of the social workers. This is, of course, not taken to be equivalent to the number who may hold the belief;

Chart 6. Medical Indigency and OPD Use

 Proportion of staff saying some patients could afford this care privately

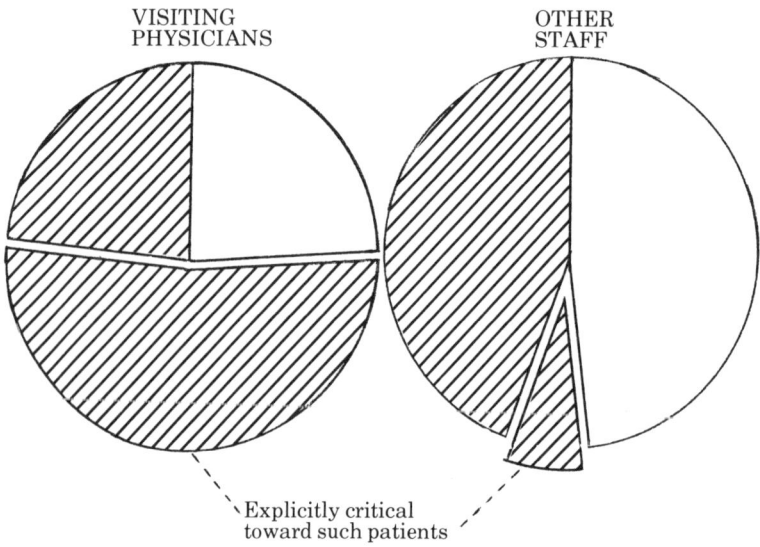

VISITING PHYSICIANS

OTHER STAFF

Explicitly critical toward such patients

but, as in other instances, its very expression is perhaps indicative of its prominence in the individual's mind.

To the physician who in his private practice is accustomed to dealing with patients who are on a higher economic, educational, and social level, the clinic population may well appear in abrupt contrast. The implications for doctor-patient communication are all too evident. That this is recognized as something of a problem within the medical profession seems abundantly clear from this recent item in *Medical Economics:* "Many a private practitioner who devotes time to dispensary or clinic work treats clinic patients with the same courtesy and finesse he gives his private patients. But there are a few notable exceptions to the rule. You may, for instance, have seen a clinic doctor skip all conversational pleasantries. Or disregard some of the niceties in applying dressings, local anesthetics, and such...."[1] The situation is not limited, however, to the *doctor's* withholding from an effective interpersonal relationship. Reader and his associates describe the phenomenon of the patient's passivity in the clinic setting.[5] Seeing this as two sides of a coin emphasizes the importance of interrelating patients' and staff's perceptions as we seek to understand how the outpatient department is used.

SUMMARY AND CONCLUSIONS

How people use a hospital outpatient department—for what basic purposes and with what specific patterns—must be in part influenced by the attitudes and behavior of the staff with whom the patient interacts. The institution is perceived through its functionaries.

Interviews with the staff of the outpatient department at Beth Israel Hospital in Boston, directed toward gauging patients' patterns of use, disclose additional enlightening information: the staff's perceptions of the patients and their use-patterns.

Rather distinct differences in perceptions and attitudes appear among the physicians, nurses, and social workers. These may be related to the values and experience situations which characterize the respective professional groups. In general, the physician seems to display the most critical attitude toward patients and various practices and use-patterns, apparently identifying primarily with his private practice. The social worker, although administratively engaged by the institution, makes it her professional task to identify with the patient. The nurse, in the investigators' observations, appears to articulate her concern for the patient with a strong organizational identification.

These differences among the staff can be functional or dysfunctional, depending on how the elements are blended. They can cause confusion and conflict in the institution's operations or, conceivably, serve a useful function in supplying balancing forces necessary to keep the institution in equilibrium. In many outpatient departments today, optimal blending of the differences is undermined by lack of clarity about the proper purposes and functions of the institution in its current setting.

The functions of the outpatient department may be said to have two dimensions. One is definition of the population eligible for its services. The other is the uses to which the services available in the OPD are put. Along both these dimensions, the functions of the institution studied are only loosely defined, and the limits of acceptable practice are not sharply drawn.

The expectations of *staff members* are consequently shaped more by the individual's or each professional group's own definitions than might be the case if the *institution* drew the lines more sharply. However, if the hospital is to delineate its policies rationally, it must first reevaluate the purposes and functions of the outpatient department in the light of current practices and values, both medical and social.

REFERENCES

1. Anonymous. Clinic Courtesy, Medical Economics, 34:86, 1957.
2. Bigley, L. I. Community Clinics: The Hospital Outpatient Department and Nonhospital Clinics, p. 30. Philadelphia: J. B. Lippincott Company, 1947.
3. Burling, T., Lentz, E. M., and Wilson, R. N. The Give and Take in Hospitals: A Study of Human Organization in Hospitals, p. 282. New York: G. P. Putnam's Sons, 1956.
4. Lee, S. S. A Fresh Look at Outpatient Department Problems. Presented at the American Public Health Association annual meeting, Medical Care Section, Atlantic City, N. J., November 14, 1956.
5. Reader, G. G., Pratt, L., and Mudd, M. C. What Patients Expect from Their Doctors, The Modern Hospital, 89:88-94, 1957.

Part III

Transportation and Communications

INTRODUCTION

The upsurge in emergency room utilization has been accompanied by renewed attention to the problem of transporting victims of automobile accidents, heart attacks, poisonings, and other accidents and sudden illnesses from wherever these events occur to a source of primary medical care. It has been estimated that 25% of the permanent disability sustained by 166,000 annual traffic accident victims could have been prevented by rapid medical intervention. New technologies, such as remote-controlled physiologic monitoring, early life-supportive care, and the use of paraprofessionals, can help to effect the recovery of victims of various emergency conditions. The degree to which communities will be able to minimize the morbidity and mortality associated with accidents and sudden illness depends upon their ability, on the one hand, to predict the demand for emergency medical services and, on the other, to utilize advanced medical, transportation, and communications technologies most effectively and economically.

Two articles in this section attempt to determine the nature of demand for emergency medical services and the characteristics of supply under varying conditions. Aldrich, Hisserich, and Lave (1971) indicate the desirability of predicting the type and frequency of medical emergencies for given areas in order to "optimize the location of ambulances and emergency treatment facilities as well as the training of ambulance attendants and of the equipment carried in ambulances." Despite certain limitations in data representing Los Angeles during 1964-1967, they were able to develop a predictive model that explains with a high degree of accuracy variations in the use of a public emergency ambulance system by persons suffering automobile and other accidents, illness due to cardiac arrest and poisoning, and other illnesses involving acute distress symptoms. That variables indicating low socioeconomic status best predict total demand for public ambulance services is consistent with the findings of studies presented in the previous section. In contrast, socioeconomic variables are not as powerful in predicting demand due to specific kinds of accidents and illness. For example, the data suggest that serious automobile accidents tend to occur outside the city on freeways and suburban and rural roads. Since public ambulances handle nearly all automobile accidents involving injuries, socioeconomic status has no way in this situation of mediating demand for ambulance service as it apparently does in cases involving poisoned children and other sicknesses.

The article by Noble, LaMontagne, Bellotti, and Wechsler (1971) adds the factors of weather and social ritual to the equation explaining demand for a variety of emergency medical services. It also explores the relationship between these factors and certain fluctuations in available medical manpower. Analysis of Boston Police Department ambulance runs, emergency unit visits to three Boston hospitals located within a six-block radius of one another, and weather conditions during 1968 allowed both a micro- and a macroview of the influence of ritualistic and meteorological factors on the demand for hospital emergency unit services and for transportation by means of both police and private ambulances. Nonetheless, integration of the micro- and macroviews led to the rueful conclusion that demand for ambulance service "cannot be translated by any simple calculus into demand for care in the emergency unit of any single hospital." The analysis raised many more questions than it answered about the interactive properties of the whole emergency care system in Boston and surrounding communities. For example, "How does case origin, type, and urgency status influence its destination after it comes to the attention of the police?" "How do existing policies, customs, and agreements between participants in the emergency care system affect the process of case distribution?"

The next two articles deal with the interactive properties of the emergency medical care system by using mathematical models to simplify and explain the complex relationships that exist between policies concerned with the recovery of emergency victims and treatment en route to the hospital and the outcome of these efforts. In Hanitzsch and Hall's view (1969), the cost-effectiveness of a medical care recovery system can be influenced by manipulation of two sets of variables:

(1) policies that establish the basic structure of the system, such as the type of recovery vehicle selected for use, the equipment carried on board, the level of attendant training required, the number of vehicles deployed, etc.; and

(2) policies that govern day-to-day operations, such as decisions about the location of vehicles, dispatch procedures, hospital selection rules, and rules prescribing what medical treatment may be given by ambulance attendants.

On the assumption that these major controllable policies approximate a Markov-renewal process in which the conditional probability that the system is in any given state depends entirely on the previous state occupied, Hanitzsch and Hall illustrate how costs can be partitioned and allocated within each state of the recovery system and how it is possible to minimize total costs over some time period.

Dunlap and Associates, Inc. (1968) use queuing theory to determine what size ambulance service is needed to meet the demand of a population for some required level of service within a specified response time. They give a number of concrete examples showing how operations research techniques can assist in planning cost-efficient ambulance systems that provide services within response times acceptable to the community. The article contains a number of charts, graphs, and tables that can be applied by local emergency medical care planners to their own situations in estimating the required size of ambulance service to satisfy demand. Four case studies take the reader step-by-step in applying the model and the associated estimating procedures to different environments. The model's one basic limitation is its tendency to underestimate the benefits that may be derived from other ambulances in a multiple location system during times of peak emergency load.

The next two articles in this section are concerned with the application of systems analysis and computer simulation techniques in judging the *potential* cost-effectiveness of innovative responses to emergencies. Jacobs and McLaughlin (1967) take a hard look at the role that helicopters might play in a community's emergency medical care system. Levine evaluates by means of a computer simulation a new emergency command system designed to provide "fail-safe and errorless" communication and dispatch of medical personnel within a hospital environment. Systems analysis of the feasibility of using helicopters to transport ill or injured patients makes clear that they can only be considered a "graft" to the total medical transportation system. Because helicopters "may prove to be of very limited applicability in densely populated areas, are susceptible to weather conditions, and are expensive to acquire and operate," it becomes necessary to identify the frequency and temporal distribution of those emergency events that could benefit from their use. After specifying what information is needed to estimate the availability of a multi-purpose helicopter to respond to emergencies, Jacobs and McLaughlin recommend computer simulation of local conditions in order to "generate a clear picture of machine availability and its impact on the service rendered to the community."

Levine's simulation study (1969) of a hospital emergency command system shows how far one must go beyond systems analysis to collect baseline data on existing conditions in order to make valid comparisons by means of computer simulation of the "new" versus the "old" system. The Hospital Emergency Command System (HECS) is an integrated electromechanical system that takes over and automatically executes a number of functions now performed by hospital personnel when an emergent situation is detected in their midst. The system mobilizes and controls communications, personnel, equipment, and the means of mobility. Computer simulation of HECS revealed an almost 100% improvement over the current system's response time in getting required medical staff and equipment to cardiopulmonary arrest emergencies. One can appreciate the clinical significance of this achievement only with the realization that irrevocable nervous system death occurs within four minutes after cessation of cardiac and respiratory activity.

The last article, by Struxness (1972), tells how existing telecommunications and transportation technologies can be joined to provide more effective life support both at the site of the emergency and in transit to a specialized facility offering "the spectrum of services needed specifically by the critically ill or injured person." In the interest of economic feasibility in a medical care system characterized by ever-increasing costs, Struxness argues, on the one hand, against proliferation of numerous specialized vehicles capable of responding to only one type of emergency and, on the other, for development of statewide plans for the use of special categorical emergency care facilities. In principle, telemetry by means of satellite can link a patient being assisted by a well-trained paramedic in the remotest area of the country with an appropriate source of medical advice. In some places, ordinary ambulances linked to hospitals by portable equipment for voice and E.C.G. telemetry have begun to reduce the mortality of heart attacks.

As previously mentioned, communities will be able to take advantage of existing and new technologies in reducing morbidity and mortality due to accidents and sudden illness to the extent that they can obtain an understanding of the regularities and dynamics of current systems. The articles in this section, in the main, point the way by offering and applying some useful conceptual tools to real transportation and communication problems of the emergency medical care system.

12. An Analysis of the Demand for Emergency Ambulance Service in an Urban Area

Carole A. Aldrich, M.S.

John C. Hisserich, M.P.H.

Lester B. Lave, Ph.D.

Although true medical emergencies are rare events for a given family, they occur frequently in a sizable city. Residents expect prompt, competent treatment of these emergencies. Medical emergencies arise from automobile accidents, poisonings, heart attacks, and a number of other accidents and sudden illnesses. In true emergencies, time is a crucial factor in treatment; protection from shock and further injury is important.

A number of other medical conditions arise which, though less severe, are emergency-like in their sudden onset and aura of anxiety. Such conditions may be resolved by first-aid, by a family physician's care, or in the event that these are unavailable, in an emergency treatment facility. Due to a variety of circumstances, the growing volume of these nonemergency demands is placing an increasing strain on all components of the emergency system.

In most communities, a public emergency ambulance system of some type is set up to respond to calls for medical assistance. The bulk of a community's true, life-threatening medical emergencies are generally handled by this system, since real emergencies are usually of such a catastrophic nature as to leave few alternatives. Many of the demands on such a system are, of course, for less medically threatening conditions. Most calls do, however, involve cases whose associated anxiety or pain is sufficient to warrant immediate response.

The over-all task for a city is one of determining the nature of the demand for treatment of medical emergencies and emergency-like incidents. Ideally, it would be desirable to be able to predict the type and frequency of occurrences for given areas. With this information, it would be possible to determine the role of an emergency medical system and each of its components. In particular, the information could be used to optimize the location of ambulances and emergency treatment facilities as well as the training of ambulance attendants and of the equipment carried in ambulances.*

This paper represents an attempt to solve one part of the problem. Using data collected on a currently operating public emergency ambulance system, we have attempted to estimate the nature of the demand for the service. Our results are limited and must be qualified. While the predominant number of true, life- or function-threatening, medical emergencies are handled by the public system, the vast majority of emergency-like conditions, which represent latent demands on the public system, are handled by other means. Therefore, relatively minor changes in the nature of the public system might lead to quite signifi-

---

*See Andrews (1969), Jacobs and McLaughlin (1967), and King and Sox (1967).

cant changes in the demand for it. Also, we were unable to obtain data on a number of factors, such as weather, that might be important.

In spite of these problems, we were able to develop a model which explains virtually all of the variation among census tracts in the demand for publicly dispatched ambulances. Given socioeconomic data about a census tract, we can predict with great accuracy the number and type of medical emergencies that the public system will be called upon to handle during the course of a year.

THE LOS ANGELES PUBLIC AMBULANCE SYSTEM

Los Angeles is an appropriate case study since the public system differs among the areas of the city. During the period of this study, three modes of service were utilized. In the western and harbor areas, the city contracts with private ambulance services to respond to public calls and transports the victim to a specified contract hospital emergency room. The San Fernando Valley section of the city is served by ambulances of the Los Angeles Fire Department. The balance of the city, including the downtown area, is served by ambulances of the Los Angeles Central Receiving Hospital Department. Some changes took place in the public system over the period of study. For most of the first three years, no charge was made for ambulance service. Late in the third year, a fee system was instituted which stipulated that all people transported to a hospital were to be charged for this service. The billing procedures for this fee system were not fully operational during 1967; hence, its impact on demand was somewhat attenuated.

Finally, Los Angeles is a sizable city of great diversity. We investigated 632 census tracts which exhibited vast differences in size, income, employment, and demographic characteristics. Population per census tract ranges from 0 to 10,108 with a mean of 3,920; the size of the tracts ranges from 63 to 7,842 acres. White population per census tract has a mean of 82.4 percent with a standard deviation of 6.8 percent; population aged over 65 has a mean of 10.5 percent with a standard deviation of 6.8 percent. The median age across census tracts for men is 32.7 and for women 34.9, while the range goes from 8.9 years to 60 years. Median income shows even more variation since it has a mean of $7,148 and standard deviation of $2,928 with a range from $2,345 to $35,000. As another measure of income, the percentage of families whose income was less than $4,000 averaged 5.7 percent with a standard deviation of 3.3 per cent. Finally, employment per census tract ranged from 0 to 46,543 with a mean of 1,308.

Two possibly important factors which could not be studied were the effects of weather and the training of ambulance attendants. A climate of greater extremes than that found in Los Angeles could be expected to produce a different mix of injuries and a seasonal shift in the nature and level of demand. The level of ambulance attendant training is relatively good throughout the city. The effects on demand of very poor attendants or considerably more skilled personnel such as registered nurses or physicians could not be evaluated.

DATA

Records of public ambulance trips were collected from the files of the Los Angeles Central Receiving Hospital, where data from the entire city are stored. Tickets, which are filled out by ambulance attendants, include information on the time required to respond to a call, the nature of the emergency, and its location. The information was coded by census tract, year, and type of incident according to the following classification: automobile accidents, other accidents, suspected cardiacs, possible poisonings, other illnesses, and dry runs. Not all calls involved transportation to an emergency room; in some cases, the attendant rendered first-aid and left the patient at the scene. Dry runs refer only to those cases in which the attendant could not locate the victim or found that the situation had been handled before he arrived. A 4 percent sample of public ambulance trips for the years 1964-1967 was collected. Each observation was weighted to reproduce the original data. A total of approximately 14,000 trips was tabulated.

Data describing the socioeconomic characteristics of the area were derived from 1960 census records. The data describe the population by age, sex, income, education, occupation, employment, marital status, and racial characteristics. The tract itself is described by various land use variables, including number of housing units, and by employment within the tract.

THE MODEL

The model focuses on the *per capita* demand for public ambulance service. Although a geographical unit (such as a census tract) is the relevant focus from a policy viewpoint, geographical units complicate the analysis. The explanatory power of a census tract model is made artificially high by the natural association between calls and population. There are also statistical reasons for preferring the *per capita* model.

Our model specifies demand as a linear function of socioeconomic characteristics of the census tract, the type of public service, and the availability of alternative sources of care. The functions are estimated by least squares regression analysis. We regard the linearity of the model as a reasonable approach to a much more complicated specification. The assumption of linearity over the relevant range is supported by the high percentage of variance explained and the similarity of the parameter estimates to *a priori* expectations.

We expected that demand would be highest in tracts with a concentration of people of low socioeconomic status.* These people may use the emergency system even in the absence of real emergencies because they generally do not have a regular physician. Low socioeconomic status is defined in terms of income (families whose 1959 income was less than $4,000), race, unemployment, age (people over 65), employment in low-status jobs, and crowded living conditions (a high number of people per housing unit). It is assumed that areas with high mobility will generate more calls than low mobility areas, as new residents are unlikely to be aware of private medical care facilities. Areas with a high proportion of commercial land and high employment within the tract are likely to generate calls due to the large inflow of people who might be injured while away from home. It seems plausible that many incidents which would be treated by a family physician or with first-aid become demands on the public system when the individual is away from home. Finally, the presence of a freeway within a tract is likely to increase the traffic volume and generate more frequent automobile accidents.

*See Alpert, et al. (1969), Lavenhar, et al. (1968), and Weinerman, et al. (1966).

An indication of the efficiency of an ambulance service is the average response time (the elapsed time between the receipt of a request for an ambulance and its arrival on the scene). This time is determined by the dispatch procedure, the availability of an ambulance, and travel time to the scene.

A long response time could lead people to choose an alternative means of transportation. Although most users are probably not aware of average response time, many, such as the police, have had direct experience and have a feeling for whether or not the ambulance arrived promptly. A variable indicating mean ambulance travel time for each census tract was included in the analysis as a partial indication of this factor. No data were available to indicate the total response time.

Within the Los Angeles system, alternate dispatch procedures are employed and an attempt was made to isolate their effect on demand. In most areas of Los Angeles, calls are screened by a registered nurse, who makes a decision as to whether the call warrants an ambulance. However, in the area where firemen handle dispatching, essentially no screening takes place. Unfortunately, the screening factor is confounded with other aspects of the service. Thus, it is impossible to isolate the effect of screening.

Total demand for public ambulance service is categorized by type of incident. By knowing whether incidents are automobile accidents, other kinds of accidents, cardiac cases, or other types of illness, one can make changes in the type of equipment carried in ambulances and the type of training given to drivers. These categories are analyzed with subsets of the variables used to predict total demand. Table 1 presents a list of the variables used in the analysis.

Table 1
List of Variables

Variable	Mean	Standard Deviation	Description
1. Total demand*	144	241	Number of calls per capita (×1,000) by public ambulances in this census tract during 1964-1967
Auto accidents	38	52	Number of calls arising from automobile accidents
Other accidents	30	82	Number of calls arising from accidents other than auto
Cardiac	7	6	Number of calls involving heart attacks
Poison	5	4	Number of calls involving poison
Other illness	49	116	Number of calls involving an illness other than heart attack or poison
Dry runs	14	19	Calls where the driver could not locate the patient or where the incident was handled before the ambulance arrived
2. Housing density	.382	.129	Number of housing units per capita in tract
3. Recently moved	.151	.075	Percentage of individuals who moved into the tract during the two years before the census was taken
4. White population	.824	.290	Percentage of population which is white
5. % over 65	.105	.966	Percentage of the population older than 65
6. % single females	.190	.084	Percentage of the population who are females (over 14) who are unmarried, separated, divorced, or widowed
7. % single males	.113	.058	Percentage of the population who are males (over 14) who are unmarried, separated, divorced, or widowed
8. % poor families	.057	.033	Percentage of the population whose family income is less than $4,000
9. % males unemployed	.019	.014	Percentage of population who are unemployed males
10. % males employed	.262	.949	Percentage of population who are working males
11. % females in labor force	.158	.059	Percentage of population who are females reporting either that they are employed or are looking for a job
12. Total employment	.576	2.833	Total persons employed in census tract divided by number of people residing in tract
13. % children	.251	.111	Percentage of population aged under 15
14. % single white males	.139	.095	Percentage of population who are white males who are unmarried, separated, divorced, or widowed

* When each year's demand is divided by population and the years are pooled, the result is 36 (mean) and 28 (standard deviation).

Table 1—Continued

Variable	Mean	Standard Deviation	Description
15. % married whites	.466	.074	Percentage of population who are white and married
16. % male farmers	.009	.027	Percentage of working males (who reside in tract) who are employed as farmers
17. % male managers	.513	.090	Percentage of working males (who reside in tract) who are employed as managers, clerks, salesmen, craftsmen, farm, or other laborers
18. % male household	.084	.057	Percentage of working males (who reside in tract) who are employed as household workers or in other service
19. % female professional	.912	.074	Percentage of working females (who reside in tract) who are employed as professional, manager, clerk, craftsmen, operative, in household service, or in other service
20. % female farmers	.034	.040	Percentage of working females (who reside in tract) who are employed as farmers or farm managers
21. % female laborers	.005	.010	Percentage of working females (who reside in tract) who are employed as general laborers
22. Acres/capita	.156	.825	Total tract acreage divided by tract population
23. % commercial land	.077	.092	Percentage of tract acreage in commercial use
24. % industrial land	.039	.080	Percentage of tract acreage in industrial use
25. % transportation land	.012	.051	Percentage of tract acreage in transportation use
26. Freeway	.316	.465	A variable taking on a value of 1 if a freeway runs through the census tract (and 0 otherwise)
27. Response time	1.004	.297	The average time (in minutes×.1) between when an ambulance was called and when it arrived
28. Area #1	.028	.045	San Fernando Valley (served by LAFD who do not screen incoming calls) ×.1
29. Area #2	.002	.014	Baldwin Hills (served by a contract ambulance company) ×.1
30. Area #3	.005	.021	Canyon area (sparsely populated, served by contract ambulance company) ×.1
31. Area #4	.002	.015	Westchester (area served by contract ambulance company) ×.1
32. Area #5	.005	.022	Harbor (area served by contract ambulance company) ×.1
37. Area #2 in 1967	.001	.011	

DATA PROBLEMS

Before presenting the results of the analysis, some problems in the data should be noted. The most significant problem concerns the socioeconomic data. Since Los Angeles is a rapidly changing city, data from the 1960 census are not likely to be perfect descriptions of what prevailed in 1967. Nearly a decade elapsed between the census data collected in 1959 and the ambulance demand data gathered in 1967. There are some indications that the data are a reasonable description, e.g., the results appear to be stable over the period 1964 to 1967. Nonetheless, we express some reservations about the socioeconomic data and suggest that these data be analyzed again when the 1970 census is available.

Data were collected on alternative sources of medical care. These data included the number of physicians practicing in a tract, the distance to the nearest hospital with an emergency room set up to handle medical emergencies, and the distance to the nearest contract emergency hospital. The distance data have the undesirable characteristic of giving a zero distance when a hospital is located in a census tract. For hospitals located close to an accident, the distance measure tends to be only a remote approximation to the notion of how convenient it is to get to the hospital. It was not surprising that the distance variables contributed nothing to the analysis and so were dropped. Similarly, data on the number of physicians whose offices were in the tract did not add to the analysis.

There are approximately 75,000 calls each year which are answered by public ambulances. Since our data cover four years (1964 to 1967), it was impossible to collect 300,000 records. Given limitations on time and expense, only a 4 percent sample could be taken. While this sample is quite an adequate representation of the total demand for all four years, it begins to have large sampling variation when analyzing disaggregate categories, such as demand by type of incident or by year.

Some notion of sampling variation can be gained by assuming that calls come from a random process which generates 36 calls per 1,000 people per year. The average census tract will generate 141 calls, but the random nature of the process means that from 118 to 164 calls can be expected in any year. This sampling variation is sufficiently large that it is difficult to estimate the demand model. Sampling variation for the various categories are shown in Table 2. For those categories where the coefficient of variation is 8 or greater, sampling variation is likely to obscure estimation.

To circumvent this problem, we aggregated census tracts together to get 157 areas (each comprising about four census tracts). This pooling of data has a significant effect in reducing sampling variation. For example, the coefficient of variation for cardiac calls falls from 20 for census tract data to 9 for the larger area data. We estimated the model with both sets of data and tended to find similar estimates.

An important problem with the ambulance call data is that during the second half of 1967, the private ambulance company which was responsible for one section of the city failed to report all of its calls. Thus, there is an underestimate of the demand for ambulance service for this period in this part of the city. The area in question is only a small portion of the city. Therefore, the results of the four-year analysis were quite similar to the results obtained from analyzing 1964-66 and 1967 separately. We also formulated a

292 Emergency Medical Services

Table 2
Sampling Variation

Category	Probability of Occurrence*	Expected Calls Per Area*	Standard Deviation*	Coefficient of Variation*
Total calls:				
per year (within a census tract)	.036	141	11.6	8
per 4 years (within a census tract)	.144	565	22.1	4
per year (within larger area)	.143	561	22.0	4
Automobile accidents				
per 4 years (within a census tract)	.038	149	11.9	8
Other accidents				
per 4 years (within a census tract)	.030	118	10.7	9
Cardiac				
per 4 years (within a census tract)	.007	26	5.1	20
per 4 years (within larger area)	.028	110	10.3	9
Poisonings				
per 4 years (within a census tract)	.005	20	4.5	23
per 4 years (within larger area)	.020	78	8.7	11
Cardiacs and poisonings				
per 4 years (within a census tract)	.012	47	6.8	14
Other illness				
per 4 years (within a census tract)	.049	192	13.5	7
Dry runs				
per 4 years (within a census tract)	.014	55	7.4	13

* Probability of occurrence is the probability, per capita, of a call being phoned in under the specified conditions. (p).

Expected calls per area is the number of calls phoned in from an area, on average (np); we assume that all census tracts have population 3,920.

Standard Deviation about the number of expected calls $[np(1-p)]^{1/2}$; sampling variation means that we might expect to observe $np \pm 2[np(1-p)]^{1/2}$ calls actually being phoned in from the given area.

Coefficient of Variation: the standard deviation divided by the mean; $(100[np(1-p)]^{1/2}/np)$. Note that aggregating years together, census tracts together, or both, greatly reduces the coefficient of variation.

model which allowed for the underestimation in this one area during 1967; it confirmed a significant amount of underreporting.

We attempted to estimate the effect of charging for public ambulance service. From 1964 to the second half of 1966, there was no charge for using public ambulance service. During the last months of 1966, a charge of $15 was instituted for cases where the victim was transported to a hospital. Collection of this fee began in 1967. Unfortunately, our data do not note whether a victim was transported to the hospital; there is casual evidence that the proportion of cases which involved transportation to the hospital fell in 1967, but there is no quantitative evidence.

Finally, we want to stress that the relevant question for analysis is the nature of demand for *all* emergency medical care. Public ambulance service is a small part of this demand. Our data were not such that we could attack the larger problem and so we are forced to assume that the characteristics of other ways of handling medical emergencies did not change over this period.*

RESULTS

A number of similar models were estimated, using least squares regression analysis. First, we added all four years and estimated a demand relation for each category, combining the cardiac-poison cases. To look at underreporting bias, we fit separate relations for 1964-66 and 1967 separately. To lessen the importance of sampling error, we aggregated the 632 census tracts into 157 contiguous areas. Using these "aggregated" data, we refit the 1964-67 relations and found similar results. We extended the analysis with the aggregated data by analyzing cardiac and poison categories separately. Finally, we took data for each year for the 157 areas and pooled it to get 628 (4 × 157) sample points with which to examine changes in demand over time. Since these analyses replicate one another, we have presented only a few of the estimated relations in Table 3.

*Excluded variables, such as the characteristics of emergency medical care outside the public system, will not bias the estimated parameters if they are uncorrelated with the included variables. Since we couldn't get data on the characteristics of these other ways of handling medical emergencies, we must assume that they did not change over time or that they changed in such a way that the change is uncorrelated with the included explanatory variables.

294 Emergency Medical Services

Table 3
The Total Demand for Public Ambulances

	$\bar{R}^2$ Degrees of freedom	Total* Demand .927 600		Pooled† Years .904 592	
1.	Constant term	161	(3.14)‡	−1	(−.07)
2.	Housing density	−534	(−6.30)	−43	(−1.74)
3.	Recently moved	593	(5.74)	151	(5.40)
4.	White population	−98	(−5.09)	−19	(−4.64)
5.	% over 65	838	(7.19)	131	(4.82)
6.	% Single females	−455	(−2.45)	−120	(−2.77)
7.	% Single males	929	(4.92)	206	(4.91)
8.	% Poor families	705	(4.12)	160	(3.35)
9.	% Males unemployed	1,563	(4.61)	346	(3.11)
10.	% Employed males	1,324	(10.88)	216	(5.58)
11.	F. in labor force	−143	(−1.17)	−164	(−6.82)
12.	Total employment	49	(37.24)	9	(14.13)
13.	% Children	519	(3.46)	14	(.62)
14.	% Single white M.	428	(3.79)	−27	(−1.38)
15.	% Married whites	125	(1.01)	−26	(−1.39)
16.	% M. farmers	−417	(−2.46)	−56	(−1.38)
17.	% M. managers	179	(3.01)	17	(1.16)
18.	% M. household	−44	(−.50)	106	(4.08)
19.	% F. professional	−180	(−3.00)	−6	(−.28)
20.	% F. farmers	1,313	(4.60)	34	(.21)
21.	% F. laborers	220	(.72)	−209	(−2.08)
22.	Acres/capita	36	(2.66)	12	(2.69)
23.	% Comm. land	170	(3.03)	11	(.87)
24.	% Indust. land	−129	(−3.07)	11	(1.33)
25.	% Trans. land	−137	(−2.36)	−1	(−.11)
26.	Freeway	7	(1.22)	−1	(−.26)
27.	Response time	−13	(−1.23)	−1	(−.78)
28.	Area #1	104	(1.07)	39	(2.34)
29.	Area #2	−161	(−.77)	−64	(−1.93)
30.	Area #3	−41	(−.28)	13	(.53)
31.	Area #4	27	(.13)	−35	(−.43)
32.	Area #5	258	(1.75)	−4	(−.15)
33.	1964			−35	(−3.46)
34.	1965			−28	(−2.75)
35.	1966			5	(.52)
36.	1967			0	
37.	Area #2 in 1967			−104	(−2.78)

* Total ambulance calls per capita for each census tract (×1,000) summed over 1964–7.
† Totals calls per capita for 157 areas, all years pooled (×1,000).
‡ The figure in parentheses is the t statistics.

The model explains total demand with a high degree of accuracy: the coefficient of determination ($\bar{R}^2$) when adjusted for lost degrees of freedom is .927, indicating that 92.7 percent of the variation is explained by the regression. The F statistic is 275 with 31 and 600 degrees of freedom (F must be greater than 1.70 for a level of confidence of .99). The regressions explaining subcategories are nearly as good since the lowest coefficient of determination (for dry runs) is .598. In all of the regressions reported, the F statistic implies that one can be confident at extremely high levels (considerably beyond .99) that the regressions explain a significant amount of variation in the dependent variables. One might further note that $\bar{R}^2$ rises with the mean of the dependent variable across regressions. We concluded that this result follows from sampling variation, as discussed above.

The regression coefficients and their t statistics (the coefficient divided by its standard error) are presented in Table 3. Each coefficient indicates the marginal effect of a variable, other factors held constant. For example, in the first regression, a one percentage point increase in the proportion of the population which is white will decrease ambulance calls per capita by .1 per cent. This effect might seem small, but one must realize that income, housing density, and many other factors are being held constant. Thus, whites call the public ambulance system less than nonwhites even when they are poor and are living in slum neighborhoods.

For the first regression, the set of variables indicating low socioeconomic status are all significant and indicate, as hypothesized, that the disadvantaged use the public ambulance system more often. Demand increases with housing density,* nonwhite population, low income, male unemployment, and females in the labor force. We also note that additional employment within the census tract increases demand.

The fact that we have estimated a multivariate regression means that great care must be taken in interpreting many of the estimated coefficients. For example, we include measures of the proportion of children and of the aged, but must exclude the proportion of people aged 14-65 in the estimation. This means that the other two coefficients are relative to the excluded category. Thus, the positive coefficients for children and the aged mean that these groups generate more calls than those aged 14-65. In particular, the aged generate more calls than either of the other groups. Similarly, relative to married people, single women (including those separated, divorced, and widowed) generate fewer calls while single men (including those separated, divorced, and widowed) generate more calls. Whites generate fewer calls than nonwhites; in addition, as with the total population, single white women generate fewer calls than married white people while single white males generate more.

Some of the less populated recreational areas within the city seem to generate more demand, primarily from auto accidents. As a consequence, the first land use variable indicates that demand rises as acreage *per capita* increases. Relative to residential land, commercial land generates more calls per acre; as the percentage of land devoted to commercial use rises, demand increases. Commercial areas have considerably more pedestrian and auto traffic with a consequently greater opportunity for injury or illness to occur on a

*Housing units per capita; the inverse of housing density is actually used in the analysis.

public street. Industrial land generates fewer calls than residential land. Industrial settings are now relatively safe due to the influence of Workmens' Compensation laws and many industrial firms have set up procedures to handle accidents without calling the public system. The imposition of the fee schedule in 1966 had its most immediate impact in eliminating calls from the few industrial firms who continued to take advantage of the free service for many minor illnesses and injuries. Similarly, land devoted to transportation generates fewer calls than residential land. Transportation acreage is devoted to airports, train yards, and docks which have little public traffic and which are often served by special ambulance services.

Automobile Accidents

Nearly all automobile accidents involving injury result in a call for a public ambulance. Thus, in predicting the number of calls for public ambulances to handle automobile accidents, one is really predicting the number (and location) of automobile accidents involving injury. This job is quite different from that of predicting the demand for public ambulances to handle illness.*

Socioeconomic variables are not as powerful in this analysis as in the other categories. Housing density has a negative effect, while acreage *per capita* and land devoted to transportation have positive effects. The results suggest the hypothesis that serious automobile accidents tend to occur either on freeways or suburban and rural roads, rather than in urban areas.

The positive coefficients for total employment within the tract and for the percentage of land devoted to

*See King (1968).

Table 4
Public Ambulance Demand by Category of Incident

	Auto Accidents		Auto Accidents		Other Illness		Dry Runs		Cardiac*		Poison†	
$\bar{R}^2$	.672		.672		.865		.597		.731		.444	
Degrees of Freedom	600		600		600		600		125		125	
1. Constant term	5	(.20)‡	72	(2.94)	67	(1.99)	9	(.96)	6	(.47)	−6	(−.45)
2. Housing density	135	(3.48)	−273	(−6.80)	−391	(−7.04)	31	(1.95)	29	(1.77)	−11	(−.70)
3. Recently moved	−206	(−4.38)	283	(5.78)	451	(6.67)	−11	(−.56)	10	(.59)	24	(1.66)
4. White population	−15	(−1.70)	−38	(−4.12)	−39	(−3.11)	−5	(−1.41)	−4	(−1.30)	1	(.30)
5. % over 65	−78	(−1.46)	262	(4.73)	598	(7.82)	11	(.50)	38	(1.94)	4	(.25)
6. % Single females	−188	(−2.22)	140	(1.59)	−308	(−2.54)	−129	(−3.70)	−15	(−.38)	28	(.77)
7. % Single males	−233	(−2.72)	398	(4.44)	716	(5.79)	41	(1.16)	−25	(−.81)	8	(.30)
8. % Poor families	139	(1.78)	259	(3.14)	177	(1.58)	43	(1.35)	16	(.53)	125	(4.47)
9. % Males unemployed	28	(.18)	279	(1.73)	1,129	(5.09)	214	(3.36)	−86	(−1.18)	−80	(−1.22)
10. % Employed males	−175	(−3.15)	669	(11.59)	789	(9.90)	−36	(−1.56)	−5	(−.20)	57	(2.62)
11. F. in labor force	98	(1.77)	−146	(−2.53)	−61	(−.77)	11	(.50)	−51	(−2.52)	36	(1.94)
12. Total employment	12	(20.34)	13	(20.67)	17	(19.52)	4	(16.16)	2	(4.77)	1	(2.27)
13. % Children	−219	(−3.20)	323	(4.53)	−416	(−4.23)	−21	(−.74)	−11	(−.44)	46	(2.00)
14. % Single white M.	57	(1.11)	64	(1.19)	258	(3.49)	46	(2.15)	9	(.45)	22	(1.13)
15. % Married whites	−97	(−1.73)	112	(1.93)	117	(1.45)	−9	(−.37)	−2	(−.10)	11	(.56)
16. % M. farmers	−24	(−.31)	−228	(−2.84)	−155	(−1.34)	−3	(−.11)	−44	(−1.53)	57	(2.62)
17. % M. managers	−174	(−6.61)	171	(6.07)	190	(4.88)	−24	(−2.17)	5	(.48)	−44	(−1.69)
18. % M. household	−218	(−5.40)	90	(2.13)	104	(1.80)	−35	(−2.11)	8	(.46)	11	(1.21)
19. % F. professional	94	(3.40)	−147	(−5.14)	−127	(−3.22)	20	(1.75)	−7	(−.42)	2	(.10)
20. % F. farmers	−917	(−7.04)	1,059	(7.82)	1,317	(7.04)	−170	(−3.18)	24	(.21)	210	(2.07)
21. % F. laborers	539	(3.86)	−550	(−3.78)	122	(.61)	99	(1.71)	0	(.03)	−213	(−3.51)
22. Acres/capita	41	(6.62)	−2	(−.30)	−5	(−.61)	7	(2.67)	0	(.0)	3	(1.18)
23. % Comm. land	76	(2.97)	−5	(−.20)	88	(2.39)	2	(.20)	−4	(−.49)	−8	(−1.02)
24. % Indust. land	−1	(−.04)	−40	(−2.02)	−83	(−3.01)	1	(.19)	10	(1.85)	1	(.23)
25. % Trans. land	35	(1.30)	−60	(−2.16)	−93	(−2.45)	−7	(−.61)	−2	(−.28)	−5	(−.79)
26. Freeway	16	(5.90)	−3	(−1.20)	−7	(−1.73)	2	(1.78)	0	(.0)	−1	(−.23)
27. Response time	−6	(−1.32)	−1	(−.97)	−3	(−.42)	−1	(−.21)	−2	(−1.31)	0	(.0)
28. Area #1	36	(.78)	−16	(−.34)	−44	(−.66)	77	(4.06)	29	(2.37)	28	(2.52)
29. Area #2	−37	(−.38)	−14	(−.14)	−68	(−.50)	−39	(−.98)	10	(.48)	−10	(−.53)
30. Area #3	−15	(−.22)	−1	(−.00)	11	(.12)	−52	(−1.92)	12	(.77)	19	(1.31)
31. Area #4	−172	(−1.79)	78	(.78)	117	(.85)	−24	(−.61)	10	(.38)	25	(1.08)
32. Area #5	148	(2.20)	66	(.95)	27	(.28)	6	(.20)	−12	(−.74)	6	(.34)

* Cardiac calls per capita for the aggregated data (157 areas).   † Poison calls per capita for the aggregated data (157 areas).   ‡ The figure in parentheses is the t statistic.

commercial activity indicate that these are good surrogates for high traffic volume.

The sociological variables of importance are difficult to interpret. One would hypothesize that the percentage of single males would have a positive effect, but the opposite result occurred in this study. The negative effect of a high percentage of children is understandable, because children tend to reside in tracts with neither freeways nor rural roads. The positive influence of female employment probably coincides with central city residence.

The coefficient of determination of .671 is lower than that for total accidents, although still quite significant.

Other Accidents

This category included injuries resulting from fights, falls, and other miscellaneous accidents. One would suspect that males are particularly likely to be involved in this category. These injuries probably involve broken bones and hemorrhage and are likely to involve a call for a public ambulance. Falls and similar accidents are more likely to occur among children and the elderly than in the population at large; they are also more likely to occur in areas such as slums. Fights generally involve young men.

The results tend to support these hypotheses. The coefficients of all variables indicating low income neighborhoods are of the expected sign and, with the exception of unemployment, are significant. Children and the elderly are related to higher demand rates, along with single males. Surprisingly, employed males have a larger and more significant effect on demand than do unemployed males. Single women have almost no effect. The land use variables indicate that these accidents occur more frequently in residential areas than elsewhere.

Sickness: Cardiac and Poison

Cardiacs and poison cases were analyzed using the aggregated areas. An attempt was made to analyze the two categories together; however, the obvious differences in the kinds of individuals likely to be victims of these types of emergencies complicated interpretation of the aggregate estimate. Thus, we used the aggregated data (each observation represents calls from four census tracts over four years) to estimate each category separately.

One would hypothesize that socioeconomic data would predict public ambulance demands arising from cardiac cases quite well. Males over age 45 are more prone to coronary attacks and the poor would tend to rely more heavily on the public system in this type of case. Difficulties arise, however, in this analysis because of a small sample of such cases.

The positive effects of low density housing and the Fire Department response area probably reflect to some degree a reliance by the suburban San Fernando Valley dwellers on the Fire Department for quick response to heart attacks. The percentage of the population over 65 has, as expected, a positive effect.

Many cardiac calls involve employed males at work. In fact, total employment and females in the labor force are the only variables that are statistically significant. Surprisingly, the data do not suggest that particular kinds of employment are more likely to generate heart attack calls than others, although the results indicate that unemployed males are less likely to have heart attacks than employed males. Despite the weakness of the individual variables due to collinearity, the $\bar{R}^2$ is .731, which is quite respectable.

As with the cardiac category, the sample size for poisoning cases was quite low, thereby reducing the predictive ability. The fact that children are a strongly positive influence certainly coincides with expectations. The positive effects of low-income variables probably reflect a greater reliance on the public system due to decreased alternatives. Children are much less likely than adults to be transported by ambulance when an emergency occurs because they can more easily be fitted into a private car. Low socioeconomic status families have fewer private autos available, especially during working hours when children are liable to get into difficulty. It is possible that the negative effect of unemployed males and the positive effect of employed males indicate this decreased availability of alternatives, i.e., if the man is home with some type of vehicle, he will transport the child to the hospital.

Sickness: Other

Illness with some acute distress symptoms is an extremely common event; a very small percentage of these cases come into the public system. In general, these cases will go to the family physician unless he cannot be reached or is otherwise unavailable. Stable, high-income families are more likely to handle these cases through a private physician; transient, recently moved people, or older people are more likely to call the public system for assistance. In this study, this category included a number of cases of drunkenness and unconscious individuals found to have no evidence of trauma.

The results showing that older people are likely to generate calls accords with our expectations. The negative effect of children probably indicates that families with small children are likely to have access to a physician and so do not rely on the public system. People who have recently moved are likely to call the public system when such an emergency occurs, as are people of low income. The reason for both is that neither of these groups is likely to have readily available alternatives, such as a family physician. Similarly, whites call the public system less often than nonwhites. Single females exert a substantial negative influence while single males have substantial positive effect. Single females are more likely to have a regular physician and the high demand generated by single men probably reflects the many downtown habitués who are high utilizers. The factor for total employment in a tract has a positive effect, again indicating highly commercial areas. As the percentage of males in the labor force increases (whether they are employed or unemployed), ambulance calls increase. Perhaps the explanation is that these males are away from home and unable to provide transportation to a physician.

Land use variables show that commercial property generates many calls, while industrial and transportation land generates fewer calls than residential land. As indicated earlier, industrial firms handle their calls outside the public system and areas devoted to transportation generate few calls.

Dry Runs

A dry run occurs when the ambulance driver either cannot locate the patient, or when he sees that the situation is being handled without any need for him. Area number one is extremely significant. This is the area where no screening of calls is done; thus, as one would expect, automatically dispatching an ambulance for every call leads ambulances to go on more dry runs than in areas where the dispatcher must be satisfied that a medical emergency is involved. The influence of income variables in this equation is not clear, probably due to collinearity among the explanatory variables (the San Fernando Valley area is of a uniformly higher income level than the unscreened areas).

The Effect of Price

In order to isolate the effect of the charge added in 1967, the data were regrouped so that each point represented the total calls from four census tracts for a given year. All four years were pooled and a variable was added to allow for under-reporting in one area in 1967. There were significant increases in demand from 1964 to 1966 (the 1964-65 increase is 23 per cent and the 1965-66 increase is 11 percent). Demand actually fell from 1966 to 1967 (by 1.7 percent) which is a significant departure from the trend and from our expectations, since Los Angeles continued to grow. Ambulance demand in Los Angeles has been growing over time; this growth was slowed through the $15 charge. Additional data are needed before the precise effect of the charge can be estimated. It seems plausible that there might be a lag between the institution of the charge and its effect on demand; people may not be aware of it for some time.

CONCLUSION

The demand for public ambulances appears to be highly predictable, using a simple linear model employing socioeconomic variables, quality of service variables, and land use variables. Low-income families and nonwhites tend to use the public ambulance system more often than others. Areas with elderly people or children also generate many calls. Estimates of demand are stable over time and tend to be similar across type of incident giving rise to the call.

REFERENCES

1. Alpert, J. J., Kosa, J., Haggerty, R. J., Robertson, L., and Heagarty, M. C.: "The Types of Families that Use an Emergency Clinic." Medical Care 7:55, 1969.
2. Andrews, R. B.: "Criteria Selection in Emergency Medical System Analysis." EMS Working Paper No. 1, 1969 (EMS-69-1-W). Paper presented at Annual Meeting, Western Section Operations Research Society of America, February 1969.
3. Jacobs, A. R., and McLaughlin, C. P.: "Analyzing the Role of the Helicopter in Emergency Medical Care for a Community." Medical Care 5:343, 1967.
4. King, B. G.: "Estimating Community Requirements for the Emergency Care of Highway Accident Victims." A.J.P.H. 58:1422, 1968.
5. King, B. G., and Sox, E. D.: "An Emergency Medical Service System—Analysis of Workload." Pub. Hlth. Rep. 82:995, 1967.
6. Lavenhar, M. A., Ratner, R. S., and Weinerman, E. R.: "Social Class and Medical Care: Indices of Nonurgency in Use of Hospital Emergency Services." Medical Care 6:368, 1968.
7. Weinerman, E. R., Ratner, R. S., Robbins, A., and Lavenhar, M. A.: "Yale Studies in Ambulatory Medical Care: V. Determinants of Use of Hospital Emergency Services." A.J.P.H. 56:1037, 1966.

13. Variations in Visits to Hospital Emergency Care Facilities: Ritualistic and Meteorological Factors Affecting Supply and Demand*

John H. Noble, Jr., Ph.D.

Margaret E. LaMontagne, M.S.N.

Carole Bellotti, B.S.N.

Henry Wechsler, Ph.D.

In the past decade, studies of hospital emergency care facilities have documented generally increasing utilization, and an apparent shift in function denoted by the population's greater propensity to rely upon these facilities for treatment of nonurgent conditions.[1-7,9,11-16,18-20,21] Depending upon the hospital, period of time studied, and the definition of urgency applied, investigators report varying increases in utilization, as well as differences in the ratio of nonurgent to urgent visits. Tables 1 and 2 present in order of magnitude the major published statistics in this regard. It is noteworthy that investigators typically cite

*Reprinted from *Medical Care,* September-October 1971, Vol. IX, No. 5.

Table 1
Percentage Increase in Emergency Unit Utilization by Hospital, Investigator, Years Studied, and Time Interval Involved

Hospital	Investigator	Years Studied	Time Interval In Years	Percentage Increase in Visits
Charleston County Emergency Room	Bradham, G. B.	1965-1967	2	16
Ottawa Civic Hospital	Barth, N. K.	1962-1966	4	48
Grace-New Haven Community Hospital	Weinerman, E. R., and Edwards, H. R.	1953-1963	10	76
Baylor University Medical Center	Bryant, L. G.	1956-1966	10	110
265 hospitals in nationwide stratified sample	Skudder, P. A., et al.	1945-1958	13	120
90 hospitals in East and Middle West	Shortliffe, E. C., et al.	1940-1955	15	400
St. Luke's Methodist Hospital	Gitchell, D.	1950-1965	15	487
Hartford Hospital	Barry, R. M., et al.	1938-1957	19	950*
Children's Hospital Medical Center	Bergman, A. B., and Haggerty, R. J.	1947-1960	13	1,472*

* Calculated from presented data.

Table 2
Percentage of Emergency Unit Nonurgent Cases by Hospital, Investigator, Year, and Time Period Represented

Hospital	Investigator	Year	Time Period Represented	Percentage Nonurgent Cases
Genesee Hospital	Kluge, D. N., et al.	1964	1 mo.	30
Baylor University Medical Center	Bryant, L. G.	1966	1 year	34
Beth Israel Hospital	Lee, S. S., et al.	1957	4 weeks	38
265 hospitals in nationwide stratified sample	Skudder, P. A., et al.	1958	1 week	42
Ottawa Civic Hospital	Barth, N. K.	1966	1 mo.	42
New York Hospital	Reed, J. I., and Reader, G. G.	1965	1 year	54*
Children's Hospital Medical Center	Bergman, A. B., and Haggerty, R. J.	1960	6 weeks	55

* Calculated from presented data.

unpublished sources and each other in support of these trends.

Many of the same studies have attempted to discover and to interpret periodicity in the utilization of hospital emergency care facilities.[1-7,9,12-13,15-16,19-20] Table 3, summarizing the findings of 15 such studies, shows that reduced volume (-) during the first shift of duty in the hospital (12M-8 am) is the only constant. Although higher volume (+) occurs in most hospitals during the second shift (8 am-4 pm), weekends, and during spring and summer months, marked departures from these tendencies are found in some places. No pattern emerges which can be related to type of hospital control, inpatient bed size, total annual volume of visits to the emergency unit, or even to various time periods represented by the studies. In consequence, health care administrators and planners cannot generalize about periodicity in utilization of the hospital emergency unit in reaching decisions about appropriate staffing patterns or other matters dependent upon such knowledge without first checking their immediate situations.

With few exceptions, explanations for periodicity in the utilization of hospital emergency care facilities cite formal and customarily repeated patterns of behavior which mark occupational and/or social ritual. Unavailability of the physician because of days taken off in the course of the week, weekends, or vacations was the most frequent explanation for increased emergency unit volume noted during certain time periods.[1-2,4,13,15] Daily alcohol ingestion patterns,[12] weekend and vacation recreational activities of children and adolescents,[2,19] vacations and travel by all age groups during the summer months,[2] all of which relate to increased risk of accident and injury at certain times for different segments of the population, have also been offered as reasons for heightened emergency unit activity. One investigator considered it significant that daily peak periods of emergency unit activity occurred during the postcibal hours of 9 am, 1 pm, and 6-7 pm, although more precise hypotheses accounting for these phenomena were not given.[13]

Efforts to link hour of visit and patient characteristics and/or case circumstances such as race, social class, type and severity of illness, length of residence in the community, third-party subsidy, means of transportation, and distance from hospital have not been successful.[3] On the other hand, there is evidence that a relationship between day of visit and type and severity of illness exists. The largest percentage of nonurgent visits at Baylor University Medical Center in Dallas, Texas was recorded on Sundays, while the majority of patients treated on Wednesdays were classified as medical emergencies.[7] The ratio of injury to disease among ambulance patients is highest weekends in San Francisco, California.[12] Theoretically, these differences in the temporal distribution of injuries vs. disease and emergent vs. nonurgent conditions treated in the hospital emergency unit are reducible to variations in levels of risk experienced by various segments of the population pursuing activities prescribed by occupational and/or social ritual.

In conjunction with ritualistic factors, biometeorological phenomena may influence the volume, types, and seriousness of conditions seen at different times in hospital emergency care facilities. Many studies have demonstrated the influence of weather and climate on human diseases, drug action, reaction speed, working efficiency, and accidents.[17] Weather and climate have both short and long periodic effects on a variety of physiologic processes, including the physi-

Table 3
Daily, Seasonal, and Shift Variations in Emergency Unit Volume by Hospital, Investigator, Year, AHA Control Code, Inpatient Bed Size, Annual Emergency Unit Volume, and Time Period Represented

Hospital	Investigator	Year	AHA control code	Inpatient bed size	Annual No. E.U. Visits*	Time period represented	Day of week M T W T F S S	Season Jan.-Mar. Winter	April-June Spring	July-Sept. Summer	Oct.-Dec. Fall	Shift 12 M-8 am 1	8 am-4 pm 2	4 pm-12 M 3
Baylor Univ. Med. Center	Dallas, Texas	Bryant, L. G.	1966	Church	794	24,075	1 yr.	− + +		+	+		−	+
Griffin Hosp.	Derby, Conn.	Bonner, P. A.	1967	Nonprofit	199	17,263	1 mo.	− + + +			+		−	+
Ottawa Civic Hospital	Ottawa, Canada	Barth, N. K.	1966	City	1,081	56,156	1 mo.	− + −			+		−	+
St. Luke's Methodist Hosp.	Cedar Rapids, Iowa	Gitchell, D.	1965	Church	432	18,943	1 mo.	− + +						
Genesee Hospital	Rochester, New York	Kluge, D. N., et al.	1964	Nonprofit	300	28,616¹	1 mo.	+ + −					−	+
Charleston County Emergency Room	Charleston, S. C.	Bradham, G. B.	1965	County	NA	34,473²	1 mo.	+ +						+
Charleston County Emergency Room	Charleston, S. C.	Bradham, G. B.	1955-1958	County	157	36,800	3 yrs.	+ +					−	+
Hartford Hospital	Hartford, Conn.	Barry, R. M., et al.	1965	Nonprofit	804	21,000³	1 yr.	+ +		+	+		−	+
New York Hospital	New York, N. Y.	Reed, J. I., & Reader, G. G.	1965	Nonprofit	1,217	31,710	1 wk.	− + +					−	+
265 Hospitals	Nationwide stratified sample⁴	Skudder, P. A., et al.	1958	NA	NA	649,189⁵		+ +					−	+

TABLE 3. (cont.)

Hospital	Location	Reference	Ownership		Volume	Period					
Vancouver Gen. Hosp.	Vancouver, B. C.	Robinson, G. C., 1965-1966	Nonprofit	2,000	c. 50,000	1 yr.				++	+
4 units of San Francisco Emer. Med. Ser.	San Francisco, California	King, B. C., et al.	City-County	NA	c. 53,372[a]	13 mos.	−			++	− +
Roosevelt Hospital	Manhattan, N. Y.		1964	Nonprofit	558	50,477	5 mos.	−		+		− +
St. Luke's Hospital	Manhattan, N. Y.	Torrens, P. H., and	1964	Nonprofit	713	64,657	5 mos.	− +		−		− +
Queens Hosp. Center	Queens, N. Y.	Yedvah, D. C.	1964	City	1,363	76,170	5 mos.	−	+	−		− +
Long Island Jewish Hosp.	New Hyde Pk., N. Y.		1964	Nonprofit	268	15,645	5 mos.	+ −		−		− +
Children's Hosp. Med. Center	Boston, Mass.	Bergman, A. B., and Haggerty, R. J.	1960	Nonprofit	354	c. 15,000+	6 wks.					− +
Boston City Hospital	Boston, Mass.		1968	City	1,132	135,874	1 yr.		−	++	+	− +
Beth Israel Hospital	Boston, Mass.		1968	Nonprofit	356	24,523	1 yr.	+		− −		+ − +
Charles Choate Memorial Hosp.	Woburn, Mass.	Noble, J. H., et al., reported in Hess, I., & Bronstad, G. W.[10]	1968	Nonprofit	130	16,623	1 yr.			− ++	+	− +
Saugus General	Saugus, Mass.		1968	Profit	125	5,256	1 yr.			++	+	− +

[1] 1963; [2] 1964; [3] 1958; [4] 6% of 5,364 short-term, non-federal, general hospitals in U. S. having emergency facilities; [5] total for 265 hospitals in sample; [6] 13 months volume of 57,820 (April 1963-April 1964) minus 1/13 of total. * For the year listed, unless otherwise specified; + higher volume; − reduced volume.

cochemical state of the blood, kidney function, the autonomic nervous system, diastolic blood pressure, capillary resistance and membrane permeability, cerebral hemorrhage and capillary fragility, and ductless gland functioning. Similarly, they effect primary and secondary causes of disease in the central nervous system, heart, lungs, pancreas, liver, kidneys, stomach, ductless glands, eyes, joints, and teeth.

Sudden cooling, accompanied by falling barometric pressure and rising wind speed, increases the incidence of asthmatic attacks. Coronary thrombosis, myocardial infarction, and angina pectoris occur more frequently after sudden strong cold or heat stress. Infectious diseases, such as the common cold and influenza, are favored by sudden weather changes affecting the thermoregulatory and membrane permeability mechanisms of the body.

The relationship between traffic accidents and passage of atmospheric depressions accompanied by sudden changes in the temperature-humidity environment is well-established. Interestingly, fog, slippery roads, glazed frost, and other seemingly menacing weather are less significant causes of accidents than sudden changes in atmospheric conditions having simultaneous impact on the human body. The *Survey of Human Biometeorology* adds the following general explanation of the action of weather on human functioning:

> Short-term aperiodic weather changes act as stimuli on the human body. If a person is unable to adjust to these stimuli their effect is disturbing. He may at first be affected by subjective disorders—general complaints, depression, over-excitability, insomnia, headaches, palpitation of the heart, etc. If his regulating capacity becomes lowered still further, he may become really ill. The decisive factor is the individual's

proneness to disturbance or illness. The effects will be accelerated in biologically unfavourable weather and retarded in biologically favourable weather. (1964:70)

Insofar as ritualistic and meteorological factors may influence variations in emergency unit utilization conjointly, exploration of the relationships between these variables appears warranted. The present study analyzes data for 1968 derived from three Boston hospitals located within a six-block radius of one another, the Boston Police Department, and the U. S. Weather Bureau to determine the relationship between daily, holiday, travel, and meteorological patterns, and 1. emergency unit visits, 2. traffic accident injuries, and 3. "sick assist" injury cases served by ambulances of the Boston Police Department. Virtually all persons suffering from traffic accident injuries and slightly more than 96 percent of "sick assist" injury cases are conveyed to emergency care and/or inpatient facilities located principally in municipal Boston. The remainder, in order of frequency, involve cases wherein police ambulance services were refused, patients were brought to a physician's office for treatment, deceased persons were transported to municipal mortuaries, etc.

PROCEDURES AND DEFINITIONS

Total daily emergency unit visits to Beth Israel Hospital, Peter Bent Brigham Hospital, and Children's Hospital Medical Center for 1968 were classified by type of transport (police ambulance, private ambulance, and "other") and coded by reference to occurrence on 1. specific day of week, 2. Catholic, Jewish, or secular (national, state, or local) holiday, and 3. day on which pre- or post-holiday travel customarily takes place. In a similar fashion, records of the Boston Police Department for 1968 involving daily tallies of traffic accident injuries and total police ambulance runs were merged and coded.

Subtracting cases involving traffic accident injuries from total police ambulance runs yielded a residual of "sick assist" calls to the Boston Police Department consisting of an unknown mix of injuries unrelated to traffic accidents and acute and chronic disease conditions, plus slightly less than 4 percent of cases transported to some other place than an emergency care and/or inpatient facility. One and six-tenths percent of all Boston Police Department ambulance runs terminated at an inpatient facility lacking an identifiable emergency unit. The aggregate character of the available data made it impossible to reduce these conceptually-distinguishable categories of the "sick assist" caseload to empirical measures subject to statistical analysis.

Information on daily local weather conditions gathered by the U. S. Weather Bureau at Logan International Airport, Boston, Mass.,[21] including maximum temperature (Fahrenheit degrees), total 24-hour precipitation (inches), total 24-hour snow fall (inches), snow depth on ground (inches), total sunshine (hours), and the occurrence of fog, thunder, sleet, hail, rain, snow, glaze, dust storm, smoke and/or haze, blowing snow, and heavy fog were merged with the aforementioned data on emergency unit visits, traffic accident injuries, and "sick assist" police ambulance runs. An index of over-all daily weather conditions[8] was computed according to a formula which gave approximately equal weight to its three component measures:

$$I_0 = W_1 T_x + W_2 S - W_3 R$$

where T_x = daily maximum temperature (Fahrenheit

degrees), S = total sunshine (hours), R = total 24-hour precipitation (inches), and $W_1 = 1.0$, $W_2 = 4.0$, $W_3 = 54.9$, so that $W_1 \sigma_{T_x} = W_2 \sigma_S = W_3 \sigma_R$.

All variables in the respective sets of data were normalized by z-score conversion, and zero-order Pearsonian linear correlation coefficients were computed. Statistically significant ($p < .05$) zero-order correlates of the criterion variables of this study were subjected to step-wise regression analyses which placed the index of over-all daily weather conditions first in the equation, thereby estimating its predictive power before selecting from the remaining correlates in a step-wise fashion the best set of predictors. This permitted assessment of the unique contribution of each predictor to the explanation of variance on the criterion variables.

Unfortunately, the aggregate character of the available data made it impossible to replicate studies showing a relationship between traffic accidents and abrupt climatological changes[17] or to assess the influence of these changes upon hospital emergency unit visits and "sick assist" calls. However, the available measures of weather conditions are expected to reveal crude temporal variations in levels of mobility, visibility, and comfort in the population of the Boston area during 1968 which, in turn, may have influenced the onset of conditions resulting in increased emergency unit utilization, traffic accidents, and "sick assist" calls to the Boston Police Department.

WEATHER CONDITIONS

The U. S. Weather Bureau station at Logan International Airport, located 42° 22′ North in latitude, 71° 2′ West in longitude, and 15 feet above sea level, reported for 1968 an average monthly temperature of

50.4 F, ranging between a 98 F high on July 16 and a −4 F low on January 9.[21] Ten days had maximum temperatures of 90 F and above, while minimum temperatures of 32 F and below were recorded for 94 days.

Total precipitation for the year was 42.28 inches, with a 4.13 inch 24-hour maximum falling on March 17-18. There were 118 days on which 0.01 inch or more of precipitation fell. Total precipitation in the form of snow and sleet was 33.4 inches, with an 8.6 inch 24-hour maximum falling on January 6-7. On 10 days, 1 inch or more of snow fell. Thunderstorms occurred on 14 days.

Sunrise to sunset, there was 62 percent possible sunshine and 60 percent average sky cover. The skies were clear on 105 days, partly cloudy on 105 days, and cloudy on 156 days. Heavy fog obscured visibility on 21 days. Average wind speed was 13.4 miles per hour.

During the year, the average relative humidity was 70 percent at 1 am EST and 57 percent at 1 pm EST. The index of over-all daily weather conditions, based upon maximum temperature, total sunshine, and amount of precipitation, yielded values ranging from −149.6 to 153.6, with a mean of 81.0 and a standard deviation of 40.8.

Utilization Patterns

In 1968, Beth Israel Hospital, a 356-bed, nonprofit general hospital, had 24,529 visits to its emergency unit, averaging 67.2 per day. As shown in Table 4, daily averages by type of transport were: 5.6 cases by police ambulance, 2.7 cases by private ambulance, and 58.6 cases by all other means of transportation.

Visits to Emergency Care Facilities 317

Table 4
Daily Distribution of Emergency Unit Visits by Type of Transport in
Three Boston Hospitals during 1968

Type of Transport	Beth Israel Hospital		Peter Bent Brigham Hospital		Children's Hospital Medical Center	
	Mean	S.D.	Mean	S.D.	Mean	S.D.
Police ambulance	5.6	2.8	5.2	2.6	5.3	2.6*
Private ambulance	2.7	1.7	0.3	0.7	0.7	0.8
All other visits	58.6	10.4	51.9	13.1	163.6	26.7†
Total visits	67.2	10.7	57.4	13.5	170.8	27.0

* Boston Police Department Ambulances only. † Excluding all ambulance and fire/rescue squad cases.

In the same year, Peter Bent Brigham Hospital, another nonprofit general hospital containing 321 beds, had 19,954 emergency unit visits, averaging 57.4 per day. Daily averages by type of transport were: 5.2 cases by police ambulance, 0.3 cases by private ambulance, and 51.9 cases by all other means of transportation.

Children's Hospital Medical Center, a 343-bed, nonprofit general hospital for children, had 66,313 emergency unit visits during 1968, averaging 170.8 per day. Daily averages by type of transport were: 5.3 cases by Boston Police Department ambulance, 0.7 cases by private ambulance, and 163.6 cases by means of transportation other than ambulance.

In 1968, the Boston Police Department made 37,515 ambulance runs, averaging 102.6 per day. The average number of "sick assist" calls per day was 93.5, while traffic accidents involving personal injuries requiring a police ambulance averaged 9.0 per day. Table 5 presents the daily distribution of these traffic accidents by the number of persons injured. Counts for the less frequently occurring accidents involving several casualties are as follows: 47 traffic accidents involving 4 injured persons, 24 accidents injuring 5 persons, 11 accidents causing 7 casualties, and 6 accidents injuring 8 persons.

Table 5
Daily Distribution of Traffic Accidents by
Number of Persons Injured, Total Traffic Accident
Ambulance Runs, and "Sick Assist" Calls to the
Boston Police Department during 1968

Variable Traffic accidents injuring:	Mean	S.D.
1	6.4	3.5
2	1.9	1.8
3	0.4	0.7
4	0.1	0.4
5	0.1	0.3
Total traffic accident ambulance runs	9.0	4.6
Total "sick assist" calls	93.5	16.1
Total ambulance runs	102.6	16.5

VISITS BY TYPE OF TRANSPORT

The degree of relationship between emergency unit visits by type of transport at Beth Israel Hospital, Peter Bent Brigham Hospital, and Children's Hospital Medical Center and daily, holiday, travel, and meteorological patterns during 1968 is expressed as beta coefficients. The beta coefficients were derived from the final equation of the step-wise regression analysis, thus indicating the degree of unique relationship between each predictor variable and the criterion—all other predictor variables held constant (partialled). It is apparent that different combinations of ritualistic and meteorological factors predict variations in total daily emergency unit visits, as well as type of transport, for each of the three hospitals. Similarly, these different combinations explain differing amounts of total variance, as measured by the coefficient of determination (R^2). In general, analyses of police and private ambulance cases explained significantly less total variance than did analyses of cases arriving by all other means of transportation and total daily emergency unit visits.

No combination of factors predicts cases transported by police ambulance to Peter Bent Brigham Hospital, while at Beth Israel Hospital and Children's Hospital Medical Center different patterns of police ambulance activity emerge (Table 6). Increased activ-

Table 6
Relationship (Beta Coefficients) between Emergency Unit Visits by Type of Transport in Three Boston Hospitals and Daily, Holiday, Travel, and Meteorological Patterns during 1968

Predictor Variables ($0 =$ No, $1 =$ Yes)	Police Ambulances BI PBBH CHMC[1]			Private Ambulances BI PBBH CHMC			All Other Visits BI PBBH CHMC			Total Daily Visits BI PBBH CHMC		
Days of Week												
Monday					−.14†	.12°		.25†	.06			.23†
Tuesday						−.14†					.12°	
Wednesday		−.11°					.10°	−.16†		.07	−.15†	
Thursday								−.07			−.08°	
Friday				.07				−.06			−.04	
Saturday	.12°						−.20†	.44†	−.13†	−.17†	.45†	−.14†
Sunday			−.15†	.14†			−.32†	.31†	−.16†	−.27†	.33†	−.18†
Holidays												
Catholic		−.12°						.06			−.12°	
Jewish								.11°				.07
Secular				−.12°	−.17†	.18†	−.15†	−.15†	.16†	−.16†		
Travel Patterns												
Pre-holiday travel												
Post-holiday travel								.10°			.10°	
Indices of Weather Conditions												
Thunder	.11°											
Smoke/haze												
Fog	.13°											
Heavy fog												
Rain								.01			.02	
Sleet					−.06	−.09					−.09	
Glaze	.09						.10°					
Snow				−.10				.04			.04	
Blowing snow					−.09°		−.10°				−.09	
Over-all weather index ($+ =$ warm, fair)	−.19†	.12°		.04	−.02	.11°	.13†	.30†	.09	.13°	.30†	
R^2	.09	.06		.05	.04	.24	.48	.26	.18	.46	.28	

° $p < .05$.
† $p < .01$.
[1] Boston Police Department ambulances only.

ity occurs at BI when weather is less favorable and on Saturdays. Police ambulance runs are fewer on Catholic holidays and on Wednesdays. At CHMC, on the other hand, dissimilar weather conditions—favorable weather and thunderstorms—are associated with increased police ambulance activity. Few police ambulances arrive on Sundays.

With respect to private ambulance runs, none of the factors are predictive at BI, while they do predict increase at PBBH in contrast to decreases at CHMC. Increased activity occurs at PBBH on foggy days and Sundays. At CHMC, on the other hand, ritualistic factors alone—Mondays and secular holidays—mark reduced private ambulance runs.

A great many variables predict both heightened and reduced volume of visits by patients reaching the emergency unit primarily by private car and public transportation. Ritualistic factors are dominant predictors at BI and PBBH, while at CHMC weather plays almost as important a predictive role. Mondays, favorable weather, and Wednesday are, in order of magnitude, the best predictors of nonambulance cases at BI. Reduced volume occurs on Saturdays and Sundays, secular holidays, and days on which there is blowing snow. In contrast, the best predictors of increased nonambulance activity at PBBH are Saturdays and Sundays, secular holidays, favorable weather, days on which post-holiday travel occurs, and glaze. Volume is down Tuesdays and Wednesdays.

The pattern at CHMC is identical to that at BI in every respect except that Wednesdays at CHMC are not marked as they are at BI by increased nonambulance activity. Of course, the order of magnitude of the predictors differ in the two places; favorable weather and Mondays have greatest predictive power at CHMC.

When total daily visits to the emergency units of the three hospitals are considered, the patterns and power of the predictor variables remain relatively stable. Some shifting occurs at Beth Israel Hospital wherein statistically significant predictors of increased non-ambulance activity—Mondays, Wednesdays, and favorable weather—lose significance as predictors of total daily emergency unit volume, while Jewish holidays become a significant predictor in this regard.

TRAFFIC ACCIDENTS VS. "SICK ASSIST" CASES

There are striking differences between sets of predictive variables for traffic accident cases and "sick assist" calls, which combined equal total demand on the Boston Police Department for ambulance service (Table 7). By far, the strongest predictor of the majority of traffic accidents causing injury to 1-3 persons is Saturday, followed by Friday. In all likelihood, most of these accidents occur late Friday night and early Saturday morning. Accidents injuring 3 persons most frequently happen on Saturdays, followed by days on which pre-holiday travel occurs. Friday through Sunday, secular holidays, days on which pre-holiday travel occurs, and Jewish holidays are high risk periods for traffic accidents causing injury to 5-8 persons. Thunderstorms and heavy fog are also significant predictors of accidents injuring 7-8 persons and probably involving several cars.

Considering total daily ambulance runs made by the Boston Police Department in response to traffic accidents involving personal injuries, the single predictor of increased volume is Saturday. Tuesday through Thursday are the best predictors of reduced volume. In contrast, the accumulation of snow from successive snow storms best predicts the volume of "sick assist" calls to the Boston Police Department. Significantly reduced volume occurs on Sunday.

DISCUSSION AND CONCLUSIONS

The data upon which this study relies allow both a micro- and a macroview of the influence of ritualistic and meteorological factors on hospital emergency unit utilization in municipal Boston. Integration of

Table 7
Relationship (Beta Coefficients) between Traffic Accidents by Number of Persons Injured, "Sick Assist" Cases, and Daily, Holiday, Travel, and Meteorological Patterns in 1968

Predictor Variables (0 = No, 1 = Yes)	Traffic Accidents by Number of Persons Injured								Total Traffic Accident Ambulance Runs	Total Daily "Sick Assist" Cases
	1	2	3	4	5	6	7	8		
Days of Week										
Monday				-.08					-.10	
Tuesday	-.09	-.05							-.17†	
Wednesday		-.05							-.13°	
Thursday	-.05								-.12°	
Friday	.14†	.16†					.13°		.10	
Saturday	.30†	.27†	.24°					.14†	.32†	
Sunday					.10	.15†				-.18†
Holidays										
Catholic										
Jewish						.12°				
Secular					.11°					
Travel Patterns										
Pre-holiday travel				.15†	.12°					
Post-holiday travel										
Indices of Weather Conditions										
Thunder									.21†	
Smoke/haze										
Fog	.08									
Heavy fog						.11°				
Rain	.11	.09							.05	
Sleet										.05
Glaze										.09
Snow									-.08	.02
Blowing snow										
Total snow fall (inches)										.05
Total snow depth (inches)									-.10	.48†
Total precipitation (inches)									.14	
Over-all weather index (+ = warm, fair)	.03	-.08	-.02	.04		.06	.08		.07	.05
R²	.16	.13	.08	.01	.07	.01	.03	.07	.26	.30

° p < 0.5; † p < .01.

the two views makes clear that demand on the Boston Police Department for ambulance service cannot be translated by any simple calculus into demand for care in the emergency unit of any single hospital. This is true despite statistically significant zero-order correlations, ranging from .14 to .27, between daily totals of police ambulance runs to the emergency units of the three specific hospitals investigated and those of the entire Boston Police Department.

Although police ambulances carrying traffic accident victims peak on Friday and Saturday, these cases are not distributed uniformly throughout the hospital network. Some of them are showing up Saturdays at Beth Israel Hospital and Fridays at Childrens Hospital Medical Center but not in significant numbers on either day at Peter Bent Brigham Hospital. In a similar fashion, the decrease in total daily "sick assist" calls to the police department on Sunday seems to be reflected by a dip that day in police ambulance activity at CHMC but not at PBBH or BI. Again, increased police ambulance activity at BI but not at CHMC or PBBH during unfavorable weather probably stems from the jump in "sick assist" calls to the police department when accumulated snow causes transportation difficulties.

The tendency discovered in each of the three hospitals to have an increase in nonambulance traffic during favorable weather is noteworthy. It may indicate increased probabilities that persons with nonurgent conditions will seek attention when the weather is fair, although this is a hypothesis requiring additional information about the ratio of urgent to nonurgent conditions at such times. If confirmed and generally applicable, the tendency for persons with nonurgent conditions to present themselves at hospital emergency care facilities for treatment during favorable weather has some relevance to staffing decisions. Of course, there is need for replication of these findings on a larger, more diversified sample of hospitals, together with measurement of organizational structures and policies which may also contribute to differences in utilization.

Theoretically, it would be possible for hospital administrators and emergency unit supervisory personnel to check the short-term weather forecast, anticipate an influx of nonurgent cases on favorable days or, conversely, a slacking off during bad weather, and plan accordingly to increase or decrease staff coverage of the emergency unit. Similarly, if the emergency unit happens to be affected by police ambulances bearing "sick assist" cases when snow accumulates on the ground, an appropriate plan, dependent upon the ratio of urgent to nonurgent conditions, could be devised. Such a plan might seek to make special provision for increased incidence of heart attacks due to overexertion or snowshoveling, or do nothing beyond accommodating the usual flow of patients with nonurgent conditions who, because of adverse travel conditions, may have turned to the police department for transportation to the hospital.

The discussion thus far makes clear that an understanding of the relationship between fluctuations in visits to hospital emergency care facilities and ritualistic and meteorological factors does not offer alone sufficient information upon which to base staffing decisions. There is need for information about the interactive properties of the whole emergency care system in Boston and surrounding communities as it is affected by ritualistic and meteorological factors affecting supply and demand. On a small area basis, what is the ratio of urgent to nonurgent cases originating at different times and under varying meteorological conditions? How does case origin, type, and urgency status influence its destination after it comes to the attention of the police? How do existing policies, customs, and agreements between participants in the emergency care system affect the process of case distribution? Until such questions are answered, hospital administrators will have to continue to guess the average expected volume of visits to the emergency unit and the ratio of urgent to nonurgent conditions among them in order to maintain the proper level and mix of staff.

Finally, it should be noted that from the standpoint of predictability, utilization patterns related to ritualistic factors are less variable phenomena than those coincident with weather. However, control of phenomena associated with both kinds of factors may be equally difficult. Longstanding habituation and expectations related to occupational and/or social ritual are not easily put aside in the effort to improve the organization and delivery of services in any sector of the health care system. Although the impact upon hospital emergency care facilities of the unavailability of physicians on weekends and on the "doctor's day off" is generally known, the suggestion that physicians stagger their practices over all seven days of the week or that hospitals provide increased coverage weekends raises eyebrows—to say the least—among the health professionals concerned.

Solutions to these problems may lie in incentive salaries for weekend and night duty by nurses and other hospital personnel, development of emergency care facilities open 24 hours per day with graduated capabilities for treating the range of nonurgent to urgent conditions, and provision of hospital-employed physicians and/or partnership arrangements of physicians devoted exclusively to coverage of emergency care facilities. Reorganization of the community emergency care system will require, of course, the financial support and encouragement of Federal and state government and the private health insurance industry, all struggling to limit the fast-rising costs of medical care in the United States.

REFERENCES

1. Barry, R. M., Shortliffe, E. C., and Wetstone, H. J.: Case study predicts load variation patterns. *Hospitals* 34:34, 1960.
2. Barth, N. K.: Examination of selected characteristics of emergency department activity: Ottawa Civic Hospital. M.A. thesis, School of Hospital Administration, Univ. of Ottawa, Ottawa, Canada, 1967.
3. Bergman, A. B., and Haggerty, R. J.: The emergency clinic: A study of its role in a teaching hospital. *Amer. J. Dis. Child.* 104:36, 1962.
4. Bonner, P. A.: The application of computer simulation techniques to an emergency room service. M.A. thesis, Dept. of Epidemiology and Public Health, Yale Univ., New Haven, Conn., 1968.
5. Bradham, G. B.: An analysis of 2,418 emergency room admissions. *J. S. Carolina Med. Ass.* 61:127, 1965.
6. Bradham, G. B.: Follow-up analysis of emergency room admissions. *J. S. Carolina Med. Ass.* 63:323, 1967.
7. Bryant, L. G.: Characteristics of emergency unit patients. M.A. thesis, Washington Univ. School of Medicine, St. Louis, Mo., 1968.
8. Davis, N. E.: An optimum summer weather index. *Weather* 8:305, 1968.
9. Gitchell, D.: "Mutual convenience" visits—what are the trends? M.A. thesis, Graduate School of Business Administration, Univ. of Michigan, Ann Arbor, Mich., 1966.
10. Hess, I., and Bronstad, G. W.: The design and selection of a sample of emergency unit visits to hospitals in the

Boston metropolitan area. Unpublished report, Sampling Section, Survey Research Center, The University of Michigan, 1970.
11. Hospital Area Planning Committee, Inc.: *Summary of a Report on Outpatient and Emergency Services in Milwaukee, etc.,* p. 49.
12. King, B. G., and Sox, E. D.: An emergency medical service system—analysis of workload. *Public Health Rep.* 82:995, 1967.
13. Kluge, D. N., Wegryn, R. L., and Lemley, B. R.: The expanding emergency department. *JAMA* 191:801, 1965.
14. Lee, S. S., Solon, J. A., and Sheps, C. G.: How new patterns of medical care affect the emergency unit. *Mod. Hosp.* 94:97, 1960.
15. Reed, J. I., and Reader, G. G.: Quantitative survey of New York hospital emergency room, 1965. *New York J. Med.* 67:1335, 1967.
16. Robinson, G. C., and Klonoff, H.: Hospital emergency services for children and adolescents. *Canad. Med. Ass. J.* 96:1304, 1967.
17. Sargent, F., and Tromp, S. W. (Eds.): *A Survey of Human Biometeorology.* Geneva, World Meteorological Organization, 1964.
18. Shortliffe, E. C., Hamilton, T. S., and Noroian, E. H.: The emergency room and the changing pattern of medical care. *New Eng. J. Med.* 258: 20, 1958.
19. Skudder, P. A., McCarroll, J. R., and Wade, P. A.: Hospital emergency facilities and services, a survey. *Bull. Amer. Coll. Surg.* 46:44, 1961.
20. Torrens, P. R., and Yedvab, D. G.: Variations among emergency room populations: A comparison of four hospitals in New York. *Med. Care* 8:60, 1970.
21. U. S. Dept of Commerce: *Local Climatological Data: Annual Summary with Comparative Data, 1968,* Boston, Massachusetts. Washington, D. C., U. S. Government Printing Office, 1969.
22. Weinerman, E. R., and Edwards, H. R.: "Triage" system shows promise in management of emergency department load. *Hospitals* 38:55, 1964.

14. Cost-Effectiveness Analysis for Evaluating Alternative Emergency Medical Care Recovery Systems*

Erik Hanitzsch

William Hall

The development of effective methods for transporting the victims of emergencies to the hospital is a problem of much concern to modern society. Each year 100,000 Americans die of accidental injuries and 400,000 more suffer permanent disability.[1] Thousands more are afflicted by sudden acute illness requiring immediate medical attention.

While the prevention of such trauma is a desirable national goal, it is reasonable to assume that medical emergencies will not be eliminated from our society in the near future. Consequently, the development of rapid, effective recovery and treatment procedures is critical if we are to reduce the morbidity and mortality caused by such emergencies.

The improvement of ambulance service offers one such opportunity. Although the reduction of suffering which can be attributed to such an improvement is un-

*Presented at The Operations Research Society of America Thirty-fifth National Meeting, Denver, Colorado, June 17-20, 1969.

certain, it has been estimated that 25% of the 166,000 annual traffic accident victims now suffering permanent disability would have been saved from this fate had rapid care been provided.[2]

Unfortunately, ambulance service in this country has suffered from a severe lack of planning and coordination. Funeral homes have traditionally provided such service. However, in recent years many of these agencies have found that their ambulance services were unprofitable and have subsequently dropped such services. Thus, in some areas the ambulance service has been absorbed by the police department, the fire department, or some hospital-related agency. In others, private ambulance services have been developed, and in some communities, neighborhood volunteer groups have been formed to provide emergency medical recovery services. This evolution has been so poorly planned and implemented that a doctor of the American Academy of Orthopedic Surgeons estimates that two-thirds of the 300,000 ambulance crews are not "truly and totally competent."[3]

Fortunately, national, state, and local agencies are becoming increasingly concerned about the magnitude and severity of this problem. Hence, systematic approaches to the recovery system problem are currently being developed at all governmental levels.

The purpose of this paper is to present some concepts useful in developing systematic cost-effectiveness analyses of alternative recovery systems. We shall develop these concepts by formulating a simplified mathematical model of the problem which relates changes in the controllable parameters to costs and measures of effectiveness.

Ideally, one would like to choose some index of victim mortality or morbidity as the measure of effectiveness. Unfortunately, no indices have been developed which have the precision necessary for analyses of this type. In addition, mortality and morbidity are affected by many factors independent of changes in the recovery system. For instance, the victim's pre-emergency medical condition, the severity of the emergency, and the quality of hospital emergency room care all affect the ultimate outcome of the case. Hence, the effects of recovery system modifications on morbidity/mortality are confounded with these factors. Figure 1 depicts this problem.

In order to alleviate this problem, we have chosen to utilize intermediate measures of effectiveness. Two such measures are appropriate: (1) the time consumed by the recovery operation, and (2) the quality of medical treatment rendered by the recovery crew. The model we shall develop will consider the relationship between recovery system modifications and these two measures.

The system modifications we consider consist of two types—those affecting the basic system structure and those affecting the system operating policy. The basic system structure is determined by specifying the type of recovery vehicle to be utilized, the emergency equipment to be carried onboard, the level of attendant training to be required, the number of recovery vehicles in the system, and the organizational and administrative structure of the system. We assume that these five parameters can be combined into a finite set of P feasible basic policies.

The system operating policy can be determined by developing decision rules which control system operation. Hence, this policy includes vehicle allocation rules, vehicle dispatch rules, hospital selection rules, and rules governing the dispensation of medical treatment by the ambulance attendant. Clearly, the selection of a policy should vary depending upon the condi-

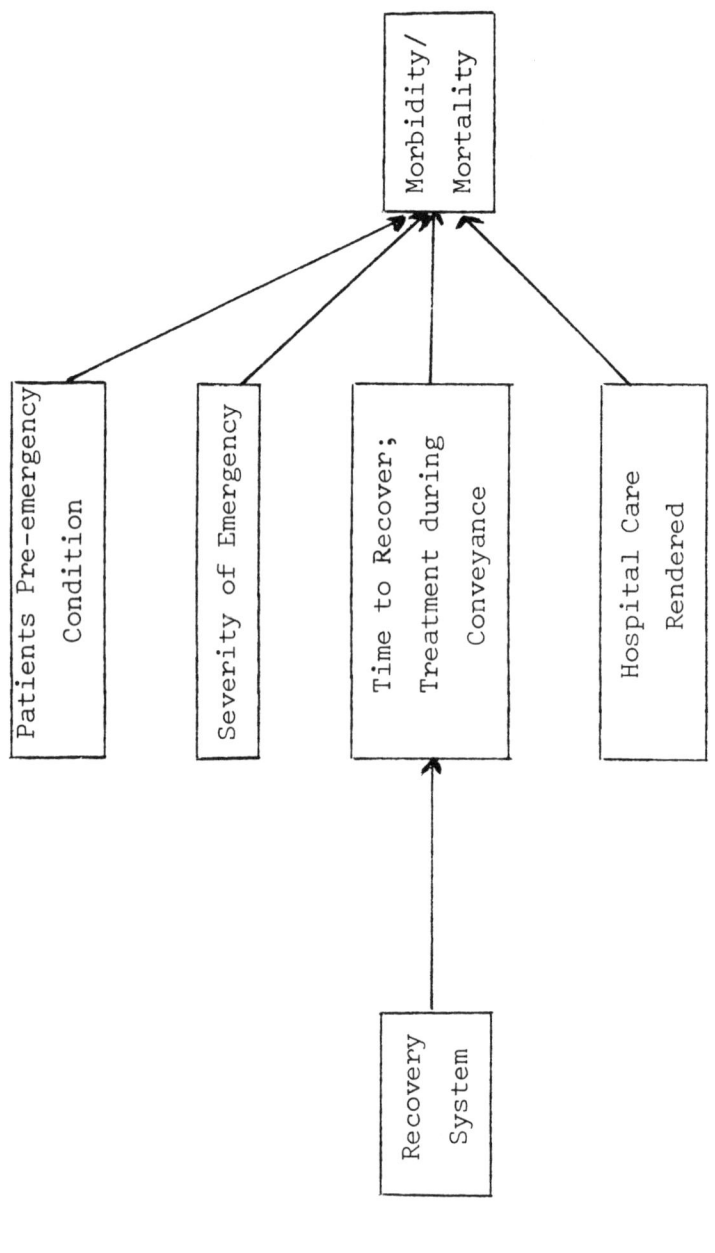

Figure 1: Some Factors Influencing Patient Morbidity/Mortality

tions which prevail in any state of the system. That is, the appropriate policy should be state dependent. We shall explore this in more detail in the next section.

It is also important to notice that the basic policies and the operating policies are interdependent. For instance, if a basic policy is chosen which gives no attendant training, then the operating policy will be constrained to include only rapid transit of the severely injured patient to the hospital. Hence, any attempts to develop optimal system configurations must consider the simultaneous effects of basic and operating policies. Figure 2 presents a schematic view of these two types of policy.

MODEL FORMULATION

In this section we shall develop a model of the system which allows us to study the effects of alternative basic and operating policies. This model is purposely oversimplified to clearly show the basic techniques and relationships. However, the insights and principles derived from this model should be useful in extending these concepts to more realistic situations. These extensions will be briefly discussed in the next section.

We first assume that the system service area can be divided into m distinct geographical regions which are denoted L_i; i = 1,...,m. We further assume that the activity of each recovery vehicle can be represented by five states (denoted S_j; j = 1, ..., 5) which change over time: (1) idle, (2) serving a false alarm, (3) serving a minor medical emergency, (4) serving a major medical emergency, and (5) transferring a patient to the hospital. The state of each of the R vehicles in the system at any time can then be represented by a two-

BASIC POLICY DECISIONS
{
- Type of Recovery Vehicle
- Type of Onboard Rescue & Medical Equipment
- Level of Attendant Training
- Number of Recovery Vehicles
- System Administration
}

OPERATING POLICY DECISIONS
{
- Allocation of Recovery Vehicles (Static and/or Dynamic)
- Vehicle Dispatch Procedure
- Medical Treatment Rendered
  (a) At the emergency site
  (b) In transit to the hospital
- Hospital Selection Procedure
}

Figure 2

Controllable Policy Parameters in an EMC Recovery System

Alternative Emergency Care Recovery Systems 335

tuple consisting of the regional location of the vehicle and the activity of the vehicle. We shall represent this state by the vector (L_i, S_j). For instance, (6, 3) means that an ambulance is in region 6 serving a minor emergency. Similarly, (7, 1) means an ambulance is idle in region 7. The state of the system at any time then consists of a sequence of R of these vectors, with each element in the sequence representing the state of an individual ambulance in the system. For instance, the state of a system which utilizes two ambulances can be represented by $(L_i, S_j)_1, (L_i, S_j)_2$; $i = 1, \ldots, m$; $j = 1, \ldots, 5$. There are a finite number N of such states.

We shall assume that system transitions from state to state follow a Markov process. That is, the conditional probability that the system is in any given state depends entirely on the previous state which was occupied. This Markovian assumption is valid for certain state transitions in the system. For instance, the transitions from idle states $(L_i, 1)$ to states $(L_i, 2)$, $(L_i, 3)$, and $(L_i, 4)$ and the subsequent transitions from these states to states $(L_i, 5)$ are Markovian. Unfortunately, the transitions from transferring a patient at a hospital to an idle state or to serving another call are not Markovian, for these depend on the number of unserved calls in the system when service on the present call commenced and on the number of emergency occurrences during this service interval. Hence, these transitions depend on those transitions made during the service interval of the previous emergency. In this analysis we shall assume that these non-Markovian transitions are such that a constant, one-step conditional Markovian probability adequately approximates the underlying stochastic process. This assumption is likely to be good if the service intervals and emergency occurrence rates are not highly variable, or if the system is operating in a steady-state condition. The one-step transition matrix for a single vehicle can then be represented in the format shown in Figure 3.

The transition matrices for the system, which consists of R emergency vehicles, can be derived by taking the Kronecker products† of R matrices of the form shown in Figure 3, one for each vehicle.

Notice that the time spent in any state of the system is a random variable which depends on both the present state and the succeeding state. It is reasonable to model these random state-occupancy times as renewal processes (sequences of independent identically distributed random variables). Under these assumptions the recovery system obeys a Markov-renewal process[4,5] defined on the underlying Markov chain.

The random state-occupancy times are described in more detail as follows. The idle time is the time a vehicle spends waiting for an emergency. The time spent responding to an emergency [in states $(L_i, 2)$, $(L_i, 3)$, $(L_i, 4)$] is the convolution of the random time spent in transit to the scene and the random time spent on the scene. Notice that this random interval depends on the number and allocation of recovery vehicles and on the actions taken at the emergency scene. The time spent transferring a patient to the hospital consists of the convolution of the transit time to the hospital, the time at the hospital, and the transit times from the hospital to the next state (either idle or serving a subsequent emergency). Notice that this random interval

---

†Recall that the Kronecker product of two matrices B and A is
$$\left\{ \begin{array}{ccc} b_{11}A & \ldots & b_{1n}A \\ & \vdots & \\ b_{n1}A & & b_{nn}A \end{array} \right\}$$

Figure 3
Transition Matrix for Single Vehicle

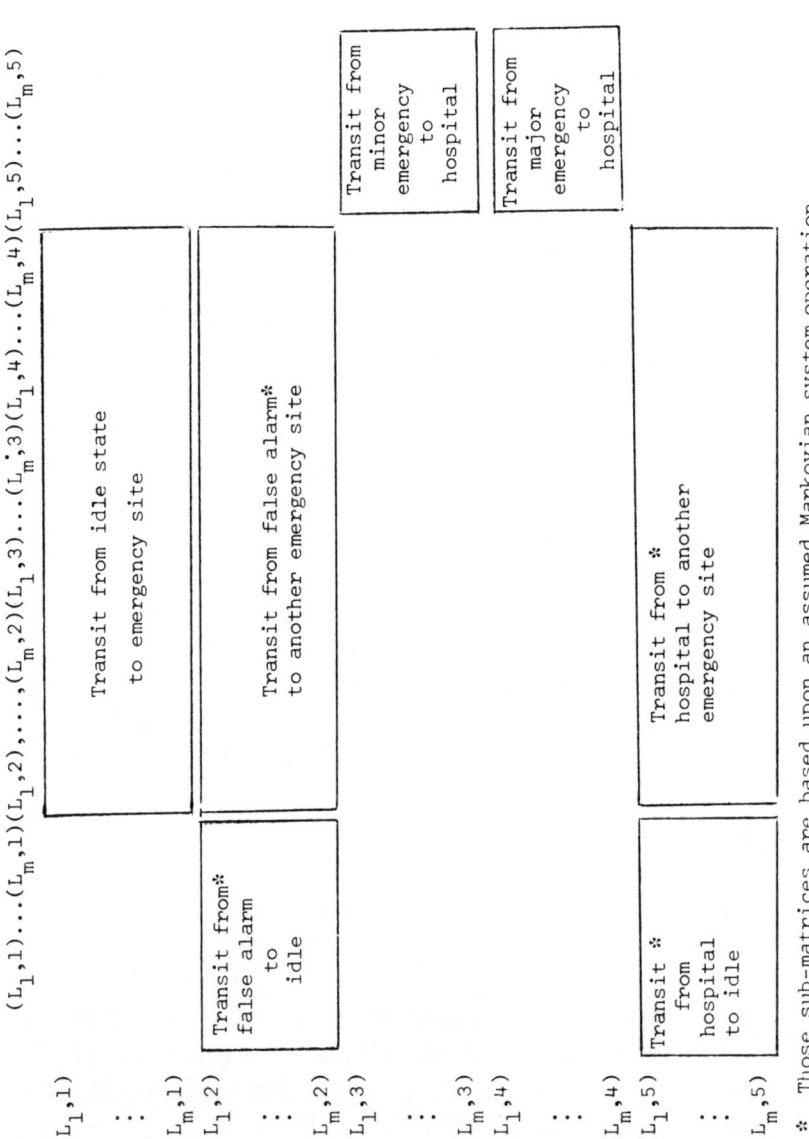

* Those sub-matrices are based upon an assumed Markovian system operation.

depends on the hospital selection decision and on the vehicle control procedure.

We now are able to model recovery system operation utilizing this Markov renewal process. In each state costs are accrued which depend on the state and on the time spent in this state. The nature of these costs can be described as follows. The cost incurred in an idle state consists of the opportunity cost due to incomplete utilization of recovery system resources. The cost accrued in the false alarm state consists of the variable real cost of making the run and the opportunity cost of inefficient resource utilization. The cost incurred in either emergency state consists of the variable real cost of making the run and the cost due to residual victim suffering given any treatment or combination of treatments by the recovery attendants. The cost incurred in the hospital transfer state consists of the variable real costs incurred in making the hospital run and the cost due to residual victim suffering in transit to the hospital.

These costs, the underlying Markov chain, and the random state-occupancy times are clearly functions of the basic policy and the system operating policy. For instance, consider the state $(L_i, 2)$—serving a minor injury in location L_i. The time spent in this state depends upon vehicle availability, vehicle allocation, and the on-the-scene emergency care rendered, all of which are policy variables. The cost incurred depends upon this time, and in addition, it is dependent upon the quality of care and the effect of this care in alleviating suffering; these latter depend upon the basic system policy regarding attendant training and equipment.

The objective, then, is to select a basic policy and an operating policy which minimize the total cost over some time period. There are p basic policies, p = 1, . . .,

P. We have seen earlier that there are N possible system states, each denoted $\{(L_i, S_j)_1, (L_i, S_j)_2, \ldots, (L_i, S_j)_R\}$, where R is the number of vehicles in the system. For notational simplification, we denote two general state realizations by the symbols α and β. The operating policy or decision made in any state α is denoted $Z_P(\alpha)$. This decision depends on the basic policy p because of the interdependencies mentioned earlier.

One may perform this minimization by utilizing Markov-renewal programming. The techniques underlying this optimization procedure are well documented [6,7,8] and we shall not review them here. Instead we state the basic recursive relation, which can be readily derived using the principle of optimality of dynamic programming.

Let

$C^\alpha(p,n)$ = Total cost incurred for n system transitions when a basic policy p is selected, the system starts in state α, and an optimum operating policy $Z^*_p(\alpha, n)$ is followed.

$P_{\alpha\beta}$ = Pr {System State (n+1) = β | System State n = α} when decision $Z_p(\alpha)$ is made.

$F^Z_{\alpha\beta}(t)$ = Pr { System State (n+1) = β, Time spent in State (n+1) $\leq$ t | System State n = α } when decision $Z_p(\alpha)$ is made.

$\phi^Z_{\alpha\beta}(t)$ = Cost incurred when state n is α, State (n+1) = β the time spent in β = t, and decision $Z_p(\alpha)$ is made.

$C(p)$ = Fixed cost incurred in implementing basic policy P.

Then, by the principle of optimality,

$$C_\alpha(p,n) = C(p) + \min_{Z_p(\alpha)} \left\{ \rho_\alpha^Z + \sum_{\beta=1}^{N} P_{\alpha\beta}^Z \, C_\beta(p,n-1) \right\} \quad (1)$$

$$\alpha = 1,...,N$$
$$n = 1,2,3,...$$

where

$$\rho_\alpha^Z = \sum_{\beta=1}^{N} P_{\alpha\beta}^Z \int_0^\infty \phi_{\alpha\beta}^Z(t) \, dF_{\alpha\beta}^Z(t),$$

which is the expected immediate cost starting in state α and making decision $Z_p(\alpha)$.

From this one can immediately calculate $C_\alpha(n)$, the minimum total cost when the system starts in state α and operates for n transitions:

$$C_\alpha(n) = \min_P C_\alpha(p,n) \quad (2)$$

The optimal basic policy p* is then that policy which satisfies (2), and the optimal operating policy is $Z^*_\alpha(p^*,n)$, which has been derived in (1).

Solution procedures for deriving the optimal p and $Z_p(\alpha)$ from this recursive relation are well known. These rely on dynamic or linear programming techniques. Computerized solution algorithms exist for these techniques at most computing centers. Rather than discussing these algorithms, we choose to discuss some problems and procedures for implementing this model with real data.

MODEL IMPLEMENTATION

One of the basic problems in implementing this model is in the large number of states which must be considered. In the present formulation this number is $(5m)^R$. When $m = 10$ and $R = 3$, reasonable values for certain applications, the number of states is 125,000. Clearly, the resulting solution algorithm, even if computationally feasible, would have to rely heavily on sophisticated storage techniques. In reasonable applications, additional states of injury type and/or severity may be necessary. In these cases the extent of the service region and the number of vehicles in this region may have to be constrained to improve computational feasibility for the model.

The parameters which must be estimated for model implementation include the transition probabilities $P_{\alpha\beta}^Z$, the probability distributions of state-occupancy times, $F_{\alpha\beta}^Z(t)$, and the costs associated with the Markov renewal process defined by these, $\phi_{\alpha\beta}^Z(t)$.

Transition probabilities can be estimated from time series data on the occurrence of emergencies and from sampled data on the geographic distribution of such emergencies. The distribution of state occupancy times can be estimated from the analysis of ambulance runs in the existing system, or possibly from theoretical or empirical arguments relating distances and emergency procedures to such times.

The estimation of costs can be accomplished through the analysis of economic data on alternative system operations and through careful determination of the effects of appropriate medical treatments on patient condition. This latter problem is probably the most difficult, although various medical groups are currently conducting research to develop a solution.

Since our primary objective in this paper is rational system selection rather than the estimation of costs of operating this system, the estimation of the *relative* costs—not absolute costs—for different policies is appropriate, and this may be an easier task.

In the end, the utility of this model must be determined by the system insights which can be obtained from its application. Hence, it may be useful to analyze the explicit alternatives under consideration by utilizing a simplified set of states and distributional assumptions. The model can then be parameterized to determine the sensitivity of the optimal basic and operating policies to these assumptions. In this way, the agency charged with decision-making responsibility can rationally consider all available alternative policies and the joint effects of these on recovery system operations. Such a systematic approach should provide insights which yield an emergency medical recovery system responsive to the needs of the community under consideration.

REFERENCES

1. "Checklists for Emergency Health Services Workshops," U. S. Public Health Service, Department of Health, Education, and Welfare, undated.
2. Ross, Sid, and Rogers, J. G., "Our Ambulance Crisis," *Parade Magazine,* p. 10, March 2, 1969.
3. *Ibid.*
4. Pyke, R., "Markov Renewal Processes: Definitions and Preliminary Properties," *Ann. Math. Stat.,* v. 33, pp. 1231-1242, 1961.
5. ———, "Markov Renewal Processes with Finitely Many States," *Ann. Math. Stat.,* v. 33, pp. 1243-1259, 1961.
6. Jewell, William S., "Markov Renewal Programming,

Parts I and II," *Operations Research,* v. 11, pp. 938-971, 1963.
7. deGhellinck, G. T., and Eppen, G. D., "Linear Programming Solutions for Separable Markovian Decision Problems," *Management Science,* v. 13, pp. 371-394, 1967.
8. Denardo, E. V., and Fox, B. L., *Multichain Markov Renewal Programs,* Rand Corporation Memorandum, RM-5208-PR, 1967.

15. Ambulance Service Size and Level of Service*

Dunlap and Associates, Inc.

The level of emergency ambulance service available depends upon the environmental demands and upon the size of the service. In this paper, we describe methods for estimating the number of ambulance locations needed to service an area and the number of ambulances needed to answer most emergency calls without delay. In developing these methods, we used certain mathematical techniques to describe the general relationships between the demands for service, the numbers of ambulances, and the chances that an ambulance will be available when an emergency call is received.

This paper discusses the size of area that can be served with a specified level of service, the relationships between number of ambulances and environmental demands, and techniques available for defining these relationships. Two charts are provided that can be used to determine what ambulance capability will meet differing combinations of environmental demands, as well as illustrations of the use and validity of the charts and some discussion of the applicability and generality of these methods.

*Reprinted from Economics of Highway Emergency Services, Vol. I, 1968.

NUMBER OF AMBULANCE LOCATIONS

We have chosen as the criterion of the level of service for an emergency ambulance system the system's response time, which is the elapsed time from the receipt of a call until an ambulance arrives at the scene of the emergency as shown in Figure 1. The response time therefore includes any delay in dispatching an ambulance plus the time for an ambulance to travel out to an emergency.

Assuming that for a service with two or more ambulances there will be no delay in dispatch, the size of the area which can be served will include all points which an ambulance can reach within a specified response time. The longer the permissible response time, and therefore the longer the travel-out time, the larger the area which can be adequately covered from a single ambulance location. All points which can be reached within the criterion response time chosen for a region, constitute the criterion service area. Any call within a criterion service area will be answered in never more than the criterion response time. This method of determining the area to be served by one location of an emergency ambulance service allows us to "carve-up" a state, county, or whatever area is being considered into a number of such service areas. This is shown diagrammatically in Figure 2. The area to be served has been distributed between four ambulance locations. These four areas represent the minimum number of locations needed so that any point within each service area can be reached in less than the criterion service time. The example is illustrative and the diagram is not to scale. The areas served will probably not be regular because of variations in local

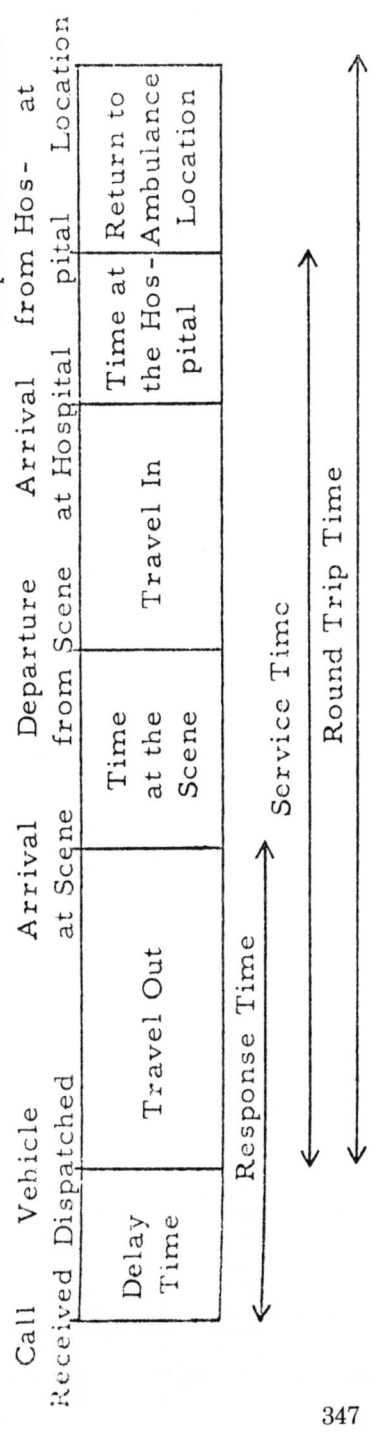

Figure 1. Bar graph of ambulance travel time

traffic and terrain conditions and the fact that they are based on travel times and not on distances from the ambulance locations. However, a first approximation of the limits of each area can be made most easily by assuming an average speed for the ambulance in each area and converting the criterion response time to the maximum distance that can be travelled in that time.

For preliminary planning purposes, each ambulance is assumed to be located at the approximate center of its service area. However, the actual location will most probably represent a compromise between being able to reach all outlying parts of the area in the criterion response time and being located near to the larger population centers. If the ambulance location is located close to most of the calls the average response time and average service time is minimized and thereby the capacity of the service is increased.

The response time that people expect in a particular area is affected by the size, the population density, and the topological conditions of the area. The level of service which would be expected in a highly dense urban area might not be expected in a rural area.

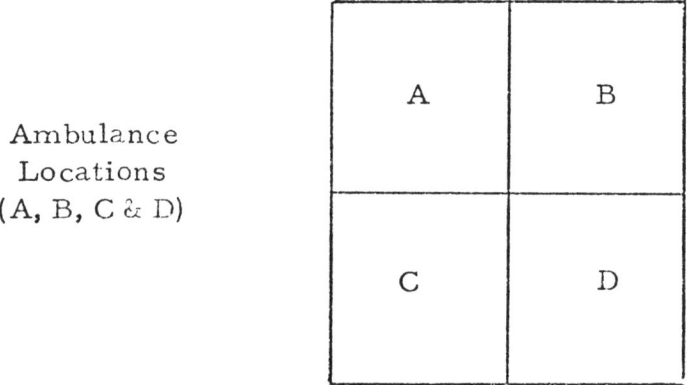

Ambulance Locations (A, B, C & D)

Figure 2. Area subdivided into four criterion service areas

The decision on a criterion response time for emergency calls is a political one with considerable economic ramifications. If the criterion response time were halved, the area which could be served by one ambulance would be quartered, and the population which could be served from one ambulance location would be reduced. As will be shown in the next section, the relationship between the number of emergency calls and the number of ambulances required to provide a given level of service is not linear, so that if the area and number of calls served by an ambulance location is quartered, the number of ambulances required would not be equally reduced. For example, if an area with a four-vehicle single location system serving 14,000 calls a year, were quartered and four ambulance locations established, each location would serve about 3,500 calls a year. The next section will show that an emergency ambulance service area with 3,500 emergency calls a year would require two ambulances to provide an adequate service if the average time to serve a call were 30 minutes. The four-vehicle, single location system, serving 14,000 emergency calls a year could be replaced, therefore, by four locations each requiring two ambulances. So by halving the criterion response time and providing a better service, four locations are required instead of one and twice as many ambulances. This increases the cost of the system considerably.

In some situations, however, a potential saving in total cost is possible by reducing the size of the area to be served. Since calls are now closer to the ambulance location, the average service time as well as the response time will be reduced. This will have the effect of increasing the number of calls that one ambulance can serve and thereby reduce the load on the system. Thus, there are situations when a second or satellite location within a criterion service area will reduce the average response time and might also reduce the number of ambulances required. This could occur in a densely populated city where each service area has a large number of emergency calls and a large number of ambulances to meet this demand. Then by establishing a satellite location within the service area the response time and the average service time would be reduced thus reducing the work load on the ambulance system and the number of ambulances required.

This idea was examined as part of a study of the New York City emergency ambulance system by the New York City Office of Administration.* The study showed that by redistributing the ten ambulances from the Kings County Hospital system between the main depot and a proposed satellite, so that six ambulances were available at the satellite and four at the hospital, there was theoretically a 19% reduction in the response time, with the number of long response times being reduced by 50%. This predicted reduction in response time was due, in this case, to there being a concentration of calls in the area of the proposed satellite location. The study showed that to reduce response times, ambulances have to be located near the probable sites of emergencies rather than near the emergency hospitals to which the patients are delivered.

The study showed that the level of service in the Kings County Hospital ambulance service area could be improved by providing a satellite location. Alternatively, the service could be maintained at the present level and the number of ambulances reduced.

*Spiegel, M. L., and Savas, E. S., "Emergency Ambulance Service," New York City, Office of the Mayor, March 1968.

Since there would be a cost involved to establish a satellite location, a trade-off would have to be made between the cost of establishing the satellite location and the saving of the cost of the ambulances. Some of the advantages of a satellite location can be realized temporarily, and with little increase in cost, by stationing ambulances on the streets near probable accident sites during peak accident periods.

The procedure of forming a temporary satellite location at busy times and thereby reducing the response time and average service time could be used by multiple location systems with the ambulances normally stationed at their home locations. When the ambulance from one location is in use, the other ambulances take up new positions to improve the service in the "busy" area. The idea is illustrated schematically in Figure 3 for the four adjacent service areas each with one ambulance referred to earlier, where the ambulances are normally located at the centers of their territories (the population of the areas is assumed to be evenly spread). From here each ambulance can best serve its area's population and reach all calls within the response time. Now assume that ambulance B is called to an emergency and there are three

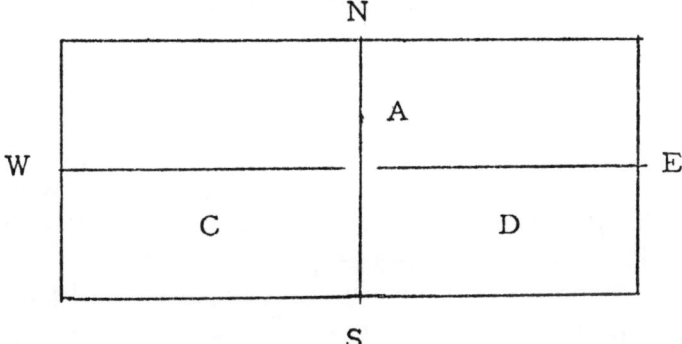

Figure 3. Combined service area covered by three equidistant ambulances

ambulances, A, C, and D, left to serve the total area. As suggested above, the three ambulances could take up new positions forming an equilateral triangle around the center of the combined service areas such that the total area is more evenly covered.

Now, if ambulance C were called to an accident, then ambulances A and D would be left to cover the whole area. A would move southwestwards and D would move north to take up new positions on the east-west axis. Similarly, if another ambulance were called while the other ambulances were still busy, then the remaining ambulance would move to the center of the area. When the ambulances return, the process would be reversed until they regained their original positions.

If, in real life, there were a four-vehicle system as in the illustration above, the points to which the ambulances might move to maintain the most uniformly complete coverage could be designated in advance. These points might be similar to those shown in Figure 3 but they would be determined also by the distribution of population in each of the service areas and the pattern of roads across all four areas. The three and then two vehicles left at their temporary locations would be positioned to be able to reach the most probable sites for emergencies in one-third and then one-half of the territory of the four service areas.

If a fifth ambulance were available in the system as a reserve emergency ambulance, this would be best located at the center of the four service areas or where it could reach the centers of population in all areas equally quickly. In this case, back-up coverage could be provided for all areas without the need to relocate the primary vehicles in all areas.

It should be apparent that the level of ambulance protection provided to a community or area is raised if the movement of ambulances in adjacent service areas is coordinated and controlled by a central dispatch service. Alternatively, a central dispatch service enables a community to achieve a criterion level of service over a large area with fewer ambulances because the number of reserve vehicles required to deal with peak load conditions is reduced.

The optimum distribution of ambulance locations could be said to be that arrangement which provided everyone in an area or region at least a minimum criterion level of emergency ambulance service with the use of the least number of vehicles and facilities. An implication of this definition is that the ambulances at every location will respond to the maximum number of emergency calls possible under the criterion of service specified.

For those services with only one ambulance, the response time will include the expected waiting time before the ambulance is available, as well as the travel-out time. If a relatively long response time is acceptable, the travel-out time is increased and the area and population which can be served are also increased. This, in turn, means that the number and frequency of calls in the ambulance service area are also increased. As the size of the area increases, the distances which an ambulance will have to travel to service emergency calls increases, thus increasing not only the response time but also the average service time, i.e., the time taken to complete a call and be available for a new assignment (see Figure 1). When both the average service time and the number of calls are increased, the service load on the one ambulance in a single ambulance service increases, which could increase the average waiting time before it becomes available. However, there will always be a size of service area for a single ambulance which has an average waiting time plus a maximum travel-out time which equals the required criterion response time. Adding ambulances can only eliminate the waiting time for a vehicle to be available and cannot reduce the travel-out time. If response time needs to be cut significantly over a large service area, additional ambulance locations must be established.

The price of a high probability that an ambulance is always available to respond to an emergency is that additional ambulances may have to be manned to take care of the calls when the primary ambulance is busy. This means that the utilization ratio of ambulances and crews will decrease when a second ambulance has to be added to a single ambulance service. In sparsely populated areas, the adoption of a uniformly short criterion response time would mean placing single ambulances at a great many separate locations. This would result in very low utilization ratios of ambulances and crews and extremely high costs per ambulance trip. In the next section, we discuss the problem of striking a balance between the size of a service area, the number of emergency calls that the area is likely to generate, and the level of service that can be provided by a single ambulance. In remote rural areas, the definitions of the optimum distribution of ambulances must also include some criterion of "reasonable" level of utilization.

NUMBER OF AMBULANCES REQUIRED

When a decision has been reached on how many ambulance locations an area needs, the next question is how many ambulances should be stationed at each location to meet the required level of service. Whenever all ambulances in a service area are already busy, there is bound to be a delay before an ambulance can be dispatched in response to another call. Conversely, an ambulance would always be available if a service area had an excessively large number of ambulances; however, since the provision of ambulances is expensive, this situation is inefficient and impractical. Thus, we need a method to determine what is the likelihood that an ambulance will not be immediately available. Fortunately, such a method is available. It has been applied by industrial engineers to a variety of related service problems, and is applicable to ambulance services. The problem of how many ambulances are needed is the same basic problem as determining for a supermarket the number of service counters needed. If there are few customers, only one service center is needed, but as the number of customers increases, the number of counters required must increase if customers are to be served without undue delay. However, the quicker the customers can be served, the fewer the counters that are necessary. Similarly, the number of ambulances needed by a community depends upon the number of calls and the length of time it takes to serve them (i.e., the elapsed time from when an ambulance is dispatched to a call till it is available to answer another call). The more customers there are and the longer it takes to serve them, the more ambulances are needed. When customers in a supermarket cannot all be served immediately, some have to wait and a queue develops; sometimes an ambulance cannot be dispatched immediately and the caller has to wait. This is the delay we wish to minimize in order to minimize response time. We would like an ambulance always to be available and for callers never to wait but this solution is impractical and we have to accept a compromise.

The first measure of ambulance system capabilities that we have chosen is the percentage of occasions when an ambulance is available to answer a call. The more frequently ambulances are expected to be available, the greater the load put on the system, and the greater the number of ambulances needed. Just what level of system capability is adequate in a particular situation must be decided with respect to local conditions and the wishes of the local community. (In the later examples demonstrating this method, we have used a 90% availability as the criterion of service capability.) The number of ambulances necessary will depend upon the number of calls and the average time taken to service a call. Irrespective of the peculiarities of different regions and conditions, if the average service time and the call frequency are the same, the same number of ambulances will be required to provide the same level of service. If a rural area has the same number of calls and the same average service time as an urban area, the two areas would require the same number of ambulances even though geographically greatly different. There is no general method to determine the average service time for any particular situation. It depends upon local conditions and the locations of the emergencies. Two areas with equal populations, one suburban with an evenly spread population and the other a densely populated area of a large city, will have very different average service times (and, in all probability, different numbers of emergency calls also). The average service time must be estimated for the particular situation with respect to the local conditions.

Call frequency is best determined from past records of emergency ambulance calls, but in the event that records of the number of emergency ambulance calls generated from a particular population or area are not available, a reasonably accurate estimate can be determined analytically. Figure 4 is based on data from questionnaires received from nongovernment ambulance service purveyors who were the only purveyors for their area and giving the number of emergency calls and the population in their areas. It shows a graph of the annual number of emergency calls generated from populations of service areas. The dashed lines on either side of the continuous line represent the boundaries of an area of confidence within which we would expect the actual number to fall. This graph can be used to estimate how many emergency ambulance calls would be expected from a given sized population. For example, if we wished to forecast the number of emergency calls we would expect from a population of 72,000, we would find the point on the graph above 72,000 on the bottom axis (Pt. 1) and read off the number of emergency calls on the left-hand axis at 820.

Calls for emergency ambulance service arrive irregularly but with a statistically discernable pattern familiar to mathematicians and known as a Poisson distribution. With this information and the average number of calls received per hour and the average service time, we can calculate for a system, the frequency of occasions when there will be no calls for a period, one call, two calls, and so on.

The proposed method of analyzing the size of service required to meet with a known probability (e.g., 90%) a demand determined by number of users, average service time, and required level of service is based on mathematics that were first developed for analyzing telephone systems and the number of lines necessary to serve the traffic. This mathematical technique (known as Queueing Theory) has been applied to other service situations where a planner has to deter-

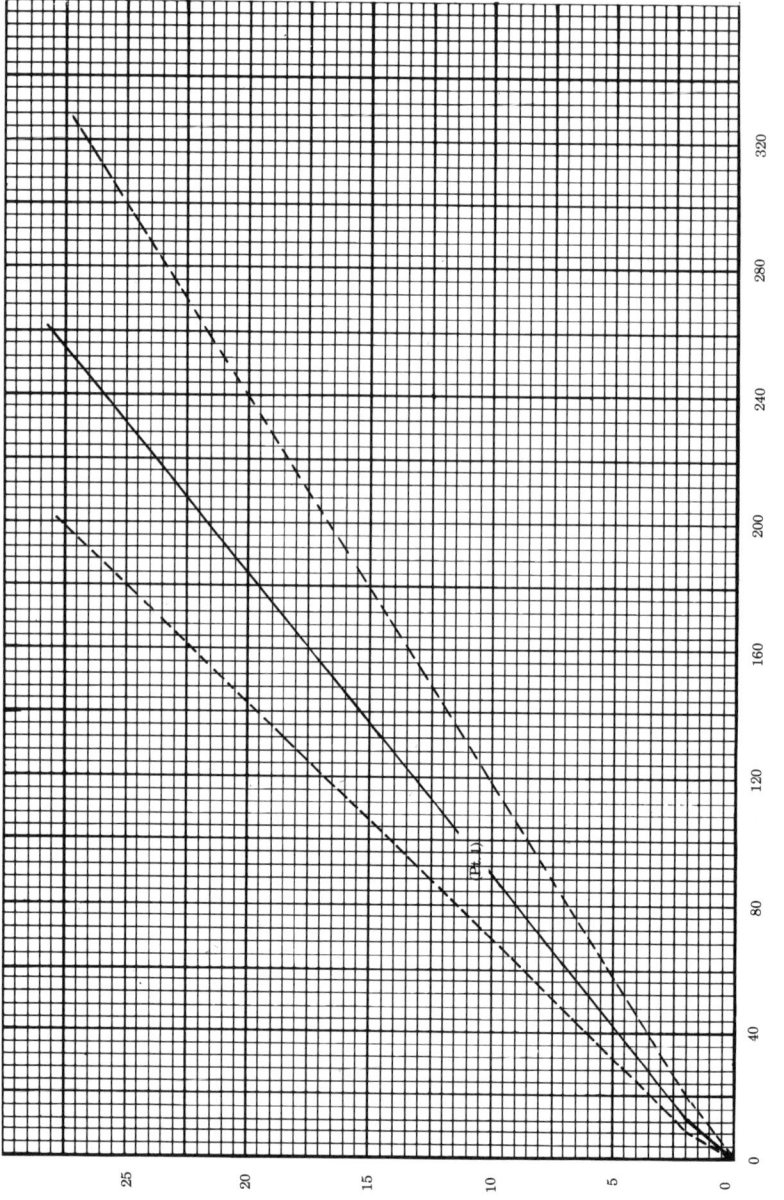

Figure 4. Annual number of emergency ambulance calls related to population of service area.

mine the size of a system needed, such as the number of highway toll booths, airplane controllers, and restaurant seats. There are many different types of service situations which can be encountered, and queueing theory mathematics has as yet developed only to the level where solutions are available for certain types of cases similar to the ones above.

A second method of assessing the adequacy of a system is to ask how long, on the average, customers have to wait before they can be served. The mathematics for applying this measure have only been developed for the case of a single server. We can therefore use this method only with a single-vehicle ambulance system to determine for number of calls and for average service time how long a delay there is likely to be before the ambulance is available. For the case of a one-vehicle ambulance system, we can specify the level of system capabilty in terms of the average waiting time that is acceptable.

Figures 5 and 6 summarize the quantitative relationships underlying these two methods. The number of calls per hour is measured along the bottom axis of the graphs. If there are daily or seasonal variations in the frequency of emergency calls, the number of vehicles required must be based on the number of calls per hour over the busiest period of the day. Whenever possible the number of calls per hour should be determined from records of number of emergency calls during the busiest season of the year. Otherwise, the estimate of number of vehicles required must be based on an average hourly frequency of calls devised from whatever records are available. The number of vehicles actually to be manned for each period of the day can be determined from Figure 5 by allowing for variations in demand from shift to shift.

Figure 5 shows the number of ambulances required

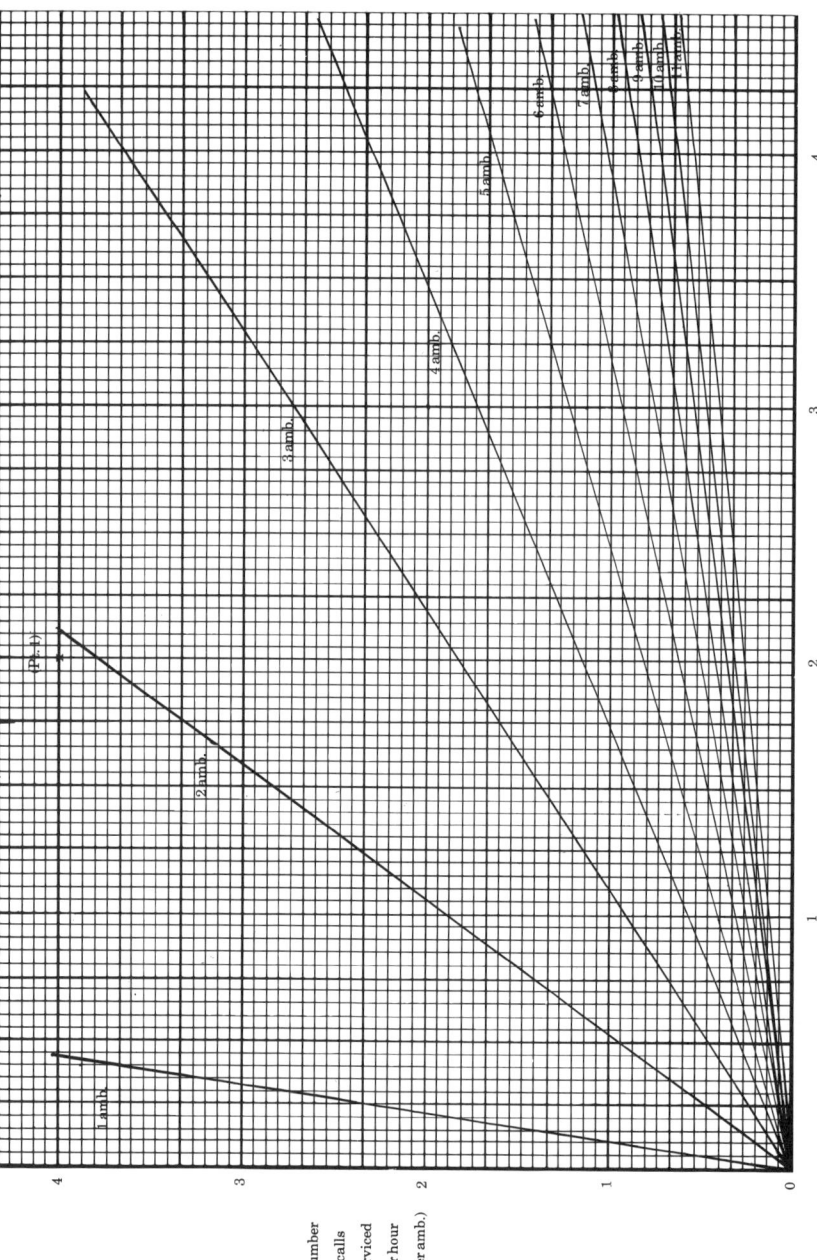

Figure 5. The relationship between the frequency of emergency calls, number serviced per hour per ambulance and the number of ambulances required (90% immediate availability).

to serve 90% of the calls immediately for call frequencies between zero and four calls an hour and service frequencies between zero and four calls serviced an hour, where the upper limit of an average service frequency per ambulance of four calls an hour would represent an average service time of fifteen minutes per call. So for a situation with a call frequency of two calls an hour and an average service time of fifteen minutes or a service rate of four calls an hour, we see from the intersection of these values on Figure 5 (shown by Pt. 1), that two ambulances would be needed. Three ambulances can serve combinations of call frequency and calls serviced that fall on the diagram to the left of the three ambulance line coming out of the origin. So, one emergency call an hour can be handled by three ambulances at a service capability of 90% providing the average service frequency per ambulance is not less than two calls an hour, i.e., the average service time does not exceed 30 minutes. Four ambulances would be needed to serve three calls an hour with an average service time of 30 minutes or an average service frequency of two calls an hour per ambulance.

Figure 6 shows the levels of demand and service combinations which can be handled by one ambulance with differing average delays before the ambulance is available to respond to a call. The average number of emergency calls an hour ranges between zero to 1.5 calls per hour and the average service time per call goes from zero to 105 minutes. The curves show combinations of service frequency and average service time which have the same average waiting time before an ambulance is available. For example, if one ambulance had 0.3 calls per hour (i.e., one call every three hours) and an average service time of 30 minutes then the callers would have to wait six min-

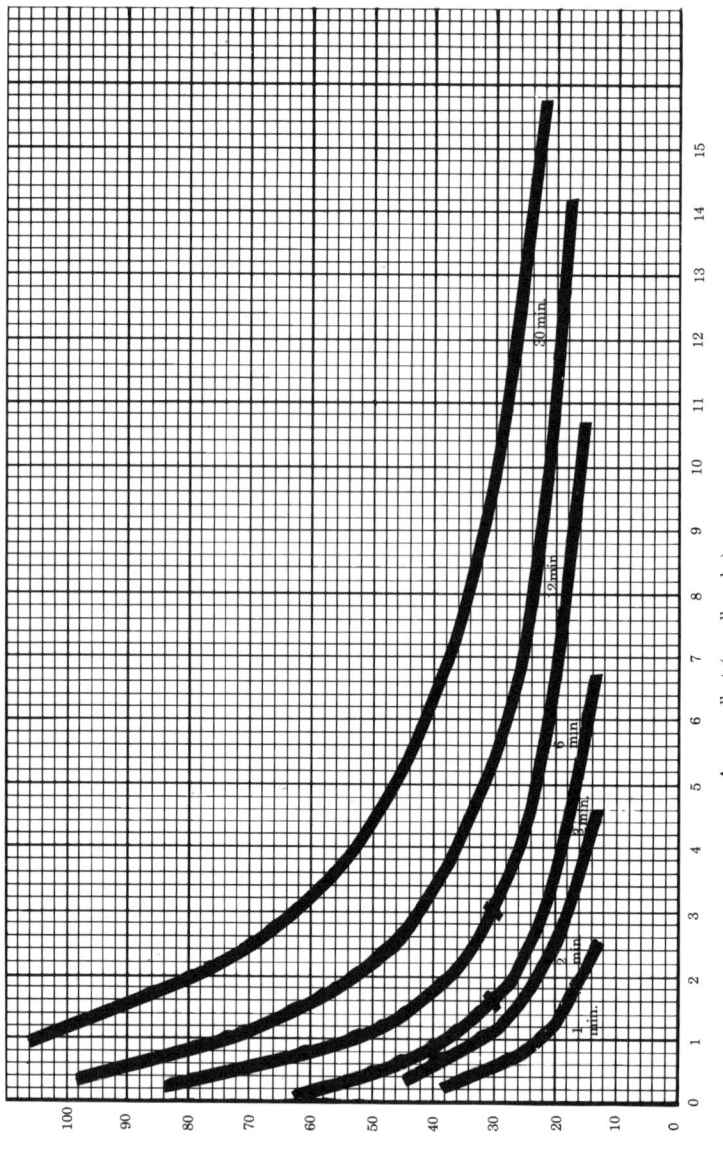

Figure 6. Average waiting line for one ambulance to become available (minutes).

utes on average (Pt. 1). If the frequency were 0.13 calls per hour with the same average service time of 30 minutes then callers would have to wait three minutes (Pt. 2) on average. This figure shows the average waiting time for different combinations of call frequencies and average service times; as the call rate increases at any average service time, the average waiting time increases, as it does also with increases in the average service time at any call frequency. With this figure, we can determine for a one-vehicle system the average waiting times for an ambulance at any call frequency and average service time combination.

DEMONSTRATIONS OF THE MODELS

In this section, we use the three charts described above to estimate the size of the emergency ambulance service required in differing environments.

Table 1 shows four examples of areas and populations served, the numbers of emergency calls generated from these areas, the criterion levels of service, and the sizes of emergency ambulance service required. The first example is of a remote rural area where the ambulance service is required to meet a criterion response time of 66 minutes. This includes waiting time before the ambulance is dispatched and the travel-out time. It has been assumed that people living in the area, because of its regional conditions, are willing to accept an *average* waiting time of six minutes. Thus, the maximum travel-out time is 60 minutes. It is assumed that the average speed of the ambulance is 60 miles per hour. The maximum distance which can be served (at 60 miles per hour) will be 60 miles, and the area served would be a circle with a radius of 60 miles and an area of 11,200 square miles or more probably a rectangular area of 120 miles by 100. If we know the population of the service area or if we can estimate the population density for the area, then we can estimate the number of emergency calls which the service could expect. If we assume a population density of six persons per square mile, then an area of 12,000 square miles would contain a population of 72,000 people. From Figure 4 we find that a population of 72,000 would generate about 820 emergency calls per year. Assuming we have no information about seasonal variations in demand we use the annual number of emergency calls to compute an average call frequency of 0.1 emergency calls per hour.

The number of ambulances required to serve an area depends, as has been said before, on the number of calls and the average service time. The average service time for this area will depend upon the location of the accidents and the times for travel to the scene of the accident and then to the hospital. In this example, we know that the time to travel from the ambulance location to the scene of the accident can never exceed 60 minutes. This provides a maximum travel-out time but it is not much help in determining the *average* service time for all the calls. This has to be estimated for each particular situation. In order to determine the number of ambulances required, we have assumed an average service time for this situation of 60 minutes (i.e., an hourly service frequency of 1) which must mean that most of the calls are at an intermediate distance to the ambulance location. Using Figure 6, which gives "Average Waiting Time," we find that one ambulance with a call frequency of 0.1 and a 60-minute service time can just about meet the criterion of an average waiting time of six minutes. It is, however, working at full capacity to maintain this level of service and in practice, this six-minute criterion

Table 1

Four environments, their demands for emergency
ambulance service and required sizes of service

Conditions	Examples			
	1	2	3	4
			(1 loc) (2 loc)	(1 loc) (4 loc)
Maximum Travel-Out Time (min.)	60	20	15 10	15 8
Maximum Distance-Out (mi.)	60	20	11 7.5	7.5 4
Area Served (sq.mi.)	12,000	1,600	500	225
Population/sq. mi.	6	50	1,000	10,000
Population ('000)	72,000	80,000	500,000	2,250,000
Number of Emergency Calls/Year	820	900	5,000	23,000
Average Call Rate/hr.	0.1	0.1	0.57 0.3 (ea)	2.6 0.7 (ea)
Average Service Time (min.)	60	30	30 20	30 20
Average Service Frequency	1	2	2 3	2 3
Number of Ambulances	1	1	2 2x2	4 2x4
Average Waiting Time (min.)	6	2	- -	- -
Criterion Response Time (min.)	66	22	15 10	15 8
Yearly Hours of Use	820	450	2,500 1,666	11,500 7,667
Percent Use/Ambulance	9.4	5.0	13 10	32.5 11.0

might have to be relaxed to allow for some inevitable periods of "down-time" for servicing the vehicle.

The second example is also assumed to be a rural area but less remote than the first with an average population density of 50 to the square mile. A maximum travel-out time of 20 minutes is assumed. At a speed of 60 miles per hour, the area served from a central location might reasonably be considered as roughly a square area of 1,600 square miles. The population served would be 80,000 persons and from Figure 4, we find that this would generate about 900 emergency ambulance calls a year or an average call rate of 0.1 per hour. If we assume an average service time of 30 minutes, we see from Figure 6 that one ambulance can handle all the emergency calls from this area if the community accepts an average waiting time of 2 minutes for the ambulance to become available. In practice, if the purveyor also handles transfer calls with a second vehicle, he could eliminate the average waiting period of two minutes for emergency calls by using the second vehicle for emergency calls when the first is already in use.

The third example represents an urban or suburban area with a population density of 1,000 to the square mile. The criterion response time is assumed to be 15 minutes and the average speed as 45 miles per hour. Assuming a roughly square-shaped service area of 500 square miles the population served will be 500,000 with approximately 5,000 emergency ambulance calls a year or an average of 0.57 calls per hour. If we estimate an average service time of 30 minutes, we see from Figure 5 that two ambulances will be able to provide the specified level of service. If two independent purveyors covered the area and had divided the area into two approximately equal zones, each purveyor would receive approximately 0.3 calls per hour. With a 20-minute service time each needs to man two ambulances in order to be able to respond immediately 90% of the time. Thus, a total of four ambulances between two purveyors are required instead of the two ambulances of a single purveyor to provide the same level of availability for emergency service to the two areas combined. However, in terms of speed of responding to a call both separate purveyors are able to provide a higher level of service (because of their smaller service areas). An efficient emergency ambulance service could be achieved for the total area if two locations were operated as a single system, possibly with two ambulances at one and only one ambulance at another location; this would risk only some small reduction in level of service and yet provide benefits from reduced response times.

The fourth example represents a city situation for which we have assumed a population density of 10,000 to the square mile and an area of 225 square miles, i.e., a total population of 2,250,000. Such a city would be expected to generate approximately 23,000 emergency ambulance calls a year or an average call rate of 2.6 per hour. Using Figure 5, and assuming an average service time of 30 minutes, we find that the city could just provide a 90% level of availability with four full-time emergency ambulances provided they operated from one central location. Assuming an average speed of 30 miles per hour, the criterion response time would be 15 minutes.

If the city were divided into four separate service areas of about 55 square miles each, the criterion response time in each would be reduced to eight minutes, and the emergency call rate in each area would be 0.7 per hour. To achieve the same level of availability as before, two emergency ambulances would now be required in each area, a total of 8 emergency ambulances. Again, some saving in numbers of emergency ambulances could be achieved if the four service areas were operated as four locations of a single ambulance system with a single central dispatching service. When one location had dispatched all its ambulances, the adjacent location could be directed to provide an ambulance. This will temporarily reduce the service capability in the donor's area. However, since it can be shown that the number of occasions when an ambulance which has been lent will be required in its home area will be smaller than the number of occasions it can aid another area, the over-all level of service for the combined areas will be improved.

The four locations of an emergency ambulance system in a city of this size could probably be operated effectively with a total of eight ambulances and a response time of eight minutes.

We have tested the mathematical model that is summarized in Figure 5 against known situations. We used as our test the 21 systems which we had surveyed, for which we knew the total number of both emergency and transfer calls for the year and also, for most, the number of ambulances they had fully manned throughout the day. From the number of calls a year an average service frequency was calculated. Assuming the calls were equally spaced over the day and the year the number of ambulances was estimated (for a 90% service availability) for three average service times; 120 minutes, 60 minutes, and 30 minutes. Table 2 shows that with the exceptions of sites 7, 14, 15, and 20, the estimates based on Figure 5 were close. Sites 7, 14, 15, and 20 were all multiple locations with 8, 4, 13, and 14 locations respectively. If the number of ambulances are computed for the multiple locations allowing equal calls at each location, then the number of ambulances are accurate. This raises a question of the applicability and generality of the model. The model helps determine the number of ambulances necessary to meet a specified demand at a required level of system capability for one location. The model can be applied separately to each location of a multiple location system and the number of ambulances determined for each location, but this provides no measure of the benefit to the system capability that results from being in a multiple location system. There is a benefit to be derived from having other locations in a system which can be called upon to assist with their vehicles at times of peak load.

The model assumes that emergency ambulance calls arrive with Poisson distribution as mentioned previously. This is a reasonable assumption for most ambulance systems. However, there will very probably be variation in the frequency of emergency calls over the day since in most areas at some periods the roads are busier than others, which increases the probability of calls during these periods. This means that the number of emergency calls for ambulances should be determined over segments of the day, and the number of ambulances that a service needs be calculated on the "call-rate" for the busiest part of the day. This calculation will provide an estimate of the number of ambulances necessary to handle the probable peak emergency load. If there are times of the day when the call rate is appreciably different, a reduction in operating costs can be effected by not manning all the ambulances all the time. The number of manned ambulances during the slack part of the day can be estimated by using the call-rate during that part of the day. Thus, it is possible to estimate the fractional numbers of ambulances manned full-time, e.g., one-and-a-half manned ambulances for a two-ambulance service that only mans the second ambulance during the day.

The definition of the average service time assumes that an ambulance is available immediately after it completes unloading patients at a hospital. (see Figure 1). If for some reason an ambulance is not then immediately available (for instance, because the hospital is far from its service area) then the average service time would have to be redefined to include travel time till the ambulance was actually available for service in its service area and could respond to a call as efficiently as if it were at its location.

Similarly, the model describes a system where an ambulance is always immediately available, except

Table

The number of emergency ambulances estimated by the model compared with actual numbers for 21 sites.

Site No.	Total Number of Calls	Average Number of Calls/ Hour	Number of Ambulances Required at 90% Immediate Availability Service Time (Min.)			Actual Number of Ambulances
			120	60	30	
1	3200	.365	3	2	2	3
2	5457	.623	4	3	2	3
3	7303	.834	4	3	2	5
4	2276	.260	3	2	2	-
5	5339	.609	4	3	2	3
6	1288	.147	2	2	1	-
7	13500	1.541	6	4	3	$12^{(1)}$
8	14000	1.598	6	4	3	4
9	4620	.527	3	2	2	3
10	1500	.171	2	2	1	1
11	2244	.256	2	2	2	2
12	3000	.342	3	2	2	2
13	4000	.457	3	2	2	3
14	1500	.171	2	2	1	$4^{(2)}$
15	72000	8.219	14	12	9	$30^{(3)}$
16	2905	.332	3	2	2	1-2
17	720	.082	2	1	1	1
19	4472	.511	3	2	2	-
20	50320	5.744	14	10	7	$17^{(4)}$
21	6275	.716	4	3	2	-

(1) Eight locations
(2) Four locations
(3) Thirteen locations
(4) Fourteen locations

for being out on another emergency call. This means that if an ambulance is not manned continuously then the time from the receipt of a call until it is manned must be included in the response time. If an ambulance is used for other duties such as transfer work, then sometimes it may not be immediately available for emergency calls and the level of system capability is thereby reduced. However, there is clearly some opportunity to use emergency ambulances for scheduled transfer calls as long as it is realized that the level of system readiness to respond immediately is no longer the same.

In general, the models outlined in Figures 4, 5, and 6 provide a method of determining the number of emergency ambulances required for any particular location.

16. Analyzing the Role of the Helicopter in Emergency Medical Care for a Community*

Arthur R. Jacobs, M.D., M.P.H.

Curtis P. McLaughlin, D.B.A.

The war in Vietnam has illustrated the technical feasibility of using helicopters for aeromedical evacuation under a wide variety of conditions. The statistics are impressive. Many have attributed the reduction in mortality among hospitalized casualties, from 4.5 percent in World War II to 2.5 percent in the Korean conflict and less than 1 percent in Vietnam, in large part to the fact that the wounded are reaching the medical facilities more rapidly by means of helicopters.[10] Can we do the same at home?

This remains a speculative question. Undoubtedly we could use the helicopter in many civilian cases, but the operational question is whether we should do so under conditions that differ markedly from those in Vietnam. A systematic analysis is required to answer

*Reprinted from *Medical Care,* September-October 1967, Vol. V, No. 5.

that question, and soon. The aeromedical helicopter may be on the way to becoming a public service without question. Witness the statement, "Helicopters are seldom employed, and landing pads are present at only a small number of hospitals, chiefly along our coasts for the use of the Coast Guard," in the February 1967 draft of the National Highway Agency standard for "Emergency Medical Services."[5] The demonstration projects to be undertaken in the near future will provide only part of the analysis that counts: Should Organization A in Region B operate an aeromedical helicopter service of size C and cost D under a set of conditions E to perform services F, G, H, etc.?

Such analyses are interesting in and of themselves because they combine technical, medical, administrative, and economic evaluations as inputs to a subsequent social decision to commit scarce resources for medical services. In the sections that follow the authors undertake to present a framework that will illustrate the magnitude and scope of the systems analysis that should precede a decision of this importance.

Like its cousin, operations research, systems analysis is a popular but little-understood term. Even though there is not a formal, accepted definition, there is reasonable agreement about what is involved. First, the term usually is reserved for approaches involving problems that are large and complex and require skills from more than one field of expertise. Second, the solution proposed is to be based on the use of existing technology to meet specific human needs. Third, these needs usually are ill-defined, seldom are consistently expressed and could be met through many alternative approaches. Fourth, once the basic problem has been defined, a model of the problem must be developed and the alternatives analyzed and rated in some objective fashion. Fifth, inconsistencies will inevitably become apparent and the final working plans will be at best a rational compromise.[2,7]

A MODEL

Decisions concerning emergency medical transportation must take into account the complex set of variables that produce the need for transportation, the request for service, and the medical care required. As a focus for further discussion a tentative, descriptive model of the community system for emergency transport is outlined below and in Figure 1. In it several alternative ways of providing services are diagrammed. It is the analysis, of course, that must determine which alternatives are to be provided in the Transport and First-care Phase.

Recognition and Communication Phase

A health emergency, a situation in which a member or members of the community feel that medical care is needed as rapidly as humanly possible, begins in the community at risk with an individual and an acute or chronic stimulus from the environment, e.g., an auto hits a child playing in the street or an obese executive suffers a heart attack. There is no emergency, however, until the individual or his peers recognize one. Perception that an emergency exists will vary with culture, age, medical severity, etc., and is subject to influence by education and availability of services. When the individual perceives an emergency, on-scene decisions, also influenced by education, are made. He may call upon the community's emergency resources or seek private care.

The individual may elect to use private or public transportation outside of the community's emergency transportation system. If so, communication time, dispatch formalities, travel time to the patient, and first care (defined as the provision of first aid or medical care during transport) are avoided. If the choice is made to utilize the community system by hailing passing police or by phone or radio communications, then a series of community judgments are made concerning method of transport, first care, and emergency department utilization.

Triage Judgment Phase

Triage judgments are made by community emergency personnel and include, but are not limited to, the triage technique adopted after wartime experiences in which casualties are sorted and priority-labelled to determine the kind of treatment needed. Complex judgments must be made among alternative sources for transport, first care, and emergency department care. If private or public transportation or a patrol car or a dual-purpose patrol car (a station wagon equipped for police patrol and stretcher transport of the injured) is on the scene, an opportunity exists to save the dispatch and travel-to-patient time. When a private car or public transportation is used, there usually is no first care. With a patrol car or dual-purpose patrol car on the scene, first care is provided at the level of police skills and equipment. Although patrol cars often are used, expert medical opinion indicates that the severely injured demand much more careful handling than is possible in such a vehicle.[8] For this reason, ordinary patrol cars are not considered as an alternative for dispatch and transport.

The introduction of the helicopter as an alternative

presents two new types of decisions: judgments about landing and flying conditions and about potential movement of more specialized personnel and equipment to the patient. It also may shift the choice of emergency departments from those geographically close to the patient to those with landing facilities. More specialized personnel for dispatch and more specialized centers for receiving and treating patients both can be considered because the speed and range of the helicopters make it possible to service and derive support from a broader population base. The Committee on Trauma and Committee on Shock, Division of Medical Sciences, NAS-NRC stated that "Within a given region, it is uneconomical and impractical to expect that every emergency department deal with all degrees of severity of injury."[1]

Because the helicopter and the more specialized personnel would not be dispatched without careful consideration of local landing conditions and the status of the patient, the communications system linking the scene, the communication center, the helicopter, and possibly the emergency department may have to be improved with quite sophisticated equipment and personnel.

Transport and First-care Phase

Triage judgments resulting in dispatch, travel to patient, and travel to the emergency department will utilize helicopter, ambulance, or dual-purpose patrol car. From a legal point of view, the same quality of first care must be provided with any given choice of transportation equipment as is maintained elsewhere in the community. This level of first care is conceptualized as "community skills and equipment." In the helicopter there may be an opportunity to utilize a

THE COMMUNITY HELICOPTER AND AMBULANCE SYSTEM FOR EMERGENCY CARE

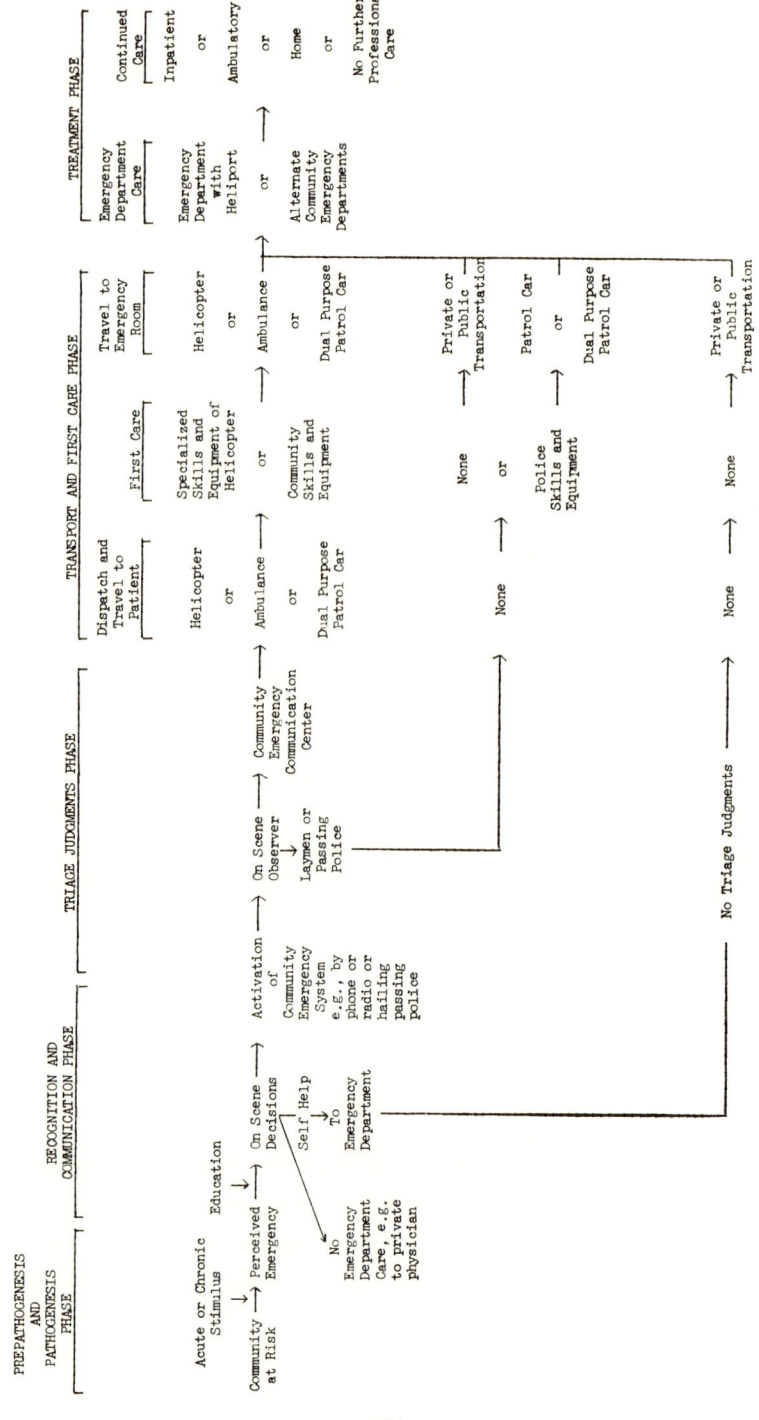

Figure 1

higher level of specialized skills and equipment, again because the cost and frequency of need for such services can be justified on the basis of a larger population base.

Treatment Phase

Triage judgment and transport and first care will culminate in care at a specific emergency department, possibly followed by inpatient care.

EVALUATING ALTERNATIVES

It becomes evident from this model that a substantial number of individual choices can be made that influence the ultimate demands for and benefit from helicopter services and that these choices can vary markedly from community to community. Knowledge that an area generated 9000 ambulance trips in a typical period will not necessarily indicate that the area will generate 9000 helicopter trips, even in the unlikely event that helicopters supplant ambulances entirely.

The model implies that the helicopter is a graft to the total medical transport system. This seems to be the realistic view. These machines may prove to be of very limited applicability in densely populated areas, are susceptible to weather conditions, and are expensive to acquire and operate. Ambulances already exist in most areas for both emergency and routine transportation. It appears, therefore, that considerable care must be exercised to identify those events that would benefit from helicopter service, their frequency, and the benefits from such service.

The cost to the community that must be justified medically or socially is not limited solely to the six-figure investment in the machine. With it must come heliports, equipment, trained crews, and a maintenance program. Helicopters do require extensive maintenance,[4] several times the basic crew costs. In many communities one must add the substantial communications system investments to support triage and aeromedical dispatch requirements. This may work effectively only if someone on the scene understands landing requirements. If the potential benefits are to be realized, the communications net will have to enable someone to acquire information and determine which alternative is warranted. With these life or death decisions come moral, ethical, and legal considerations that must be dealt with by a policy-making body. In addition, mechanisms for financial support and auspice (police, medical center, health department, etc.) within the community must be developed. Greater centralization and coordination of existing services will probably accompany these arrangements.

On the other hand, the full cost of the communications and helicopter systems may not have to be attributed to medical emergencies. Both can be used for other purposes by the community. These joint uses, however, complicate the already difficult task of identifying and evaluating the relevant alternatives for the specific community.

It is clear that the system analysis must be community specific to give a meaningful result. This fact should influence the design of any demonstration projects that are conducted in the near future. The demonstrations will fully answer the questions of only a few communities for it is doubtful that such experiments could or should undertake the full range of community requirements over the test period, or that the test period will include the full range of possible events. It seems important, therefore, that demonstrations be designed to test the feasibility of certain technical approaches and to gather data for the use of persons modeling individual community requirements, probably with the aid of a computer simulation based on local conditions. For example, if a medical helicopter test were conducted in a compact area where auto traffic delays were important, but helicopter transit time was negligible, it still would be desirable to record transit times and mileages for the benefit of those who might consider using the machines in open country.

As examples of the complexity of a meaningful system analysis for a community, consider three related topics: aircraft availability, frequency of need for service, and evaluating the resulting benefits from the service.

AVAILABILITY

In a helicopter application several factors could limit the availability of a given complement of equipment: 1) weather, 2) maintenance, 3) use for another emergency call, and 4) use for other purposes.

In adverse weather, federal regulations as well as pilot judgment constrain the use of aircraft. This is, of course, variable from community to community, but it is an important consideration. Fortunately, data for analysis can be acquired by checking Weather Bureau and airport records and FAA regulations.

Helicopters require periodic inspection and overhaul. During such activities service coverage is reduced. Where there is more than one machine available this may not be serious, but given the high initial costs of suitable machines, there will be few areas that can afford one, let alone a backup, machine. Information on maintenance requirements can be gathered with the cooperation of manufacturers, other users, or the Armed Services.

Given that there will be limits to the availability of equipment, there may be periods of the day when the equipment will be performing its intended function and be unavailable or delayed in responding to a second call. This possibility cannot be ignored in the light of all the evidence that shows peak demands at specific hours of the day and days of the week.[12] Computer models for analysis of availability of services with variable demand are quite common in the analysis of many types of community services such as maternity wards, fire trucks, post office windows, etc.[6,11] These techniques, generally called queuing models, waiting-line studies or simulations, could be applied to emergency medical transportation as well. Such studies often are useful because intuitive judgments about the intermingling of numerous events of variable frequency are highly unreliable.

Helicopters that are large enough for ambulance service involving multiple cases, or specialized personnel and equipment, are expensive, and it is likely that their existence in the community can be justified only if they perform multiple services, e.g., medical transport, traffic control, crime prevention, fire fighting, and construction work.

The indication is that the machine will be available much less than 100 percent of the time. A very rough estimate can be obtained by:

$$A = (1-P_w)(1-P_m)(1-P_e)(1-P_o)$$

where A is proportion of the time that the machine will be available,

P_w is the proportion of the time that the weather grounds the machine,
P_m is the proportion of the time that maintenance grounds the machine,
P_e is the proportion of the time that the machine is out on call, and
P_o is the proportion of the time that the machine is on other duties, e.g., fire fighting.

This would be only a rough estimate, since we are not interested in the time but in the proportion of instances that the machine is called and is available. The four events producing unavailability above are not likely to occur randomly nor independently of each other or the demand for the service. For example, the principal demand in some areas might be occasioned by motor accidents in heavy fog, a condition that might also ground the helicopters. A computer simulation generating a model of events based on local conditions would be necessary to generate a clear picture of machine availability and its impact on the service rendered to the community.

FREQUENCY OF NEED

The emergency care requirements of the community will have to be surveyed to record and evaluate the calls by time, severity, and location. Frequency of occurrence in time is important in determining the number of machines required to provide reasonable coverage during peak periods of the day or week.[12] Average demands are of limited importance, since concern must focus on the periods of peak demand and the services they require.

It is unrealistic to plan a system utilizing helicopters that will cover the entire medical transportation requirements of the community. Therefore, it will be necessary to determine the number of cases within the population of emergencies which would require or benefit from emergency helicopter transportation. Not only is such data useful in estimating need, but it is an important tool in testing out various administrative and policy alternatives for their impact on the system. Ambulances are employed for many reasons. One study indicates that only 35 percent of the calls answered might be perceived as emergencies from the point of view of the ambulance attendants.[14] Studies of emergency departments in metropolitan hospitals indicate that the perceptions of users are quite different from those of professional teams evaluating usage. The Skudder study classified 42 percent of all such visits as nonemergencies.[13] Under some circumstances lower socioeconomic groups appear to use the ambulance service in lieu of taxis.[9] On the other hand it is obvious that an emergency service should respond to a call involving an unconscious person, regardless of whether a later examination classifies the cause as drunkenness instead of diabetes. In many cities triage judgment is required before an ambulance is dispatched. In other communities all calls are answered. The cost of the helicopter system will depend on these policies, and they should be evaluated during the analysis.

BENEFITS

The helicopter has been treated as an added service for special emergency situations. Then what are the benefits that justify this added service? They do exist and they appear to derive from four sources: 1) speed, 2) accessibility, 3) use of more specialized personnel and equipment, and 4) ability to utilize more centralized and specialized emergency departments and hospitals. The latter two derive primarily from the first. Greater speed allows the machine to range over a much wider area and allows consideration of larger investments because a broader population can be serviced effectively. These latter benefits can be considerable not only in medical outcome, but also in community health costs. In a sparsely settled area fewer conventional emergency transport services may be needed, fewer hospitals will need to allocate scarce resources to an elaborate emergency department, and hospital services can be further specialized and regionalized to avoid duplication of expensive facilities such as burn centers, due to the capability to make rapid interhospital transfer of patients, personnel, and equipment.

The value of reduced elapsed times in most emergencies is not yet defined qualitatively or quantitatively. Certainly existing ambulance services will continue to make those trips that are routine. Of the remaining trips that are emergencies, some portion will appear suitable for the use of a helicopter. Two California studies indicate the significance of careful differentiation between those trips that can benefit from added speed or more specialized handling and those that cannot.[14,15] Even if the figures are not representative, they indicate the process that can be followed to arrive at benefit estimates based on data from badly needed demonstration projects.

Start with a supposed area population of one million persons to be serviced. On the basis of the Yolo County, California, figures this population would generate 35,580 ambulance trips per year. But only 13,530 would be perceived as emergencies by the ambulance driver or triage system. Thus one might argue that helicopters if available would be used 13,000-14,000 times per year. Yet that is not the relevant figure. Ambulances could service these cases. It is necessary to identify those cases where a specific helicopter system would benefit the patient through faster arrival of a better trained and equipped medical team, through faster transport to the nearest hospital, or through transport to a better staffed and equipped insitution.

Identification of the cases that will benefit will require extensive retrospective analysis of actual emergency cases for a judgment of comparative outcomes. Potential evaluators, i.e., patients, family, attendants, physicians, are not likely to agree on the criteria or the outcomes, but nevertheless retrospective evaluation is a needed information input to triage decisions, as well as benefit analysis.

What data exists indicates that a few minutes shaved off the delivery of the individual to the hospital is of value in only a small percentage of the cases.[3,15] But little is known about the delivery to the scene of specialized personnel and equipment for cardiopulmonary support, gastric lavage for poisoning, vehicular extraction, and surgery. If specialized skills and equipment are made available on the scene to stabilize the patient, transport speed may not even be a factor in the benefit calculation.

There may be drawbacks as well. Patient attitudes toward flying, altitude, dust, noise, and psychic stress, as well as costs, may mitigate against use of the helicopter. The problems of equipment availability and the greater length of trips from a central airport or hospital location may also reduce effective speed of service. Obviously the assessment of the benefits must be based in part on information to be gathered through a series of demonstrations.

Such demonstrations undoubtedly will produce a series of potentially dramatic events, but they must be carefully designed to test whether the machine influenced favorably the level of service in time, skills, equipment and, most importantly, the medical outcome (mortality, morbidity, discomfort, and functional recovery).

The demonstrations will not answer fully the questions of most communities, however. Widespread evaluation will have to await the gathering of data about each community's emergencies. Although studies have been made of patients presenting at emergency departments and utilizing ambulances, the epidemiological characteristics of a total community's health emergencies are not known. Data on the outcome of a community's emergencies prior to the addition of helicopter service is a logical precursor of any decision to add the helicopter service. This data should be the input to a system analysis necessary to determine the contributions of the helicopter to the specific community.

REFERENCES

1. Accidental Death and Disability: The Neglected Disease of Modern Society. National Research Council, National Academy of Sciences, Washington, D. C., September, 1966, p. 20.
2. Affel, H. A., Jr.: System engineering. *International Science and Technology,* November, 1964, p. 20.
3. Caldwell, L. A.: Ambulance services and traffic casualties. *Ontario Med. Rev.* 28: 172, 1961.
4. Direct Operating Costs and Other Performance Characteristics of Transport Aircraft in Airline Service. U. S. Federal Aviation Agency. Government Printing Office, Washington, D. C., 1963.
5. Emergency Medical Services, Draft Highway Safety Program Standard No. 4.4.11. U. S. Department of Commerce, National Highway Safety Agency, Feb-

ruary, 1967.
6. Fetter, R. B., and Thompson, J. D.: The simulation of hospital systems. *Operations Research,* September-October, 1965.
7. Goode, H. H., and Machol, R. E.: System Engineering. New York, McGraw-Hill Book Company, Inc., 1957, p. 24.
8. Hampton, O. P., Jr.: Transportation of the injured, a report. *Bull. Am. Coll. Surg.* 45:56, 1960.
9. Kinloch, D. R.: Personal communication.
10. Medicine battles the odds in Vietnam. *Medical World News,* November 18, 1966, p. 114.
11. Naylor, T. H., Balintfy, J. L., Burdick, D. S., and Chu, K.: Computer Simulation Techniques. New York, John Wiley and Sons, 1966.
12. Robertson, J. S., McLean, A. J., and Ryan, G. A.: Traffic Accidents in Adelaide, South Australia. Australian Road Research Board, Special Report No. 1, 1966.
13. Skudder, P. A., McCarroll, J. R., and Wade, P. A.: Hospital emergency facilities and services, a survey. *Bull. Am. Coll. Surg.* March-April, 1961, pp. 44-50.
14. Waller, J. A., Garner, R., and Lawrence, R.: Utilization of ambulance services in a rural community. *Am. J. Public Health* 56: 513-520, 1966.
15. West, I., Kleinman, G., Taylor, E. B., Majors, A., and Mitchell, H. W.: Study of Emergency Ambulance Operations. A Preliminary Report. State of California, Departments of Public Health and Highway Patrol, May, 1964.

17. Simulation Study of a Hospital Emergency Command System*

Stephen A. Levine

The inadequacy of emergency care in hospitals throughout the United States has received much attention recently. The lack of consistency, organization, and immediacy in mobilizing the emergency resources within the hospital prevents timely response to a majority of clinical emergencies, such as:
- Cardiopulmonary Arrest
- Surgical Emergency (originating in the accident ward)
- Civil Disaster (or major influx of acutely injured patients).

Determination of the weaknesses of current hospital techniques has been made by the staff of The Emergency Care Research Institute. The following description[1] of a typical resuscitation episode was compiled from more than 400 individual events studied at various hospitals:

A nurse discovers a pulseless and apneic patient and immediately institutes mouth-to-mouth respiration and external cardiac compression. She waits 19 seconds (range 5 to 112 seconds) after dialing for the

*Presented at Third Conference on Applications of Simulation, Dec. 8-10, 1969, Los Angeles, California.

telephone operator to answer. During this period she is diverted from her basic role of supporting the patient. The operator triple pages the emergency code every 20 seconds. The time elapsed from initial dialing by the nurse to hearing the first page is 31 seconds. The emergency cart arrives 175 seconds after initial dialing. Of this 175 seconds, 31 is due to telephone and paging lag. Five to seven physicians and nurses are present in the patient's room 148 seconds after dialing.

At night the situation is considerably worse. A single telephone operator must page and notify individual house staff in on-call rooms. The notification procedure alone increases from 31 seconds to over two minutes. During this period, of course, the switchboard sustains no other functions.

In our limited study of human errors in two urban hospitals, the telephone operator erred by giving no room location or the wrong room location four times in a series of 58 real resuscitation alerts. This closely approximates the experience of other hospitals.

With surgical emergencies, time is often less critical but organization becomes a major problem. Similar patterns in obstetrical emergencies and civil disasters involving mass accidents with a large influx of acutely injured persons have also indicated that the elements of time and organization are interrelated and critical.[1]

A Hospital Emergency Command System (HECS) has been proposed for installation in existing or new hospitals as a means of applying technology to provide "fail-safe and errorless" communication and resource dispatching. Since a relatively consistent set of responses are required for the emergency categories previously listed, an integrated electromechanical system would inherently permit an organized, timely, and accurate means of response. The HECS configuration is illustrated in Fig. 1.

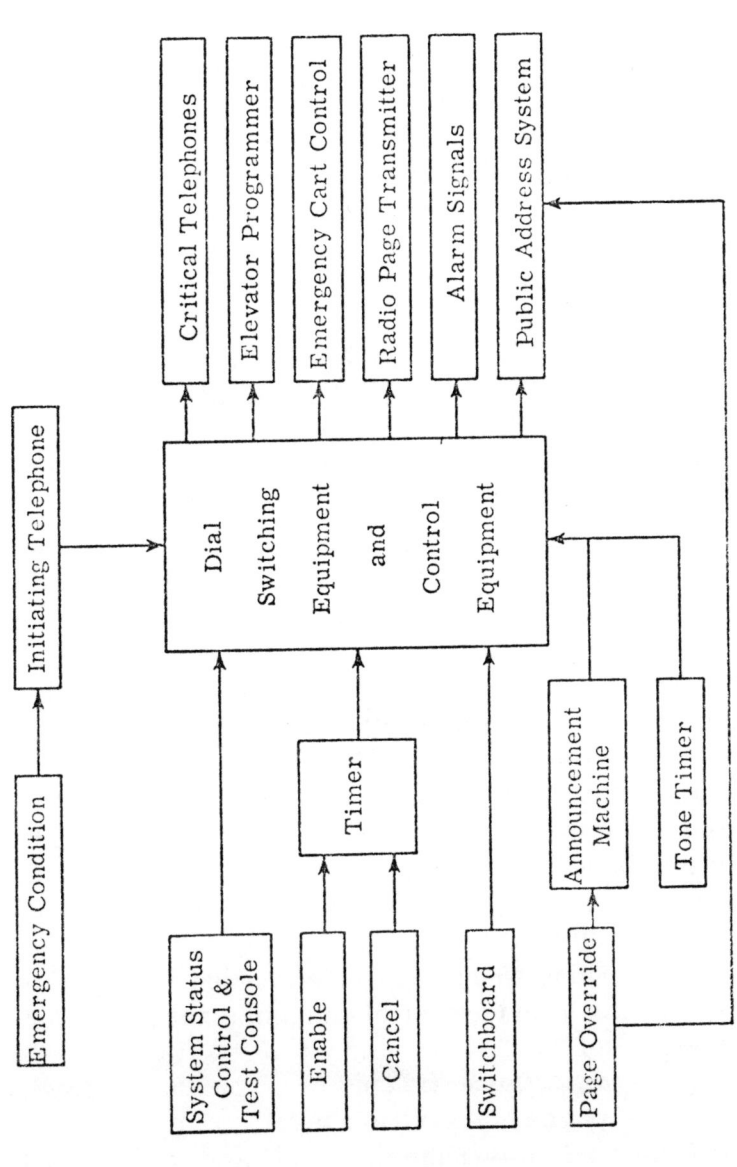

FIGURE 1. HOSPITAL EMERGENCY COMMAND SYSTEM (HECS)

Subsequent sections of this paper address the mathematical modeling, system analysis and design along with supportive statistical analyses and baseline data acquisition utilized to define existing conditions within the hospital and to evaluate the potential benefit to be gained from the HECS. A computer simulation of the system operation in its actual environment is discussed as well as a parallel simulation which permits evaluation of a hospital's present emergency care response capabilities.

THE IN-HOSPITAL EMERGENCY ENVIRONMENT

The clinical significance of the time element in responding to in-hospital emergencies has prompted its use as a yardstick in the simulation study. That is, the critical variable is the time to deliver appropriate medical personnel and equipment to support the emergency patient. This time interval is composed of a number of mission-related subintervals, which are defined in Fig. 2. A prevalent characteristic of all of these time values is their randomness, and therefore it is appropriate to describe them by probability distributions. The mission profile has also been divided into a number of phases which provided the most convenient framework for modeling the in-hospital emergency environment.

Any response to clinical emergencies within the hospital must provide control and mobilization in four areas (see Ref. 1):

(1) *Communications* (telephones, public address, pocket page system, visual page).
(2) *Personnel* (physicians, nurses and technicians on the general floors, in laboratories, offices, on-call rooms, and homes).

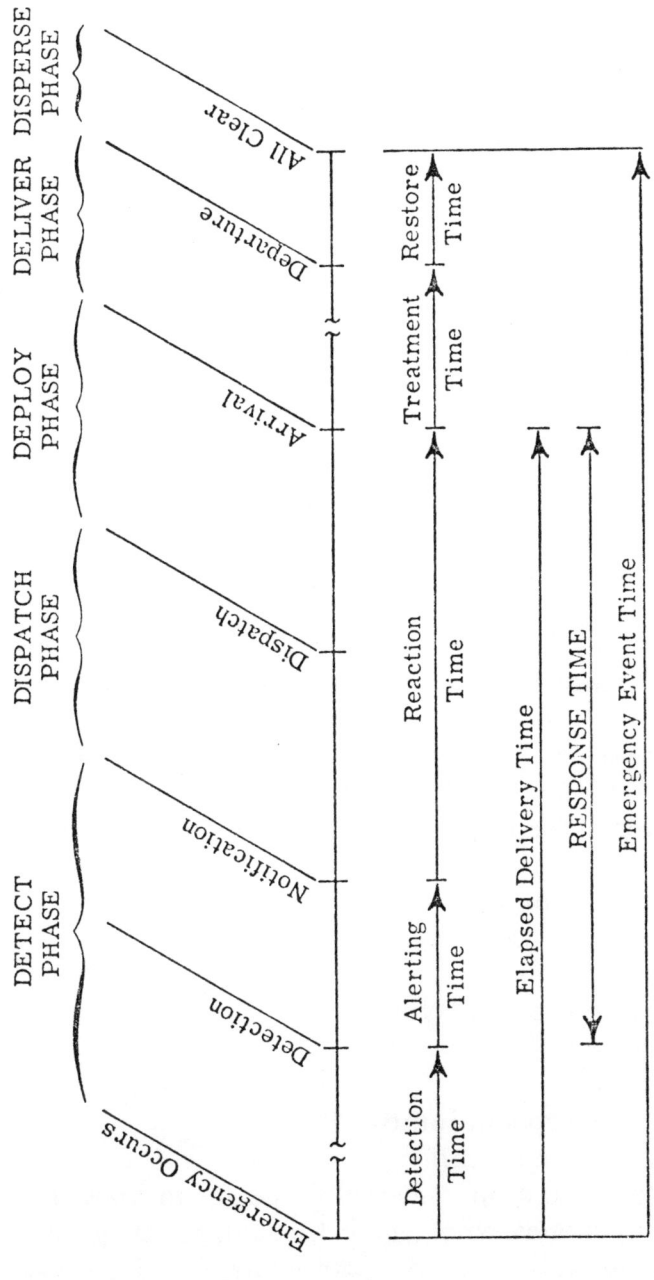

FIGURE 2. MODEL OF THE IN-HOSPITAL EMERGENCY MISSION PROFILE

(3) *Equipment* (emergency carts or cases with a broad variety of drugs and equipment).
(4) *Mobility* (elevators, doors, corridors, etc.).

To varying degrees, each of these elements are involved (in a relatively specific manner) in the five phases of an in-hospital emergency. These phases, shown in Fig. 2, exist with or without HECS, but their time values may be different. Each of these phases is discussed in what follows with regard to the actual hospital environment. These scenarios aid in model formulation, data collection specification, and computer simulation program development.

Detect Phase

This is the phase where someone in the hospital discovers that an emergency situation exists. This phase depends entirely on people, except when the patient is continually instrumented, as in some cardiac care units. The kind of person who finds a patient in cardiac arrest may be untrained, may be part of the alerting agency in the hospital, or may possess high medical competence. We can list several kinds of people who may be the ones to detect an arrest. They are, in increasing order of the amount of medical training they may have:
(1) Outside visitors or another patient
(2) Nonmedical hospital personnel
(3) Orderlies and aids
(4) Licensed Practical Nurse
(5) Registered Nurse
(6) Physicians
  (a) Not on hospital staff
  (b) On hospital staff

For the simulation, it would be useful to know the relative frequency with which these different groups of people actually discover cardiac arrests. However, we would expect these data to come only from Post-Alert Interviews which contain specific questions addressing this issue.

Three types of particular situations can arise in the process of placing an emergency call in the hospital (notification process). The first is the false alarm and the second is failure to detect the emergency until the patient is beyond medical help. The third is the situation in which inadequate information is transmitted to permit accurate identification of the location and type of emergency. These aspects are not considered in the simulation study, but have been examined and are being treated during the HECS implementation study.

The DETECT phase is also important to the simulation from the viewpoint of "generating" emergencies. For each event, we need to know date, time, location, and type of event. Extensive data for date, time, and location of cardiopulmonary arrests at several of the study hospitals were made available for this effort. It is interesting to note that in one hospital the data were obtained from telephone switchboard operator's logbook and at another hosital from medical team records. At several hospitals this information could only be generated from patient records and only for a limited number of emergency situations.

Examples of the arrest data collected on event occurrence are shown in Figs. 3 and 4 for a single hospital. The frequency of occurrence by specific locations of interest is presented in Fig. 3a and the results by specific hospital building and floor are given in Fig. 3b. Figure 4 graphically shows the frequency of occurrence by time of day. If this detail data were not available for other emergencies and/or hospitals, then appropriate random processes models could be used to generate the required case data.

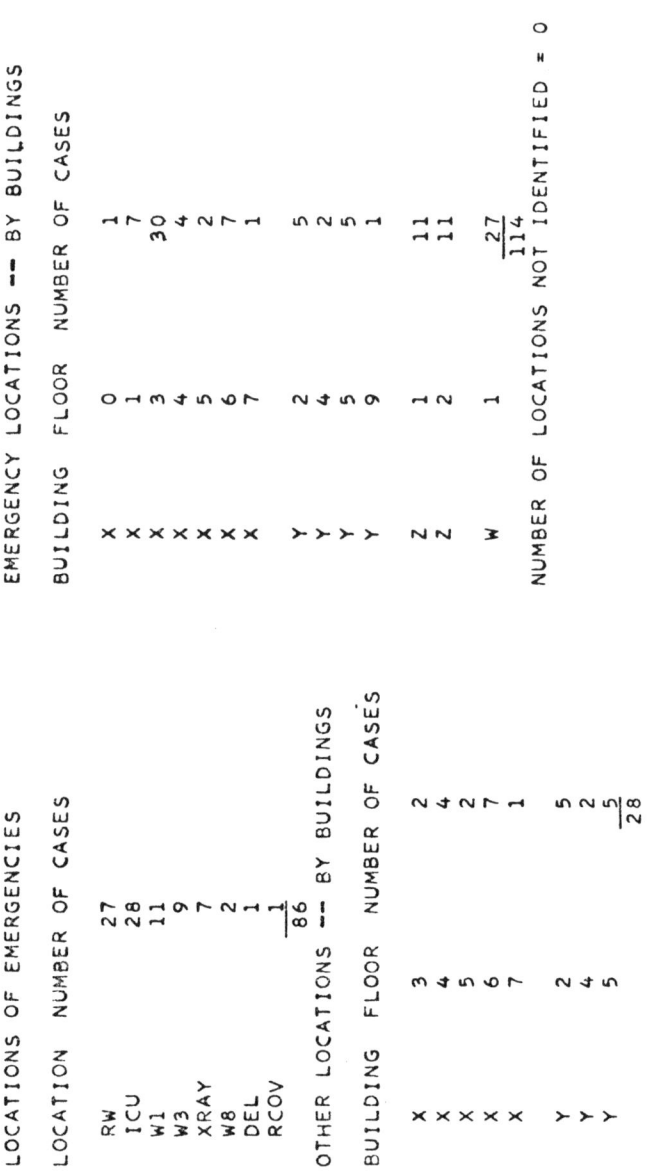

FIGURE 3. IN-HOSPITAL EMERGENCY LOCATIONS AND FREQUENCY

Dispatch Phase

The DISPATCH phase is represented by two parts. First, the person who discovered the emergency event must alert the dispatch system. The dispatch system, manual or automatic, must then alert the team members and direct them to the emergency. That is, the operations are:
- Alert the "system"
- "System" alerts the team

How these two events come about depends on the physical structure of the hospital and on the operating policy of the institution.

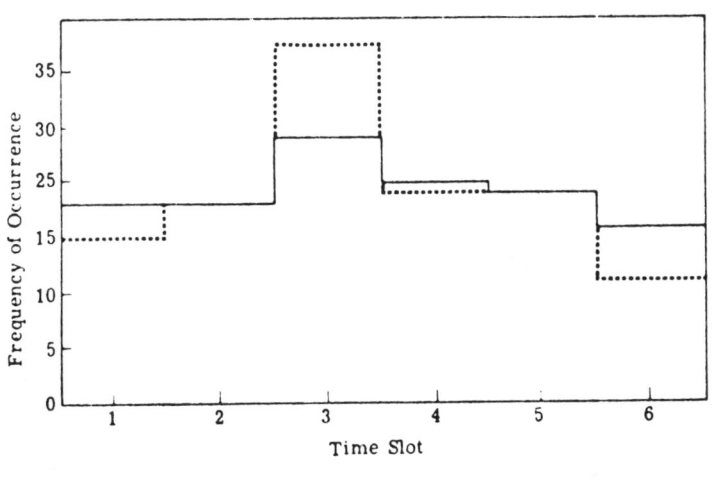

Time Slots	
1.	2AM to 6AM
2.	6AM to 10AM
3.	10AM to 2PM
4.	2PM to 6PM
5.	6PM to 10PM
6.	10PM to 2AM

1966 ———
1967 ·········

FIGURE 4. FREQUENCY OF OCCURRENCE

The alerting system, either the current hospital procedure (switchboard PBX operator) or HECS, must identify the type of emergency and location. Errors and time delays certainly occur in both systems, but the specific operational procedures associated with each approach are different and these differences must be modeled.

Once the "system" knows that there is an emergency, it must determine what kind of emergency it is and where the team must go. The task now is to call the proper emergency team and its members and give them the alerting message. Who is called and the contents of the message depend on the nature of the event and the time of day. The physical equipment also controls the procedure to use in the alert, manual or HECS.

There are two parts to this segment of DISPATCH, (a) attract the attention of the team member and, (b) give him the message. The means of attracting the attention of the team members are the following:
(1) Visual page
(2) Aural page
   (a) Public Address system
   (b) Tone signal
(3) Telephone
(4) Pocket page
   (a) Tone signal
   (b) Voice channel
(5) Messenger

Access to the alert message is more limited. The types of equipment usually used are the telephone, aural page, voice channel on pocket receiver, and messenger.

Field studies and surveys must be performed to evaluate the time delays and errors incurred in actual practice. Furthermore, the operating policies under

HECS use must be examined to permit the representable modeling of the modifications to existing practices at the hospital.

Deploy Phase

In this phase, specific medical personnel must travel to the patient treatment location, special medical equipment and supplies must be obtained and transported to specified sites, and other emergency team members must prepare certain facilities and equipment to render medical aid. DEPLOY ends when an "effective" clinical team is at the care-delivery site. In the case of cardiopulmonary arrests, this typically requires the presence of one or two trained physicians and a resuscitation cart or equipment.

For any emergency, the team members must make successive trips along corridors, on stairs, and on elevators to reach the storage place of a piece of equipment and then another series of trips to the site of the event. In specific cases, the team member may be normally stationed near the equipment or may go from alert site to event site directly. The simulation model must then take into account the following types of problems:
(1) To get from a general point in the hospital to a fixed location (equipment storage site)
(2) To get from a fixed location to a general point (any possible patient location)
(3) To travel between two general points

In each case, there are many paths which the team member may choose. The decisions are a function of experience, layout of the hospital (buildings, corridors, elevators, stairways, etc.), and personal choice. The description of the transit of heavy equipment is more restrictive. The routes are even more deterministic under HECS operation since specific elevators would be under automatic control.

Extensive field studies have indicated that one of the significant delays in responding to in-hospital emergencies is due to the waiting time required to obtain elevator transportation for facilities and staff. Therefore, a data collection and evaluation effort was performed for obtaining statistical estimates of performance for current elevator operation and various alternative HECS operating policies. The results of these studies, using actual hospital environmental data, are presented here for a selected elevator bank (having three elevators).

The HECS operating alternatives have been programmed using basic elevator travel time data and the results of probability models analyzed and implemented in the simulation program. This program allows a number of different elevator bank configurations as well as a flexible scheme for specifying travel times. Also, a variety of selection rules may be specified in the case where HECS can command any of several elevators in a bank. A comparison of arrival time delays after alerting is shown in Fig. 5 for both current and HECS operation. It is expected that actual HECS operating results may differ by about 10 percent from those obtained here, due to the data and model uncertainties.

It should be noted that the data presented for current procedures does not include an allowance for the time delay incurred from announcement of the emergency until arrival at the elevator and depression of the elevator button (or insertion of the emergency operating key). This delay may vary considerably under current operations, but would not exist under HECS operation since elevator call is initiated at about the same moment as emergency notification.

Modeling of the DEPLOY phase, as well as the phases discussed previously, requires an organized and selective collection of information. Table 1 illustrates an over-all outline of the data collection requirements which were used in the study described herein. Most of the information can be obtained easily, whereas some of the elements require a heuristic modeling effort—these are discussed in subsequent sections of this paper.

Deliver Phase

This is the time period during which members of the emergency team are treating the patient(s). The time required may vary from minutes to several hours and

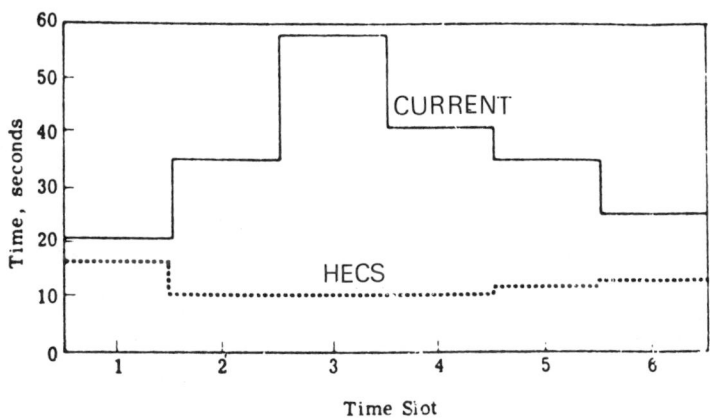

Time Slots
1. 4 AM
2. 8 AM
3. 12 Noon
4. 4 PM
5. 8 PM
6. 12 Midnight

Figure 5. Comparison of mean elevator arrival time for current and HECS operations.

TABLE 1
SIMULATION DATA COLLECTION REQUIREMENTS

Information Element	Hospital Name					
	Current Procedures			HECS Operation		
	Cardiac Arrest	Surgical Emergency	Major Patient Influx	Cardiac Arrest	Surgical Emergency	Major Patient Influx
Incident Survey (when, where)						
Detection Survey (who)						
False Alarm Survey						
Failures to Detect						
System Alert Procedures						
PBX Operator						
Alerting Equipment						
Alerting Message						
Alert Error Survey						
Emergency Team Procedures						
Equipment						
Medical Personnel						
Other Personnel						
Team Staffing and Location Survey						
Team Travel Survey						
Hospital Configuration Survey						
Buildings						
Elevators						
Equipment Storage						
Supplies Storage						
Communications						
Treatment Sites						

depends upon the type of emergency and its severity as well as many other medical and environmental factors.

Disperse Phase

This last phase occurs when the "emergency" is over and represents the time required to restore and return equipment to its standby location ready for the next event. Also, during this time period the emergency team members return to their normal activities.

The question of simultaneous emergencies must also be considered if the HECS is to be designed to meet such a contingency. Figure 6 illustrates the time between cardiac arrest emergencies at a selected hospital. In no instance did any two events occur less than ten minutes from each other. Also, we may infer from the figure that, for about 50% of the cases studied, the time between emergencies (of this class only) is about two days. Consideration of the other emergency situations HECS would handle must also be made. If HECS could not handle the multiple emergency event, it seems reasonable to expect that the current hospital procedure could be used as a back-up system. Only the case of nommultiple emergencies is treated in the simulation program.

COMPUTER SIMULATION PROGRAM DESIGN

Hospital administrators and medical staff have several alternatives to evaluate in the utilization of special equipment and trained teams for response to in-hospital emergencies. There is a policy matter as to the number and type of team members and their train-

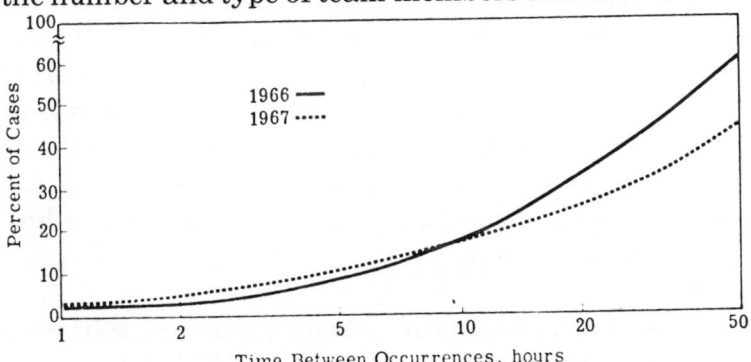

FIGURE 6. CUMULATIVE DISTRIBUTION FOR TIME BETWEEN CARDIAC ARREST EMERGENCIES

ing. The second is the capital investment in special treatment equipment and communication equipment used to alert the team and to help deploy the team to the site of the emergency. It is not enough for these managers to know that HECS equipment has worked in another hospital under some policy; they need to know the value of the device in their own environment, using a "custom-built" operating policy. The simulation developed aims at providing a flexible evaluation tool that permits decision-making before hardware purchase and installation.

The simulation encompasses two main options denoted as the CURRENT and HECS approaches; each operates in the same hospital environment. Once an emergency has been detected, either system must use its "hardware" and "software" to carry out several tasks. They are:
- Notify the warning subsystem
- Alert the emergency team
- Determine the path for the team members to get to the emergency site

The simulation program breaks each type of alerting mechanism down to elementary steps, as in a time-and-motion study. The program includes stochastic elements where they are appropriate.

The diverse nature of the stochastic elements of the problem dictated the use of simulation as the only tool which would lead to dependable results in a reasonable time. As the details show, the convolution integrals would be most difficult to evaluate, whereas the computer simulation gives large samples in a few minutes of computer time. Also, a wide variety of hospital configurations and policies can be accommodated.

In most simulations of complex human activities we find that the quality of data is spotty; this project was no exception. Within project time restrictions (this entire project was a two man-year effort) it was possible to get two years of history for the sites and times of specific emergencies and yet there was only sparse data on the time that it takes to push a resuscitation cart through the corridors. Information on elevator travel and response times was adequate, but HECS automatic control had to be modeled.

The locations and times of emergencies are read from cards punched from data furnished by the hospital. If this data was not available, it would have been necessary to devise a case-generator which would pick locations and times using an appropriate random process model.

The start of the response sequence centers around the dialing of the telephone and an answer by the alerting system. In the case of the HECS device, this operating cycle is fairly repeatable and includes dial time and the time for the recording to be made. When the alerting system involves human operators, the activity is more complex. The first action is the time that it takes to dial the PBX operator. While there was no actual data on the response times at the PBX board, the hospital personnel schedule showed the number of operators on duty during any shift. Since there is usually a line open to the board most of the time, it seemed reasonable to model the operator response by a delayed exponential distribution. The form of the probability distribution function for the delayed exponential is given by

$$p(t) = \begin{cases} 0 & 0 \leq t \leq a \\ k\exp[-k(t-a)] & a \leq t \end{cases}$$

where the mean and standard deviations are both given by $1/k$. The mean value for the exponential generating function was adjusted to take into account the service levels of each operating shift. Another factor in the response of the human operator was the time needed for her to log in the call to the PBX and to write down the information to pass on to the team members. Experiments showed that the time required was relatively constant for this element.

Having modeled the entry of a case into the alerting system, we next considered the timing in notifying the team and directing them so the site of the cardiac emergency. Again, there are differences between the automated situation and the completely manual system. Using the HECS equipment, the alert is sent over the public address system while the equipment is simultaneously ringing all the telephones on the emergency event warning list. For manual operation, the girl at the PBX board first calls a warning over the public address system and then calls the numbers on the warning list until all the team members have been notified. There is another complication in the manual system—when the operator is dialing, she cannot identify the lights on the board which refer to calls in answer to the public address summons. The simulation takes this into account and also treats the serial nature of the manual system operation. The model chosen for simulating these reductions in time response was a delayed exponential distribution. The delay assumed that it takes a fixed period of time from the time the telephone dialing starts until the person called starts to respond. The stochastic part of the process includes the time necessary to travel to the telephone from a remote location and to communicate the emergency message before responding to the emergency alert. The use of the particular stochastic models is based mainly on the criterion of "reasonableness" in comparison with timing data collected on individual phases of this event.

The time for all team members (doctors, nurses, equipment handlers, etc.) to travel along hospital corridors and through the passages between buildings is generally the same for the manual and the automatic systems. However, the goal was to simulate the entire emergency care notification and dispatching operation. Accordingly, the simulation includes means to model these similar travel times. For travel time between buildings, there was a stochastic delay superimposed on a base level travel time; the latter time was calculated from the hospital corridor geometry and average movement times for both equipment and personnel. Since there are frequent short random delays in any trip through the corridors, the simulation uses a log-normal sample to carry the weight of the travel times farther from the base level. A variable is said to have a logarithmic normal distribution if the logarithm of the variable is normally distributed. The resulting probability distribution function is[2]

$$p(t) = \frac{\log_{10} e}{\sigma t} \varphi(u) \quad 0 < t < \infty$$

where

$$u = \frac{\log_{10} t - \log_{10} \xi}{\sigma} \quad \text{and} \quad \varphi(u) = \frac{1}{\sqrt{2\pi}} \exp[-u^2/2]$$

Hald (1952) shows that the mode, median, and mean of the random variable t are determined by

mode: $\log_{10} t = \log_{10} \xi - 2.3 \sigma^2$

median: $\log_{10} t = \log_{10} \xi$

mean: $\log_{10} t = \log_{10} \xi + 1.2 \sigma^2$

The simulation of elevator travel presented a different problem from the single-floor travel time modeling. It is possible for the HECS equipment to control a number of elevators in several buildings. However, it may be desirable to control only one elevator for emergency equipment transport. The only stochastic variable is the location of the car when the HECS device commands it. Since this car is in use around the clock, a uniform distribution over the floors of the building has been used. Once HECS has acquired control, the delivery to the proper floor is deterministic. This algorithm was developed using published elevator performance data and actual statistics. Note that this situation is also representative of the case where the hospital has elevator operators, except for the delay in notification.

The control of automatic elevator cars under the current hospital alerting system was different. Here, the team members on the detail press the call button and wait for the car. A large body of data on the rate of response to the call button for the elevators in several buildings at various times throughout the day can be readily collected. The sample data collected fit the log-normal distribution extremely well. Standard statistical methods gave the proper means and variances for the various time periods.

The program to simulate both current and HECS operation has been written in FORTRAN IV. There were several reasons for choosing this language. Most important, it can be implemented readily on many computer systems with only minor changes. This is useful should one want to simulate cases from one hospital on a number of optional computers or if one desires to simulate different hospitals, geographically separated, on locally convenient systems. Also, the program consists of a main program and a number of subprogram modules. This simplified the original programming and debugging and also resulted in a more flexible simulation. At any time we can replace a subprogram module with a new version. The programmer need only write the new version in a form which is logically consistent with the rest of the program.

Figure 7 illustrates the design of the over-all HECS and current operations simulation. Each one of the major routines is designed in accord with the actual in-hospital emergency environment and thorough analytic consideration. The entire program is initiated by tape or cards documenting a given sequence of emergency alerts or by using a statistical description in conjunction with a random number generator (Emergency List Routine). The Hospital Configuration Routine is used to translate the physical structure of the hospital to a set of tables describing the transit times between any two important staff, equipment, or department locations. Actual physical design constraints are also accounted for. The Staff and Equipment Routine is intended to permit a description of the expected locations, as a function of time of day and day of week, for all members of the professional staff and equipment pertinent to any one of the possible emergency conditions. The Elevator Routine provides the information necessary in estimating the travel time incurred in using any of the hospital's elevators, for equipment or staff transportation, during the course of an emergency. This routine is depicted in

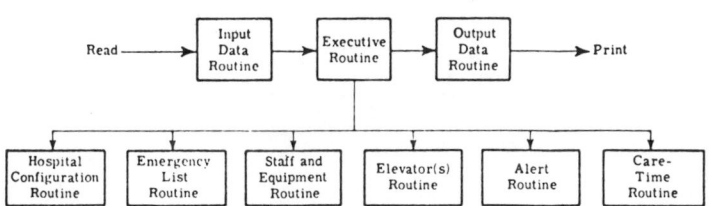

FIGURE 7. CURRENT AND HECS OVERALL SIMULATION FLOW DIAGRAM

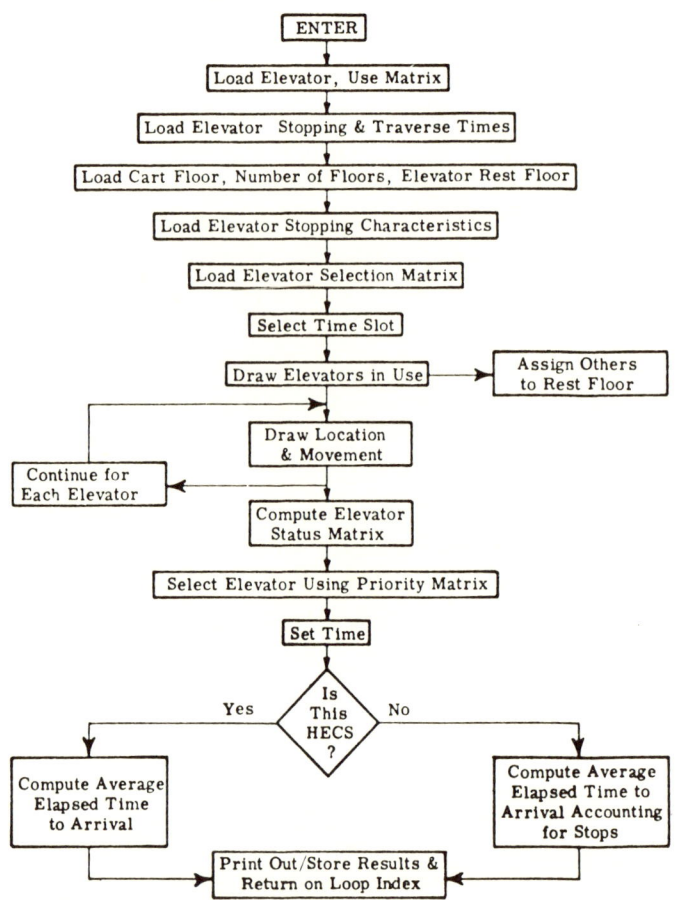

FIGURE 8. ELEVATOR SIMULATION ROUTINE LOGIC

Fig. 8 in its verbal form. The Alert Routine is incorporated to reflect the policies or operational procedures for carrying out any of the subject emergency alerts, as presently adopted by the hospital and under HECS control. The Care-Time Routine is used to collect the actual time required to deliver each element of appropriate medical care to the patient for both the pre- and post-HECS installed conditions. Summary statistics are also computed within this module. Some details of specific aspects of the simulation program are discussed in what follows.

The Input Data Routine provides control over placing all information (data, parameter values, selection rules, indices, etc.) in the appropriate subroutine description matrices. An example of the form of these information arrays is the alert table which lists the team members and equipment selection rules for each emergency category. The Hospital Configuration Routine maintains several arrays, one of which specifies the interbuilding travel times for the situation in which a hospital complex has several buildings. Wherever necessary, these arrays are stored for both current hospital procedures and HECS so that the computation subroutines can access the data pertinent to the particular case. The Executive Routine provides over-all program control and performs the necessary data transfer from one subroutine to another. As time delay information is computed for each of the personnel and equipment elements, the data is transferred to the Care-Time Routine.

The simulation development effort and experimental results were generated on the IBM360-75 via Remote Job Entry from a TASC-based IBM 1130. This provided an on-site capability for a program requiring significant computer storage. The ability to maintain all the data arrays in computer core during a simulation run permitted economical use of computer time. Of course, the core requirements and run time are a complex function of the hospital configuration, operational policies, and the number of cases treated, as well as other less important parameters. But, the results for the current and HECS case (under the conditions of a single emergency category) for a large urban hospital required less than 100K bytes of core and less than 3 minutes to execute. This actual sample situation is treated in detail in the following section.

ACTUAL SIMULATION EXAMPLE

The computer simulation of the full scale operating systems must be keyed to baseline data gathered on the existing conditions within the hospital. It is important to obtain this data so that a valid comparison may be made of the time required to bring appropriate medical care to the patient before and after HECS is in operation. Without such an approach, justification for the HECS becomes theoretical rather than proven.

The simulation example chosen is for a large urban hospital having four major buildings. The emergency event data used was obtained from hospital records only for the case of cardiopulmonary arrests occurring within the hospital (this is the same data illustrated earlier in the paper). Since no information could practically be obtained for the detection delay time, the main objective was to establish the system response times (see Fig. 2). The team data used was:

MD1: located on the 3rd floor of Y building
MD2: located on the 5th floor of X building
Emergency CART: located on the 3rd floor of X building

It was assumed that only one of the three elevator cars in the X building would be under HECS control, whereas all other ones operate under the current system. In simulating the elevator delays, the data presented in the previous section is used including appropriate adjustments for the time of day of the emergency. In addition, the elevators in the Y, Z, and W buildings are much older and assumed 20% slower than the cars in the X building. This gives an average rate of travel of 0.13 minutes per floor for the X building and 0.16 minutes per floor for the others.

The total delay which the team experiences in servicing a call has three major parts, Alert Delay, Corridor Delay, and Elevator Delay. Each of these has fixed and variable parts. The variable parts are either deterministic (e.g., elevator travel speed from floor to floor) or stochastic (e.g., waiting for an elevator). Table 2 lists the Alert Delay budget and mathematical

TABLE 2
ALERT DELAY BUDGET

Current System			HECS	
Dial Operator		10 sec	Dial HECS	10 sec
Operator Response			Record Data	10 sec
Exponential Distribution			Public Address	
11 pm - 7 am	k = 5 sec		System Page	5 sec
7 am - 3 pm	k = 15 sec			
3 pm - 11 pm	k = 10 sec		MD's Hear Page	5 sec
Operator Records Data		10 sec	Cart Nurse Responds	
Operator Calls MD's			Exponential Distribution	
on Public Address		15 sec		k = 10 sec
Operator Dial Cart		10 sec		
Cart Nurse Responds				
Exponential Distribution				
		k = 10 sec		

models used. Travel times in corridors and between buildings are not fixed. These figures are given as random trials, but always in excess of a minimum time. We do assume that travel time distributions in corridors are the same in all buildings. That is, corridor delay is independent of the building and independent of HECS. Travel on one floor of a building is a sample from a log-normal distribution with a mean of 30 sec and coefficient of variation 1.36. We do not use constant travel times, because obstructions slow down corridor travel speeds in a random manner. An exponential distribution would tend to concentrate simulated cases close to the elevators. To offset these factors and to prevent negative travel times, we chose the log-normal distribution. With the parameter values assumed, less than 1% of the trips on a floor of a building take longer than one minute. When there is travel on two floors, each is an independent sample. There is a different constant base level time between pairs of buildings. Table 3 shows these inter-building travel times.

The computer simulation results for the total of two years of emergency cases, 229 cardiopulmonary arrests, is shown in Fig. 9 for current hospital opera-

TABLE 3

TRAVEL TIME BETWEEN BUILDINGS IN MINUTES

Buildings	X	Y	Z	W
X	0	1.5	0.75	0.5
Y	1.5	0	0.75	2.0
Z	0.75	0.75	0	1.25
W	0.5	2.0	1.25	0

	CURRENT HOSPITAL EMERGENCY OPERATIONS							
	229 CARDIOPULMONARY ARRESTS							
	RESPONSE TIME IN MINUTES							
	FRACTION OF CASES							
	.95	.9	.7	.5	.3	.1	.05
MD1	2.16	2.35	2.99	4.02	4.58	5.76	6.21
MD2	1.16	1.32	3.95	4.42	4.86	5.88	6.34
CART	1.35	1.48	2.82	4.00	4.64	5.87	6.33
TOTAL CARE	3.83	3.98	4.48	4.92	5.63	6.61	7.44
PARTIAL CARE	2.35	2.48	3.32	4.18	4.67	5.98	6.42
ALERT DELAY							
MD1	0.59	0.60	0.65	0.69	0.76	1.04	1.23
MD2	0.59	0.60	0.65	0.69	0.76	1.04	1.23
CART	0.81	0.85	0.92	1.03	1.16	1.48	1.65
CORRIDOR DELAY							
MD1	0.86	0.94	1.04	1.48	1.68	2.43	2.51
MD2	0.47	0.58	1.67	1.75	1.83	2.28	2.30
CART	0.45	0.47	0.94	1.48	1.70	2.44	2.52
ELEVATOR DELAY							
MD1	0.46	0.63	1.11	1.67	2.09	2.78	3.57
MD2	0.0	0.0	1.37	1.70	2.15	3.11	3.69
CART	0.0	0.0	0.79	1.44	1.78	2.53	3.20

FIGURE 9. CURRENT OPERATIONS SIMULATION RESULTS AND DELAY COMPONENTS

HECS EMERGENCY OPERATIONS
229 CARDIOPULMONARY ARRESTS
RESPONSE TIME IN MINUTES

			FRACTION OF CASES				
	.95	.9	.7	.5	.3	.1	.05
MD1	2.00	2.12	2.44	3.57	3.87	4.76	5.07
MD2	1.01	1.08	3.52	3.83	4.04	4.32	4.47
CART	0.95	1.02	1.88	3.08	3.41	4.33	4.67
TOTAL CARE	3.48	3.58	3.86	4.02	4.22	4.88	5.16
PARTIAL CARE	2.08	2.15	2.44	3.37	3.69	4.33	4.67

ALERT DELAY

MD1	0.50	0.50	0.50	0.50	0.50	0.50	0.50
MD2	0.50	0.50	0.50	0.50	0.50	0.50	0.50
CART	0.43	0.44	0.49	0.55	0.66	0.82	0.87

CORRIDOR DELAY

MD1	0.91	0.94	1.05	1.47	1.70	2.45	2.50
MD2	0.51	0.58	1.67	1.75	1.84	2.25	2.29
CART	0.44	0.48	0.95	1.46	1.70	2.42	2.49

ELEVATOR DELAY

MD1	0.47	0.64	0.88	1.48	1.71	2.03	2.20
MD2	0.0	0.0	1.19	1.40	1.60	1.92	2.04
CART	0.0	0.0	0.43	0.96	1.14	1.44	1.64

FIGURE 10. HECS OPERATIONS SIMULATION RESULTS AND DELAY COMPONENTS

tions and Fig. 10 for HECS operation. The term "Total Care" refers to the situation in which *both* MD's and the resuscitation cart are at the emergency site. The term "Partial Care" refers to the case when the cart and only *one* MD arrive. Summary results are also given in these figures in terms of the component delays defined previously. The balance between the corridor and elevator delay components under HECS operation indicates that further improvement in elevator control would not significantly influence the results in this hospital situation. This is also true of the alert delay component. Replication of each individual year of data, 1966 and 1967, and the total cases presented was excellent. These results have also been drawn to graphically illustrate the nature of the response time distribution for total and partial care—see Figs. 11 and 12. Single case summary reports may also be computer-generated and one is shown in Fig. 13—the abbreviation CPA denotes that this is a cardiopulmonary arrest emergency.

The improvement in emergency response time afforded by the HECS approach can be readily inferred from these results, at least for the specific hospital and situation studied.

There are some features of the response curves that must be explained. Chief among these is the bimodal nature of the cumulative frequency distribution of response time. This is barely noticeable in the case of the Total Care curves, but strongly visible in the curves for Partial Care. When one examines the physical structure of the hospital and the locations of the team members in relation to the sites of the emergencies, the reason for the bimodality becomes apparent. Looking first at the Partial Care situation, we find the cart and one physician in the same building. Most of the cases are in two of the buildings. Therefore, there

Percent of Cases for which
System Responded by Time T

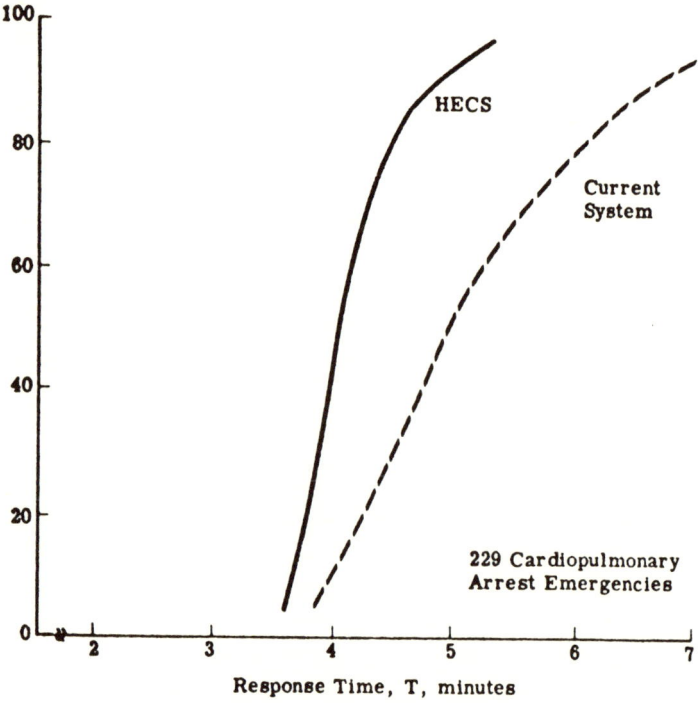

Response Time, T, minutes

FIGURE 11. "TOTAL CARE" SIMULATION RESULTS

is a distribution of times to service the local building and a superimposed distribution of times to service the other building. The bimodality is partly disguised in the Total Care situation by the need to wait for the other physician in every case.

This does not mean that the variance of the distribution is increased. In fact, the need to wait for the last team member in order to have Total Care makes the variability smaller. We can readily see this by a table of interdecile ranges—see Table 4. The interdecile range is defined as the difference between the 90th and 10th percentile values of the cumulative distribution functions given in Figs. 9 and 10. When distributions start to be markedly non-Gaussian, the standard deviation becomes quite inefficient as a measure of dispersion. On the other hand, some of the order statistics are quite efficient in this case. For that reason, we have chosen the interdecile range rather than the standard deviation. In both Partial Care and

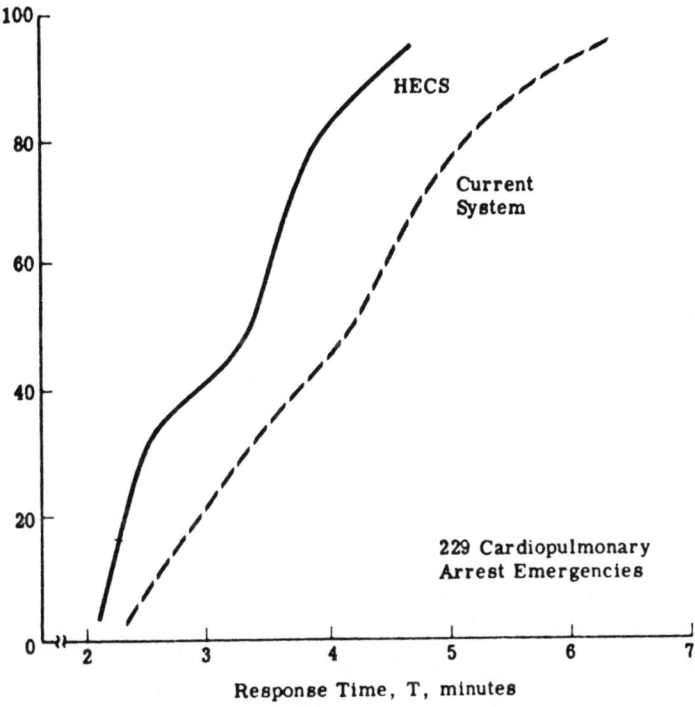

FIGURE 12. "PARTIAL CARE" SIMULATION RESULTS

CURRENT HOSPITAL EMERGENCY OPERATIONS

RESPONSE TIME IN MINUTES

CPA   5/29/66   8.25 PM   SPR BUILDING 5TH FLOOR

TEAM MEMBER	ALERT DELAY	CORRIDOR DELAY	ELEVATOR DELAY	TOTAL DELAY
MD1	0.83	2.53	2.14	5.50
MD2	0.83	1.70	2.17	4.71
CART	1.43	2.51	2.23	6.16

TIME TO TOTAL CARE   6.16
TIME TO PARTIAL CARE   6.16

FIGURE 13. INDIVIDUAL CASE REPORT

Total Care, HECS has reduced the variability by about one-third of the current system value.

SUMMARY

The in-hospital emergency simulation discussed herein has been prepared in a manner that readily permits evaluation of current procedures and HECS evaluation for any of the several thousand hospitals throughout the United States. As may be noted, the results for the situation of cardiopulmonary arrest emergencies are given in terms of response time as depicted in Fig. 2. This has been done since no reliable information is available on the time delay from occurrence to detection of this type of emergency. This is not necessarily true for the other classes of in-hospital emergencies that HECS can handle. Although response time is a fair means of comparing HECS and current operations, further clinical interpretation may

TABLE 4

INTERDECILE RANGE OF
SIMULATION RESULTS IN MINUTES

Care Case	Current System	HECS
Partial	3.5	2.2
Total	1.6	1.3

be desirable. That is, even if HECS saved two minutes on the average beyond the current system, the total delay time may still not be acceptable with regard to patient care. Nobel (1968) considers the time element in the following manner:

> Consider the clinical significance of the time element alone in resuscitation. While the commonly accepted time period for irrevocable nervous system death to ensue following cessation of cardiac and respiratory activity is four minutes, this is an arbitrary and misleading figure. The time interval is frequently well under a minute in patients with compromised cerebral vasculature or with higher than normal ambient or patient temperatures. It depends on cardiac output, respiratory gas exchange and tissue oxygen uptake prior to arrest.
>
> It is not true that once a patient is being sustained by mouth-to-mouth breathing and external cardiac compression, time becomes a less critical factor. Under such conditions, cardiac output is approximately twenty percent of normal and blood pH decreases rapidly. It is infinitely harder to defibrillate the heart at the eighth or tenth minute post arrest than it is during the first or second minute. Pacemakers are almost worthless more than a minute or two post arrest. The more rapidly these therapeutic modalities are applied, the greater is the probability that they will achieve the desired effect. Elapsed time in resuscitation is an even more critical factor than is generally appreciated.[1]

Using the time criterion itself, the results obtained in the previous section could be compared as shown in Table 5. For the particular situation examined and available data, this presentation reveals almost a 100 percent improvement provided by HECS.

A somewhat different approach is illustrated in Fig. 14. If a statistical distribution model for the time interval between occurrence of a cardiac arrest and the oc-

TABLE 5
PERCENT OF CASES FOR WHICH SYSTEM RESPONDED IN A GIVEN TIME

System Case	Three Minutes	Four Minutes
Current System	21	47
HECS	41	82

currence of an irreversible patient clinical condition could be developed, then we could derive a hazard function representing the instantaneous probability of an irreversible condition as a function of elapsed time. Such a measure would show a variance among patients, but a hazard function zone could be developed to represent such a situation. A probabilistic measure of in-hospital emergency system effectiveness is suggested then by Fig. 14, which shows the cumulative distribution function of response time for both system approaches plotted against an increasing hazard function. The effectiveness measure is the probability (P_H) that a response system (provided by the HECS) will restore the patient to a viable condition before a critical hazard level (h_c) is reached. Note the difference in the effectiveness between HECS and the current operation. The model shows that, like most statistical problems of this type, it is not sufficient for the average response time ($\bar{t}$) to be less than the critical time (t_{h_c}); the dispersion of response times is also important.

424 Emergency Medical Services

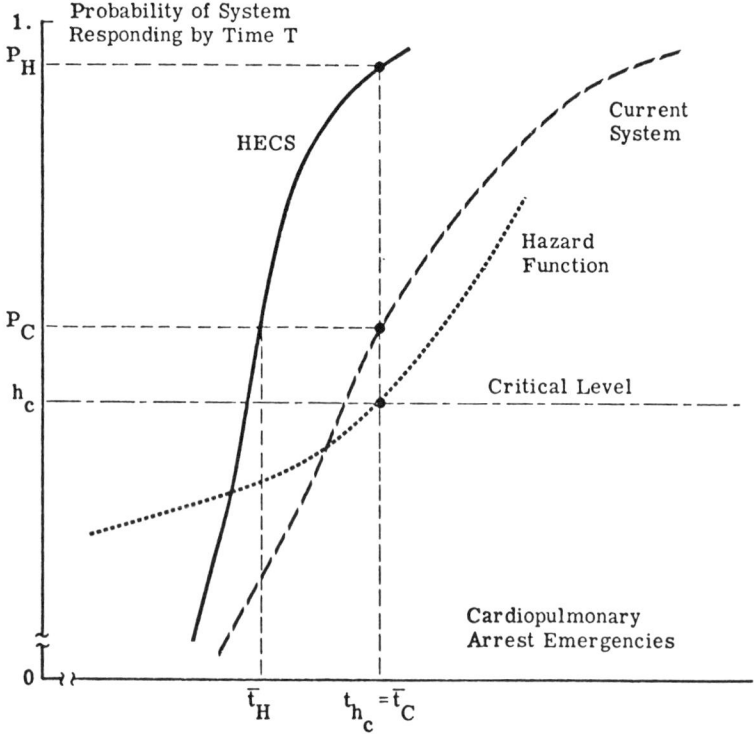

FIGURE 14. EFFECTIVENESS OF RESPONSE SYSTEMS

The over-all accuracy of the simulation results is currently being confirmed through actual demonstration projects at three large hospitals. In the ultimate analysis it is hoped that this simulation program promotes the goal of the Hospital Emergency Command System, namely providing decreased patient mortality and decreased central nervous system damage in survivors.

REFERENCES

1. Nobel, Joel J., "Hospital Emergency Command System," The Emergency Care Research Institute, 1968.
2. Hald, A., "Statistical Theory With Engineering Applications," John Wiley & Sons, Inc., New York, 1952.

18. Mobile Emergency Medical Care

E. B. Struxness, M.D.

One recent innovation in the delivery of medical services is the development of Mobile Emergency Medical Care (MEMC). MEMC can be described as that subsystem of total emergency health care which encompasses everything that happens to an emergency patient from the time of the actual emergency to the conclusion of treatment and release from an emergency facility. In sequence, an incident must have occurred, someone must have recognized the fact, a call for help must have been dispatched, aid must have been supplied on site and continued during transport to an appropriate facility, and decisive care must have been provided in that facility. Adequate life support throughout this chain of events can and will reduce morbidity as well as mortality.

Mobile emergency medical care is currently characterized by proliferation of numerous specialized vehicles—probably an unnecessary and unfortunate development. There are mobile intensive care units, mobile coronary care units, and mobile surgical care units. All have the common advantage of making possible more definitive emergency medical care at the scene of life-endangering illness or injury. All have the common disadvantage of being designed to respond to only one medical or surgical problem. It should be possible, using the medical and engineering criteria established by the National Academy of Science-National Research Council, for ambulance designers to develop one vehicle equipped to serve multiple medical and surgical purposes.[1]

The emergence of burn and trauma centers, intensive care units, coronary care units, and pediatric and geriatric specialized units has altered the basis upon which we must consider the problems associated with emergency care, including mobile emergency medical care. The economics of these specialized units limits their feasibility to those large hospitals capable of providing the facilities, equipment, personnel, and supplies necessary to serve sufficiently large numbers to warrant their establishment in the first place. It should be noted further that economic feasibility in a total medical care system characterized by ever-increasing costs dictates application of these specialized resources only to those cases of acute illness or injury that pose a threat to life or high risk of aggravated morbidity and/or permanent disability. In addition, categorization of specialized hospital emergency capabilities will result inevitably in statewide plans similar to the one developed by Illinois.[2,3] Once implemented, such plans will require transportation of patients over extended distances while using existing communications and patient monitoring technologies to link the ambulance and the ultimate receiving hospital capable of providing the spectrum of services needed specifically by the critically ill or injured person. Only by these means can the physician guide and support the care of patients by Emergency Medical Technical Assistants (EMTA) on site and in transit.

Mobile emergency medical care exists both within and outside the confines of the hospital. In-house emergencies have resulted in the development of "crash carts," "blue teams," and various other means of bringing definitive aid to the patient at the site of his need. A sophisticated example is afforded by the use of a "max" cart coupled with the Hospital Emergency Control System (HECS), developed by the Emergency Care Research Institute under the direction of Dr. Joel Nobel in cooperation with The Analytic Sciences Corporation. In this system one telephone call triggers a complete response—personnel, equipment, supplies, coordination of elevators, etc.—and directs medical personnel to the site of the emergency. The system not only provides prompt life-supportive care at the patient's bedside but can also continue it while he is being transferred to the appropriate specialized care unit of the hospital. Of particular interest is this system's potential for the kind of automated data collection that could add to our store of objective knowledge concerning appropriate management of life-threatening emergencies.[4]

Unfortunately, similar use of existing technology has not been extended to mobile emergency medical care outside the hospital. Statistics concerning in-hospital deaths from heart disease led to the development of coronary care units with a resultant reduction in morbidity and mortality rates. By comparison, the death rate from heart disease prior to hospital admission is significantly higher. Attempts are now being made to prevent the death of people with hearts "too good to die" by developing mobile coronary care units capable of aiding the patient on site. One such unit has been operative in Dublin, Ireland since January, 1966.[5] Different techniques have been employed in the United States which utilize highly-trained fire rescue personnel and E.C.G. transmissions to the hospital. Dr. Eugene Nagel of Miami, for example, has improved the salvage rate of heart attack victims by using remote E.C.G. monitoring to direct by radio the activities of these paramedical personnel.[6]

Although deaths from heart disease exceed by ten times deaths resulting from traffic accidents, automobile fatalities as well as accidental injuries occurring at home and at work constitute a grave and sizeable problem. There is recognition of the need for change and improvement in the mobile care of trauma victims, but little progress to date. Frey, et al. discovered that 18 percent of auto accident deaths could have been prevented if prompt and adequate care had been delivered on site and in transit to an emergency facility.[7] As mentioned previously, development of an adequate noncategorical ambulance would go far to advance possibilities for improved care of trauma victims.

Inherent in the concept of mobile emergency medical care is the supposition that either the patient, a vehicle, or a treatment team is on the move for the purpose of providing intensive medical care on site or in transit to a source of definitive care. Voice and E.C.G. telemetry between ambulances and emergency departments are already established modalities in some places. The technology exists to expand telemetry to other medical data. Automated data collection that surpasses the subjective judgment of an EMTA is a current possibility.

It is not necessary to invest a fortune in specially-designed vehicles to obtain the benefits of telecommunications technology. Portable equipment can, for example, convert an ordinary ambulance into a mobile coronary care unit. A modulator-amplifier can convert an E.C.G. signal into an audible tone for transmission by radio to a hospital where the demodulated signal is translatable into an immediately available E.C.G. printout for interpretation.[9] In somewhat similar fashion, a miniaturized transmitter can be used to monitor an ambulatory heart patient continuously. Any significant or dangerous alteration of the heart rhythm will produce a buzzing sound to alert the patient. He can then go to the nearest telephone to transmit the E.C.G. signal to his personal physician or to the hospital for demodulation and interpretation, and await instructions.[10]

Highly-trained EMTA's in radio communication with emergency physicians are being permitted in some places to start intravenous infusions, to give medications, and to defibrillate. In fact, the Oregon Board of Medical Examiners has ruled that defibrillation by properly trained attendants is not to be considered the practice of medicine, but an emergency procedure.[11]

Medical care—particularly emergency care in remote areas—continues to present many problems that telecommunications technology can assist in solving. A well-trained paramedical person could manage perhaps as much as 80 percent of the problems seen by primary care physicians. As telemedicine advances, paramedical personnel will be able to contact and stay in touch with appropriate sources of medical advice. This, coupled with improved transportation for patients, should go far to overcome the paucity of primary medical care and inaccessibility of remote areas. Telemetry by means of satellite will reach even the remotest areas of the country.

Although some of this thinking may seem "blue sky" and farfetched, advances in telecommunications and transportation technologies seem to offer the only proximate hope we have for providing a sizeable segment of the population of the United States with a higher standard of medical care than is currently available.

REFERENCES

1. "Emergency Help." *Red Cross Newsletter*, March 1970. "Greensburg Receives New Mobile Coronary Care Unit." *Para-Medical Journal*, 2: 6 & 11, March 1970. Kimbel, S.: "New Ambulance in Pentagon Helps Save Life in First Week." *Pentagram News*, 1 Oct. 1970. "Mobile CCU Can Help Curb Heart Deaths." *Hospitals*, 43:27, 16 Oct. 1969. Monsees, A.: "A Stroke Unit on Wheels." *Health News*, Aug. 1969. National Academy of Engineering: Ambulance Design Criteria. National Highway Safety Bureau, U.S. Dept of Transportation, 1970. National Academy of Science-National Research Council: Medical Requirements for Ambulance Design and Equipment. Division of Emergency Health Services, U.S. Dept. of Health, Education, and Welfare, 1970. "New Van for Coronary Care Unit." *Seattle Times*, 11 Oct. 1970. "Special Van Gives Babies Head Start on Survival." *JAMA,* 209:1826, 22 Sept. 1969. Wood, Q. L.: "Mobile Emergency Unit Saves Lives in Hospital-less Community." *Hospitals*, 43:59-61, 16 March 1969.
2. Commission on Emergency Medical Services of the AMA: Recommendations of the Conference on the Guidelines for Categorization of Hospital Emergency Capabilities. American Medical Association, 1970.
3. Flashner, B.A., and Boyd, D.R.: "The Critically Injured Patient: A Plan for the Organization of a Statewide System of Trauma Facilities." *Illinois Medical Journal*, 139: 256-265, March 1971.
4. Nobel, J.J.: "A Single Phone Call Mobilizes Hospital in Cardiac Emergencies." *JAMA*, 209:857, 11 Aug. 1969. ——— and Rauch, R.M.: "Emergency Resuscitation and Life Support Vehicle." *Medical Research Engineering*, 7:11-16, 4th quarter, 1968.
5. Pantridge, J. F., and Geddes, J. S.: "A Mobile Intensive Care Unit in the Management of Myocardial Infarction." *Lancet*, 2:271-273, 5 Aug. 1967.

6. Nagel, E. L., Hirschman, J. C., Nussenfeld, S. R., Rankin, D., and Lundblad, E.: "Telemetry-Medical Command in Coronary and Other Mobile Emergency Care Systems." *JAMA*, 214:332-338, 12 Oct. 1970.
7. Frey, C. F., Huelke, D. F., and Gikas, P. W.: "Resuscitation and Survival in Motor Vehicle Accidents." *Journal of Trauma*, 9:292-310, April 1969.
8. Stack, J.K.: "Emergency Squad Doctor." *Journal of Trauma*, 2:102-103, Jan. 1962.
9. "Door-to-Door Coronary Care." *Emergency Medicine*, 3:134-139, March 1971.
10. "A Walking Coronary Alarm." *Medical World News*, 12:4, 8 Oct. 1971.

Part IV
Standards and Policies

INTRODUCTION

The pressure upon hospitals and their boards, medical societies and their membership, and public officials at every level to "do something" to improve emergency medical care has been unceasing. Newspaper editorials on "First Aid—The Medical Stepchild," "Grim Diagnosis: More Americans Turn to Emergency Rooms and Receive Poor Care," and the like, have reflected increasing public concern about the apparent lack of standards and consistent policy governing emergency care facilities and personnel.

The gap between current practice and the achievement of its goals is the topic of the first three articles of this section. The recommendations of the Committee on Acute Medicine (1968) cover ten major classes of life-threatening situations that can be expected to occur with some regularity in the pursuance of everyday life. The Committee begins with the recommendation that "the total emergency medical care program of a community should be evaluated, coordinated, upgraded, and supervised through appropriate 'community councils' . . ." and offers detailed standards concerning the facilities, personnel, training, and equipment that each community should provide to assist victims of accidents and acute medical conditions.

The article by Owens (1966) presents the findings of a survey of emergency departments in seventy-two general hospitals in Colorado in the mid-1960's. Face-to-face interviews with hospital administrators, physicians, and nurses and on-site inspection of the facilities and equipment in these hospitals revealed many of the same deficiencies reported five years earlier by Skudder, *et al* (1961). Almost a third of the hospitals were lacking in emergency equipment and supplies; two-thirds or more contained immobile examining tables, or stretchers that necessitated repeated movement of fracture patients during examination and treatment; and less than one-fifth of the hospitals had emergency department committees representing the major medical services, hospital administration, and nursing. Indoctrination of nursing and paramedical staff was haphazard. Other notable deficiencies included: nurses inexperienced or poorly trained in emergency procedures, inadequate physician coverage, "a distressing number of exceptions to recognized standards of surgical, anesthesia and aseptic practice," lack of familiarity with treatment methods of airway obstructions and other critical respiratory problems, and inadequate provision for the diagnosis and treatment of poison victims.

The irreverent article on hospital "moonlighting" policies gives some idea of the conflicts that can arise in implementing standards concerned with emergency room staffing. *Resident Physician's* survey (1967) of more than 2,000 interns, residents, chiefs of service, and directors of medical education provides further evidence of the close relationship between imbalances in the wider health care system and those in the emergency medical care sector. The survey revealed that, while the majority of hospitals forbid or discourage "moonlighting" by interns and residents, the ban is seldom enforced because of the shortage of private physicians and the availability of low-paid substitutes. This and other inconsistencies between stated policy and actual practice gave rise among affected house staff to resentful cries of "hypocrisy," and moved one resident to insist: "Hospitals must make a radical change in their attitude towards residents—both professionally and financially."

The next group of articles offer practical advice and suggestions to hospital trustees, administrators, medical staff, and nurses about their professional and legal responsibilities in the emergency room. Kennedy (1966) describes the duties and types of problems facing an emergency department committee. His recommendations cover such matters as the conditions under which general anesthesia should be given; when minor operations may be performed; how to ensure physician coverage of the emergency room; how to control use of observation beds; and what professional and administrative procedures to enforce for fractures, aseptic treatment of wounds, and the like. He states his strong conviction that "physicians working in a hospital must take more responsibility for the community and must be their brothers' keepers." The physician is to subordinate his economic interests to the common good in the context of emergency medical care.

Feldman's advice (1966) on how to deal with the public and the press in providing information about emergency cases and services reinforces Kennedy's message by showing the possible consequences to the hospital's reputation and fortune if it fails to meet the community's expectations of quality emergency medical care. In its treatment of emergency victims every hospital is faced with the dilemma of satisfying the public's "right to know" while withholding medically privileged information or that which might injure the good reputation of the patient or his family. Unprivileged and privileged information are likened to a two-sided coin that must be called while it is still spinning in the air: "When you guess wrong you know it—the press pounces on you." Consequently, to eliminate misunderstanding about the functions and responsibilities of the emergency room and its resultant bad press, poor public relations, and possible lawsuits, Feldman recommends that the community's hospitals join together in a better use of the media to educate the public about their emergency medical care policies and procedures.

The evolution of case law governing tort actions that may be brought against hospitals and medical and nursing staff in case of negligence highlights the importance of strict adherence to standards in the examination and treatment of all persons who enter the "open door" of the emergency department. As Power's article (1968) points out, hospitals could refuse to treat persons in need under traditional common law which imposed liability for intentional or negligent misfeasance but none for failure to act. This harsh "no duty to act" rule has been softened, however, by numerous court decisions which coincide with a shift in societal values emphasizing the contemporary view that human life has transcendent worth. An analysis of precedent-making court decisions makes it clear that hospitals, by establishing emergency medical facilities and services known to the public, assume liability if they do not offer treatment to all who seek aid. While many legal questions remain about the extent of the hospital's duty to distinguish between emergent and nonemergent cases and the degree of care required in treating emergencies, there is little doubt that "the law should not sanction any degree of care below that generally prevailing for other medical services." The standards formulated by the medical profession are likely to become those applied by the courts. *Caveat venditor!*

The last article in this section, by Keller and Gemma (1972), offers a planning perspective on the challenges and opportunities that face communities as they attempt to fit together the fragmented components of an emergency health care system to form an integrated whole. Recognizing that each component of the system has its own culture and set of special interests and perceptions, they ask: "Who puts the whole thing together?" How can the public, hospitals and medical manpower, transport, and communications be brought together to achieve that measure of consensus and organization necessary for assessing the current status of the system and, in view of its deficiencies, setting realistic change goals? Who can be held responsible for articulating the plans, policies, and standards needed to accomplish these goals?

While public input to the planning process is considered appropriate, it is uncertain what form this input should take—given the need for considerable technical expertise in developing plans to effect changes in the emergency health care system. But, on the other hand, even if ombudsmen were appointed to record and analyze the public's complaints, questions, and demands, where would they go with the data? Nobody at the local, state, or Federal levels has "authority to speak for the system." Perhaps the emergency health systems specialist, a new breed of physician conversant with all aspects of emergency health care, and/or emergency medical services advisory councils springing up in communities across the nation will become catalysts for change by gaining the acceptability and authority needed to draw all of the system's components into an integrated whole.

Questions concerning the level and quality of emergency medical care will continue to press public officials and those organizations and professionals responsible for its delivery as long as consumers and their advocates are confronted with inconsistent policies and a gap between current practice and standards based upon available technology. The articles of this section point out the directions for change by identifying standards and policies proposed by medical authorities, documenting some major deficiencies, and offering practical advice and suggestions about professional and legal responsibilities. Although, in many ways, the emergency medical care arena is an ideal place for community groups concerned with health to gather for cooperative action, it is premature to predict what combination of volunteerism and public authority—Federal, state, or local—will produce the stimulus and capital to get on with the job.

19. Community-Wide Emergency Medical Services*

Recommendations by the Committee on Acute Medicine of the American Society of Anesthesiologists**

The need is urgent for improving emergency medical services (a) at the scene, (b) during transportation, and (c) in hospitals. Published standards [1-5] are either inadequate in scope or outdated in concept for the best management of acute life-threatening medical and surgical conditions. In such cases, survival often depends on the immediate application of special life-supporting measures at the scene, during trans-

* Reprinted from *Journal of the American Medical Association*, Vol. 204, No. 7, May 13, 1968.

** For periodic upgrading of these recommendations our Committee invites comments, criticisms, and reports on experiences with ambulance design, equipment and training programs.

Committee Members: Peter Safar, MD, *Chairman*, University of Pittsburgh School of Medicine; Frederick W. Cheney, Jr., MD, University of Washington School of Medicine; James O. Elam, MD, University of Chicago School of Medicine; William K. Hamilton, MD, University of California (San Francisco) School of Medicine, Stephen G. Kent, MD, Lake Charles, La; Eugene L. Nagel, MD, University of Miami (Florida) School of Medicine; Henning Pontoppidan, MD, Massachusetts General Hospital, Boston.

portation, and within the hospitals, and further depends on high standards of staffing and equipment.[6]

About 700,000 medical and surgical emergencies occur in the United States annually which result in death for the victims. Many of these deaths could be prevented by applying presently known and available techniques in resuscitation and intensive care.

Life-threatening emergencies, which may be detected even by paramedical or lay personnel, include (1) unconsciousness, (2) absence of breathing movements, (3) pulselessness, (4) respiratory insufficiency (cyanosis, labored breathing, suspected inhalation of gastric contents), (5) circulatory insufficiency (massive hemorrhage, shock, heart attack), (6) intracranial insufficiency (head injury, stroke, convulsions, delirium), (7) poisoning, (8) crushing injury of the chest, (9) multiple fractures, and (10) extensive burns.

THE FOLLOWING RECOMMENDATIONS ARE NOT MINIMAL STANDARDS, BUT RATHER ARE GOALS BASED ON TECHNIQUES THAT ARE PRESENTLY AVAILABLE. THE RECOMMENDATIONS SHOULD BE REVIEWED AND UPGRADED PERIODICALLY.

COMMUNITY-WIDE ORGANIZATION

The total emergency medical care program of a community should be evaluated, coordinated, up-graded, and supervised through appropriate "community councils," by members of the medical profession, public safety offices, and contributing agencies. Specifically, representation should include physicians from the specialties of anesthesiology, internal medicine, pediatrics, and surgery, as well as firemen, policemen, and ambulance personnel. Agencies which could provide assistance, sponsor courses, and establish guidelines for the community programs are the American Red Cross, American Heart Association, National Safety Council, public health agencies, medical schools, area hospitals, medical examiners, and those involved in community planning.

RESUSCITATION TRAINING

Recommendations of the American Heart Association[7-10] should be followed for teaching airway care, emergency artificial ventilation, and cardiopulmonary resuscitation to lay, paramedical, and medical groups. Courses in cardiopulmonary resuscitation should, in general, follow the outlines described in the American Heart Association instructors' manual.[8] Medical and paramedical instructors in cardiopulmonary resuscitation should, periodically, have their attendance at American Heart Association courses for resuscitation instructors certified. All physicians, nurses, dentists, inhalation therapists, and rescue personnel should be carefully trained in heart-lung resuscitation.[7,8,11] Training should be provided by either physicians or instructors who have had special courses in cardiopulmonary resuscitation under the organized programs of the American Heart Association.[7,11]

Until there is agreement that external cardiac compression should be taught to the general public, carefully controlled pilot projects with selected lay personnel are encouraged, to determine the feasibility and effectiveness of such programs.[711]

Tracheal intubation should be taught to medical students, physicians, and nurse anesthetists. The value and practicability of teaching tracheal intubation, intravenous infusion, and defibrillation to paramedical personnel should be studied.

TREATMENT AT THE SCENE

Participation in first aid courses for the lay public should be encouraged by means of audiovisual publicity and by having local newspapers show the value of this type of instruction in handling emergencies occurring at home or on the highways.[7,12,13]

First aid courses should become obligatory in high schools and for drivers' licensure.[6] Televised mass instruction in first aid measures (excluding external cardiac compression) should be considered. Local chapters of the American Red Cross should be encouraged to provide these classes under the guidance of physicians. Maximal use should be made of nonphysician instructors.

First aid courses should include training in airway care (backward tilt of the head, forcing mouth open, clearing pharynx, mouth-to-mouth and mouth-to-nose ventilation (preferably with manikin practice), the control of hemorrhage, immobilization of fractures, and moving the victim without compounding injuries.

Early treatment at the scene by trained ambulance and rescue personnel is of utmost importance. The physician at the scene should have authority over treatment, transportation, and choice of hospital.

TRANSPORTATION

Organization

Each ambulance service should have both a physician advisor who is experienced in emergency care and resuscitation and a paramedical supervisor. Minimal training standards and licensure of ambulance personnel should be state-wide. There should be annual inspection of equipment and vehicles.

"The driver's ability to drive and the attendant's competence in emergency care should be certified by a licensing authority. The employer should be accountable for the character and moral conduct of those whom he employs."[3]

In addition to the driver, there should be at least one, preferably two attendants with the patient in the ambulance.

Ideally, emergency transportation should be restricted to full-time licensed ambulance personnel, which has proved feasible in urban centers. In rural areas training of the presently prevalent part-time ambulance attendants should be upgraded. The training in acute medicine of paramedical technicians who would serve as helpers in emergency rooms, intensive care units, and inhalation therapy departments, and who would staff hospital-based ambulances when needed should be thoroughly investigated.

Patients with life-threatening conditions should be taken to major emergency hospitals, which should be made available on a regional basis (see VI). Those requiring resuscitation en route should be taken to the nearest hospital which has a physician on call. If it is not a major emergency hospital, the victim's vital functions should be stabilized, as much as possible, before an elective transfer to a major emergency hospital is begun, and the transfer should be made only after a safe airway has been established and ventilation and circulation have been stabilized. During transfer the patient should be attended by a person experienced in resuscitation and care of the intubated or tracheotomized patient.

Communication

"A dispatching office with an adequate communications system, a time recording device and adequate space for records should be set up. On all shifts, the dispatcher should have at least as much training as the ambulance personnel so that he can safely transmit reliable information as to the injury or illness."[3]

The central ambulance dispatching officer should be allowed to select ambulance vehicles and hospitals according to the needs of the patient.[13]

Ideally, the community should establish an "Emergency Medical Operations Center" (EMOC) for appraisal of everyday medical emergencies as well as disasters and to serve as a communications and ambulance dispatching center. It would mobilize resources outside of hospitals and direct the flow of patients. The EMOC[14] may be operated by the local public health service under the guidance of the community council. It should be coordinated with all other emergency services controlled by the local government (e.g., fire, police). The dispatching center, all ambulance and rescue vehicles, and all major emergency hospitals should be linked by two-way radiotelephone. Ambulance personnel in the field should be able to consult directly with hospital physicians via radiotelephone. The efficacy of data transmission by use of telemetry systems from the emergency scene to the physician should be explored.[15]

Training of Ambulance Attendants

Recommended Basic Training. The ideal minimal standard ambulance attendants' training course has not been worked out as yet. However, all initial and continuing education should be under the direction of a physician, and under the supervision of a paramedical instructor. The use of highly motivated personnel (nurses, practical nurses, inhalation therapists, or former medical corpsmen of the Armed Forces) for leadership roles in ambulance work should be explored.

"Driver and attendants should hold a current certificate of completion of an advanced First Aid course, given by the Red Cross, the US Bureau of Mines, the St. John's Ambulance Association or equivalent."[3]

The Red Cross first aid course is a basic requirement, but it does not constitute total adequate training. All ambulance attendants should be certified and annually recertified by a chapter of the American Heart Association, after they have completed one of AHA's courses in cardiopulmonary resuscitation. Manikin practice and periodic refresher courses can be continued under the instruction of a paramedical ambulance attendant. Attendants should demonstrate on manikins their ability to provide a patent airway in the unconscious patient, and proper positioning; artificial ventilation by the mouth-to-mouth, mouth-to-nose, and mouth-to-adjunct techniques and by use of their own equipment; insertion of an oropharyngeal tube: external cardiac compression; oxygen inhalation and suctioning with their own equipment; and positioning in shock and major injuries. They should practice with their own equipment on manikins or volunteers from the time the "patient" is first encountered and during simulated transportation. Resuscitation training should be followed by a written and practical test. Trainees should be instructed by physicians in various aspects of emergency care, including emergency childbirth and the management of patients with acute mental conditions.

Advanced Training in Hospitals. Experience suggests that work with patients in hospitals, under the supervision of nurses and physicians, is more effec-

tive than lectures for developing judgment and skills. Therefore, for the upgrading of full-time ambulance attendants' training, the feasibility of in-hospital training should be explored. The following over-all curriculum is suggested and should be evaluated and upgraded:
- High school or equivalent education; driver's license.
- American Red Cross Advanced First Aid Course.
- Instruction with rescue equipment and techniques.
- Course in human anatomy and physiology.
- American Heart Association Cardiopulmonary Resuscitation Course, including manikin practice to perfection.
- Instruction by physicians in various aspects of emergency care.
- In-hospital, preceptor-type experience consisting of the following:

    —Approximately two weeks' training with anesthesiologists in the operating room and recovery room (supervised practice on unconscious patients in airway management, artificial ventilation, oxygenation, positioning, general unconscious-patient care, checking of vital signs, restraining, etc.).

    —Approximately one week of training with nurses and inhalation therapists in the intensive care unit.

    —Approximately one week of training with physicians and nurses in the emergency room.

    —Observation of obstetric deliveries.

    —Instruction in newborn resuscitation with the use of manikins.

    —Training of professional ambulance personnel to perform tracheal intubation, electrocardiography, defibrillation, and intravenous fluid administration under the direction of physicians should be explored.
- Defensive Drivers' Course; instruction in emergency vehicle operation and radio communication.
- Patient transportation practice under physician guidance and initially under the direct supervision of paramedical instructors; with periodical interrogation sessions by physicians.
- Continuing education "on-the-job" by attendants in the field receiving advice from physicians via radiotelephone.
- Continuing education with periodic seminars and practice sessions by physicians and paramedical instructors.

Advanced Paramedical Education. College-linked paramedical technicians' courses of about two years' duration may cover many areas of acute medicine, including emergency transportation, and assisting physicians in hospitals in inhalation therapy, resuscitation, intensive care, and emergency room work.

Comment: The upgrading of ambulance personnel will have to be gradual. Although in-hospital training of full-time attendants has been initiated, training of part-time volunteer attendants must also be upgraded since a need for their services will continue in many areas. The National Academy of Sciences' Committee on Emergency Medical Services is in the process of submitting to the United Sates Public Health Service standards for an advanced training curriculum for ambulance attendants.

Physician Control of Emergency Transportation

While the trend has been to remove physicians from ambulance duties, the conditions of some patients may necessitate the attention of a physician resuscitation specialist at the scene and during transportation. Trial programs are proposed with physicians staffing specially equipped, hospital-stationed ambulances or aircraft to answer special calls, including those for the elective transfer of patients who require life-support en route from one hospital to another.

Physician-staffed ambulances may prove unfeasible because of the scarcity and resultant high value of physicians' time. Physician control of hospital-trained ambulance attendants during their field work may permit more definitive therapy by the attendant, such as defibrillation, tracheal intubation, and intravenous infusion. Thus, the possible use of two-way radio, telemetry of physiologic parameters,[15] television surveillance, and/or other communication systems in connecting ambulance attendants and physicians in hospitals should be explored. The physician giving remote supervision should be experienced in resuscitation and emergency care.

Transportation by Air

The use of helicopters or aircraft for the transport of acutely ill and injured patients from isolated or otherwise inaccessible sites (e.g., traffic congestion) and from smaller hospitals to major emergency hospitals should be developed. Heliports should be established, at least at the major emergency hospitals. Helicopter ambulances and aircraft for patient transportation should have the same equipment and comparable interior dimensions as those listed below for regular ambulances.

Design and Equipment of Emergency Ambulances

An emergency ambulance is for transport with life support of one or more patients on stretchers. The emergency ambulance should have sufficient storage space for equipment used by attendants and physicians. The general features include:

(1) Separate (?) driver and patient compartments with communication between the two.
(2) Illumination adequate for medical treatment.
(3) Temperature control of patient area.
(4) Two-way radio capable of clear transmission and reception over the entire community service area, among vehicles, dispatching center, and hospitals.
(5) Warning devices acceptable to state or local statute.

(6) Smooth riding characteristics.

Most vehicles presently in use are unsatisfactory for life support. The following specifications for improved design and equipment are recommended for field trial and should merely be considered as the first step toward further modification and improvement. They are based on present knowledge and existing recommendations.[2,7,16-18] Design and equipment should permit treatment of the patient during transportation including resuscitation of at least one patient, with the operator kneeling or sitting.

Internal dimensions of patient compartment for kneeling or sitting attendant.

Minimum height: 54 in (135 cm)
Minimum width: 72 in (180 cm)
Minimum length: 110 in (275 cm)

Minimum space between head of stretcher and partition is 25 in (62 cm), including seat for operator who sits at the patient's vertex for respiratory resuscitation and airway care.

Minimum space along one side of main stretcher is 25 in (62 cm) to provide space for the feet of the operator, who kneels while performing external cardiac compression or other functions.

Stretcher. The dimensions of the stretcher must allow the patient to lie at full length in the supine, prone, or lateral position. The bottom of the stretcher should be firm for external cardiac compression. In addition, a chest board, which in raising the patient's shoulders makes his head assume a backward tilted position without manual support, is desirable.

The head of the stretcher should be capable of being tilted upward to 60°. The entire stretcher frame should be capable of being tilted to 15° head down position (e.g., airway care).

The sides should be capable of stabilizing the patient in any position. There should be straps to hold the patient.

The stretcher should be equipped with a pole for supporting intravenous infusion bottles and a support for a portable oxygen cylinder.

Stretcher fasteners should be capable of securing the stretcher in any of the above positions during transport. Attachments to the frame of the vehicle should follow seat-belt requirements. There should be a safety-belt attached to the frame.

The stretcher must be light, sturdy, easy to carry, provided with wheels, and easy to load into and remove from the ambulance.

In addition to the main stretcher there should be at least one collapsible portable stretcher of the chair type (capable of being elevated at the head) for transport in narrow spaces, e.g., on staircases.

Suction. There should be one suction for stationary use in the ambulance and an additional portable one for use outside the ambulance.

The suction in the ambulance should be powerful, preferably providing a flow of over 30 liters per minute at the end of a delivery tube to which the suction tip or catheter is connected and a vacuum of -300 mm Hg (12 in of mercury) or more when the delivery tube is clamped. This powerful suction required for adequate pharyngeal clearing can be obtained from the ambulance engine manifold or from an electric motor, but usually not from a venturi type oxygen suction device. Additional features include:

a) Suction delivery tube sufficiently long to reach the airways of all patients (optionally, a second delivery tube long enough to reach to the ground outside the ambulance in the case of multiple casualties).

b) Delivery tube—thick walled, nonkinkable, but easily pinchable by hand.

Community-Wide Emergency Services 453

c) Collection bottle, preferably nonbreakable.

d) Pharyngeal (tonsil) suction tubes, metal or plastic (in clean towel) to fit delivery tube.

e) Suction catheters of various sizes (French 8-18, 3-6 mm o.d.) for nasal and tracheal suctioning, sterile, wrapped, with one Y or T piece to permit insertion of catheter without suction.

f) Bottle with water for rinsing (sterile for tracheal suctioning).

Oxygen equipment. Ample supply of oxygen, (3,000 liters) at 50 psi pressure (e.g., M, G, or H cylinder) with reducing valve, pressure gauge, flow meter, and delivery tube.

One portable cylinder for use outside the ambulance, with second small cylinder as spare (300 liters each) with pressure gauge, needle valve, flow meter, and delivery tube.

Oxygen tube connectors interchangeable for all stationary and portable inhalation and ventilation devices used.

Oxygen humidifier (heated nebulizer for long trips with intubated patient)—optional.

Oxygen bag-mask or oxygen mask, transparent, semi-open, valveless for O_2 inhalation, to be used with oxygen flow rates of about 10 liters per minute; one attached to stationary oxygen source (e.g., wall outlet), one for portable oxygen unit, others spare.

As an alternative, an oxygen demand (inhalator) unit is acceptable. A demand valve should be highly sensitive and flow rates should follow the patient's demand, even during dyspneic breathing, without excessive airway pressure fluctuations.

Resuscitation Equipment:

Artificial Ventilation Devices: Hand-operated self-refilling bag-valve-mask units, one for use inside and one for use outside the ambulance, are recommended. Face masks (preferably transparent) of adult and child/infant sizes with head strap should be available. The bag-valve-mask unit should be for use with air and for administration of oxygen. The highest possible oxygen concentration should be provided by attaching a reservoir tube to the intake valve, at least for the unit used in the ambulance. The nonrebreathing valve should permit oxygen inhalation from the bag, not only during positive pressure ventilation but also during spontaneous breathing.

Another example of an approved artificial ventilation unit is an oxygen-powered hand-triggered device. This should be able to deliver instantaneous flow rates of 1 to 2 liters per second for adults (lower flow rates for infants and small children). A safety valve release of 50 cm H_2O for adults (30 cm H_2O for children) should be provided. A manual override in case more than 50 cm H_2O pressure is needed to ventilate the patient is recommended, for use by physicians only.

Automatic pressure-cycled oxygen resuscitators are *not* recommended.

All ventilation units should have standard tracheal tube (15 mm female) and mask (22 mm male) connectors. The units should be made of material which can be sterilized.

Airways: Regular Guedel type oropharyngeal airways in adult, child, and infant sizes should be provided for use under the mask. In addition, mouth-to-mouth airways (S-tubes) in large (adult/child) and small (child/infant) sizes should be available.

Tongue blades are used to assist in insertion of pharyngeal tubes, and three blades taped together and padded are used to protect the tongue in convulsions.

A chest board (about 22 in long and 19 in wide)

should be available to be placed under the patient for external cardiac compression. It should preferably be shaped to raise the shoulders about 4 in above the level of the stretcher, thus maintaining the patient's head in a maximally backward tilted position.

The use of external cardiac compression machines is not preferred over the use of the manual method at the present time. The comparative efficacy of these machines during transport situations should be evaluated.

Splints. For exact dimensions, see American College of Surgeons *Bulletin,* May/June 1967.

Thomas splint (hinged, half ring, lower extremity splint with webbing ankle hitch).

Padded boards 4½ ft long for splinting of leg.

Splint 15 in long for fractures of forearm.

Long and short spine boards with recommended straps, tapes, head band, chin strap, and neck roll; and appropriately placed holds and strap holes.

Triangular bandages, at least 12.

Timmens splint for leg or thigh.

Inflatable splints.

Miscellaneous. Sterile gauze dressings, gauze pads, roller bandages, and adhesive tape. For hemostasis, pressure dressings and tourniquet. Pillows, short sandbags, long sandbags, emesis basin, Kleenex, bedpan, urinal, sheets, blankets, pillowcases, towels, thermometer, flashlight, stethoscope, a sterile kit for obstetrical delivery (including cotton dressings, absorbent cellulose, disposable gloves, towels, clamps, scissors, and umbilical tape).

Blood pressure cuff with aneroid manometer is optional.

Equipment for Use by Physicians. Special ambulances, for instance hospital-stationed ones, should have additional equipment needed by physicians for more definitive therapy. Equipment should be disposable or easy to sterilize.

(a) Tracheal intubation equipment (oro- and nasotracheal tubes for adults, children, and infants; sterile, equipped with 15 mm adaptors; adult tubes cuffed; laryngoscope handle with adult, child, and infant size blades; stylette; bit block; cuff inflation syringe and clamp; anesthetic lubricating jelly; appropriate adaptors; gastric tube; forceps for insertion of nasotracheal tube and gastric tube).

(b) Nasopharyngeal tubes.

(c) Cricothyrotome.

(d) Drugs, syringes, needles for definitive therapy in cardiopulmonary resuscitation as recommended by the American Heart Association ERT Manual.[9]

(e) Pleural drainage set (trocars, catheters, and Heimlich valves), sterile.

(f) Minor surgical tray for hemostasis, sterile (including one scalpel with #10 blade; three hemostats, small, straight; needle holder; one toothed forcep; three silk sutures with needles 00; 4 × 4 gauzes); Vaseline gauze pack for open chest wounds; roller gauzes; sterile gloves.

(g) Aerosol nebulizer, mouthpiece, and bronchodilator for spontaneous inhalation and use with positive-pressure equipment.

Items (a) through (g) may be carried in an "emergency kit for physicians."

(h) Intravenous infusion equipment (administration sets, stopcocks, venotubes, needles, catheter needles, tape, tourniquet) and blood substitutes (several units of 5% dextrose in isotonic saline solution or Ringer's solution and 5% albumin or dextran 75, preferably in plastic bags).

(i) Defibrillation/monitor/pacer unit or units (preferably portable, battery powered, rechargeable).

Optional:
(a) Tracheotomy tray (all sizes of tubes with 15 mm male adaptors; adult tubes cuffed).
(b) Automatic ventilator for transport of intubated patient.

Equipment for Transportation of Infants. Neonates should be transported in clean isolettes which permit oxygen enrichment, humidity and body temperature control. The baby's head should be accessible for resuscitation. There should be ventilation and tracheal intubation equipment for use by trained personnel.

Comment: The National Academy of Sciences' Committee on Emergency Medical Services is in the process of submitting to the Department of Transportation medical standards for ambulance design and equipment which incorporate most of the above recommendations.

HOSPITAL FACILITIES

Categorization and Regionalization of Hospitals

In view of the required team of specialists and the high standards of over-all hospital facilities needed for the management of life-threatening conditions, emergency services should be centralized. Hospitals should be categorized according to their emergency-care and intensive-care facilities, perhaps through regional, self-policing community councils on emergency medical services.

The following recommendations are made for total hospital facilities since emergency departments depend on backup facilities of a general hospital.[6,13,19,20] One way of categorizing hospitals is as follows[19]:

Type 1: The *First Aid Facility* does not have a physician present at all times.

Type 2: The *Emergency Hospital* is staffed around-the-clock by a physician, but not by a team of specialists and lacks the sophisticated backup facilities of a Type 3 hospital.

Type 3: The *Major Emergency Hospital* is staffed around-the-clock by a team of specialists available within minutes and will conform to the highest standards hospital-wide and particularly in emergency rooms, resuscitation services, coronary surveillance, and respiratory and general intensive-care facilities. Type 3 hospitals should be established on a regional basis and receive most patients with life-threatening emergencies (see I and V). Non-life-threatening emergencies may be taken to any hospital with an emergency room.

Special cases such as obstetric, ophthalmic, or neurologic emergencies should be directed to previously identified *specialized hospitals* or the best facilities to care for such patients in a community. These special hospitals should also fulfill the criteria of Type 3 hospitals as they apply to their special fields.

Since coronary disease is recognized as the principal cause of sudden death, a patient suspected of having a myocardial infarction should be admitted as an emergency to the nearest hospital which provides continuous surveillance with arrhythmia control and intensive care.[13]

Patients requiring prolonged artificial ventilation should be admitted to respiratory intensive care units, which should be provided on a regional basis.

The value of intensive-care units for newborn infants should be explored. Such units should provide for sophisticated respiratory care, fluid, glucose, and acid-base balance, and control of infection.

Emergency Rooms of Type 2 and 3 Hospitals

Basic requirements are those recommended by the American College of Surgeons.[4]

Organization and Staffing. The emergency room should be located on the ground floor of the hospital, easily accessible from the main hospital. Equipment should be of the same quality as provided throughout the hospital. Textbooks, printed rules and regulations, and a poison manual should be available. A poison control chart and the telephone number of the nearest poison control center should be displayed.[4]

Policy should be established by an emergency room committee representing the major medical services, hospital administration, and nursing.[4] One physician, as the director, should be responsible to the committee for implementation of policies and supervision of professional services.

The emergency room should be open 24 hours a day. At least one primary physician should be assigned to the emergency room at all times. Another physician should be on second call. Specialists should be obtainable as promptly as possible, when needed. Every patient presenting himself for treatment should be seen by a physician within 15 minutes; resuscitation cases should be seen immediately.

Nursing staff in the emergency room should consist of at least one registered nurse and one nurse's aide present at all times. Additional nursing personnel should be available in case of need.

Every patient should have a record. Periodic review of records, death, and resuscitation procedures should be made.

Operations requiring general anesthesia or major regional anesthesia should be performed in the operating suite. Resuscitative anesthesia and operations, however, may be performed in the emergency department when necessary.

Equipment. Resuscitation equipment available in the emergency room should not be used for other areas of the hospital. Recommended equipment includes the following [4,9]:

- Wall oxygen outlets (or two large mobile oxygen cylinders on carts, with reducing valves), flow meters and delivery tubes.
- Two self-refilling bag-valve-mask units with oxygen reservoir tubings.
- Oropharyngeal and nasopharyngeal airways of various sizes.
- Suction equipment as outlined in the ambulance (see V, F).
- Tracheal intubation kit[9] including equipment for gastric intubation.
- Emergency drug kit.[9]
- Injection/infusion kit[9] including needles, syringes, catheter needles, stopcocks, venotubes, administration sets, blood substitutes (e.g., dextran 75 or 5% albumin, dextran 40, isotonic saline solution, dextrose in Ringer's solution), blood (type O, Rh negative—refrigerated), blood warmer, equipment for infusion under pressure.
- Venous cut-down tray.
- Separate crash cart[9] with electrocardioscope (needle and disc electrodes), external/internal defibrillator with appropriate electrodes and battery-powered pacemaker.
- Electrocardiograph.
- Tracheotomy tray (all sizes of tube, with 15 mm male adaptors; adult tubes cuffed).
- Thoracotomy tray for open chest resuscitation.[2]
- Pleural drainage tray (with trocars and catheters of various sizes; Heimlich valves or water seal drainage bottles).
- Equipment for central venous catheterization.
- Equipment for arterial puncture and catheterization.[9]
- Tray for nerve blocks and local anesthesia.
- Trays for minor surgery (hemostasis, etc.).
- Ventilating bronchoscope (all sizes, available in hospital).
- Blood pressure cuffs and stethoscopes.
- Mechanical ventilator capable of producing assisted and controlled intermittent positive pressure ventilation with 100% oxygen, drug aerosols and heated mist, with airway pressures and tidal volumes readable.

All equipment should be suitable for adults, children, and infants. Respiratory equipment must have standard 15 mm tracheal tube and 22 mm mask connectors.

Equipment should be checked daily by responsible personnel.

General Backup Services of Type 3 Hospital

General backup services should be available on a 24-hour basis and include:

(1) Blood typing and cross matching, available within minutes.

(2) Roentgen and laboratory services within minutes by appropriate technicians, with medical consultation available in these specialties.

(3) Operating room services available within five minutes.

(4) Anesthesia services by a department of anesthesiology under the direction of an anesthesiologist. Ideally there should be an anesthesiologist in the hospital 24 hours a day.

(5) Personnel trained and experienced in resuscitation including tracheal intubation and curarization, in the hospital 24 hours per day.

(6) A cardiopulmonary resuscitation team serving the entire hospital including the emergency room, available 24 hours a day.[9]

(7) A multidiscipline approach in the management of seriously ill patients including the ability to mobilize within minutes specialists (attending staff or house staff backed up by attending staff) of anesthesiology, cardiology, internal medicine, neurosurgery, obstetrics, orthopedics, pediatrics, surgery, and thoracic surgery.

(8) Respiratory evaluation (including simple spi-

rometry and arterial pCO_2, pO_2 and pH determinations) and respiratory care (see intensive care, VI, D).

(9) Pacemaker insertion and countershocking for arrhythmias.

(10) A physician available within minutes capable of acting as triage officer in case of a disaster.

Intensive-Care Facilities of Type 3 Hospital

Organization. Intensive care is life-support and/or surveillance by specialized nurses and physicians of patients with actual or threatening respiratory, circulatory, or intracranial insufficiency. The concentration of all patients for whom these measures may be life-saving in an intensive care unit (ICU) has been widely accepted.[6,13,20-22]

Intensive care includes general intensive care, respiratory care, postoperative care, and coronary surveillance. Geographic connections and functional links between all intensive-care areas and the emergency room are desirable.

A common interdisciplinary intensive-care unit adjacent to a coronary surveillance unit has advantages over departmentalized, fragmented intensive-care facilities.

The development of intensive care should follow these steps:

(1) Organization (intensive care committee, medical director or supervisor, head nurse).
(2) Physical facility.
(3) Coverage by nurses.
(4) Coverage by physicians.
(5) Clinical research (optional).

Intensive care units in major emergency hospitals should be staffed 24 hours a day by specially experienced nurses and physicians. These personnel at any

time of the day or night should immediately be able to provide:
- Cardiopulmonary resuscitation.
- Respiratory care, including tracheal intubation; prolonged artificial ventilation; aseptic, atraumatic care of the intubated patient; tracheotomy; PaO_2, $PaCO_2$, pHa control.
- Temperature control.
- Arrythmia control.
- Treatment of "shock" including central venous and arterial catheterizations (for blood gas control and pressure monitoring).

The smooth functioning of an ICU depends on organization, well-defined responsibilities and authorities, and standardization of certain procedures.

An intensive care unit committee should establish and enforce safe policies and routines. This committee usually consists of representatives of anesthesiology, medicine, pediatrics, surgery, administration, and nursing. Ideally, the chairman of the ICU committee should be the medical director or supervisor of the unit and should be selected on the basis of responsibility, interest, availability, and competence in resuscitation and intensive care, rather than on the basis of specialty affiliation. He should be responsible for the implementation of ICU policies, administration, and teaching in the unit.

The ICU policy should clearly spell out responsibilities for medical care. These will depend on local circumstances. In specialized units (e.g., coronary care, respiratory care) it may be possible for every patient admitted to the unit to be transferred to the service of the ICU supervisor and his house staff, with the admitting physician becoming the consultant. In multidiscipline units the admitting physician usually remains in charge of his patient's general care. Respiratory care and resuscitation for all patients should be managed or guided by one service which can provide this coverage around-the-clock. The admitting physician may delegate responsibility for his patient's general care to the ICU supervisor's staff or to any other physician.

The ICU policy should include nursing coverage and training, infection control, and standardization of certain procedures (e.g., care of the intubated or tracheotomized patient, prolonged artificial ventilation, hypothermia monitoring).

Monitoring techniques are in a state of clinical appraisal. They should not distract nurses away from bedsides. Parameters, which should be monitored continuously, should be displayed at the bedside. Another set of displays and alarms should be at the nursing station (at least for the patients in enclosed cubicles). Resuscitation equipment in the ICU should be more sophisticated and more complete than in any other area of the hospital.[9]

Coronary surveillance[13,20,22] should be done in a quiet area. Patients with coronary conditions, therefore, should be admitted to a general open ICU facility only if the resuscitation and respiratory care are required (e.g., shock, pulmonary edema). In large hospitals, a separate coronary surveillance unit is indicated, and should be located as close as possible to the general ICU. The coronary surveillance unit is usually supervised by a cardiologist. In small hospitals a combined ICU and coronary surveillance unit of several single-bed cubicles is more practical, as it offers interchangeability and better staffing. Here a single medical supervisor for the combined unit would be adequate.

Staffing by Nurses. Nursing personnel should be especially assigned to intensive care without additional duties outside the unit. ICU nurses should be under the direction of a head nurse who is professionally responsible to the ICU medical supervisor and administratively responsible to the director of nursing.

ICU nurses should receive continuing education in cardiopulmonary resuscitation (American Heart Association instructors' course), respiratory care, general intensive care, postoperative care, and arrhythmia recognition and control. ICU nurses should be permitted to perform defibrillation and to administer drugs (as pre-ordered by physicians), if necessary, prior to the arrival of the physician.

Staffing by Physicians. Medical students and physicians in training in all clinical disciplines should have intensive-care experience. Intensive-care units should have 24-hour coverage by physicians who know all patients in the ICU and who are not occupied by other duties. These physicians should be experienced in resuscitation and respiratory care (including tracheal intubation and mechanical artificial ventilation) and may also function as leaders in hospital-wide resuscitation attempts.[9] These could be staff men or experienced residents in anesthesiology, medicine, surgery, or pediatrics. Ideally, they should work under the guidance of the ICU medical supervisor. Admitting physicians should make rounds to see their patients with the ICU physician on call.

Physicians experienced in acute medicine, who can act as part-time or full-time supervisors of intensive-care and resuscitation programs in hospitals and organize and teach in community-wide resuscitation programs are required.[6,13,20,21] These physicians may come from any specialty, providing they have been trained and are experienced in resuscitation, respiratory care, arrhythmia control, and treatment of shock. Interested and qualified anesthesiologists have the background for further training in acute medicine and for the role of ICU supervisor.

REFERENCES

1. Highway Safety Program Standards 4.4.11 Emergency Medical Services, US Department of Transportation: Washington, DC, June, 1967.
2. Minimal Equipment for Ambulances, *Bull Amer Coll Surg* 52:92–96 (March-April) 1967.
3. Standards for Emergency Ambulance Services, American College of Surgeons' Committee on Trauma, *Bull Amer Coll Surg* 52:131–132 (May-June) 1967.
4. Standards for Emergency Department in Hospitals, American College of Surgeons' Committee on Trauma, *Bull Amer Coll Surg* 48:112-125 (May-June) 1963.
5. *First Aid Textbook,* ed. 4, American National Red Cross, Garden City, NY: Doubleday & Co., Inc., 1957.
6. Safar, P.: "Community-Wide Emergency Care for Acutely Life-Threatening Conditions," in Wulff, H. B. (ed.): *Proceedings of the Second Congress of the International Association for Accident and Traffic Medicine,* Aug 9–12, 1966.
7. Cardiopulmonary Resuscitation, American Heart Association/National Academy of Sciences/National Research Council, *JAMA* 198:372-379 (Oct. 24) 1966.
8. *Cardiopulmonary Resuscitation, A Manual for Instructors* (EM 408), Committee on Cardiopulmonary Resuscitation of the American Heart Association, New York: American Heart Association, 1967.
9. *Emergency Resuscitation Team Manual: A Hospital Plan* (EM 439), Committee on Cardiopulmonary Resuscitation of the American Heart Association, New York: American Heart Association, 1968.
10. Cardiopulmonary Resuscitation, in National Academy of Sciences/National Research Council: *Proceedings of Ad Hoc Committee Conference,* May 1966.
11. Winchell, S. W., and Safar, P.: Teaching and Testing Lay and Paramedical Personnel in Cardiopulmonary Resuscitation, *Current Researches in Anesthesia & Analgesia* 45:441–449 (July-August) 1966.

12. International Symposium on Emergency Resuscitation, Stavanger, Norway, 1961, *Acta Anaesth Scand,* Suppl. 9, 1961, p. 203.
13. International Symposium on Emergency Resuscitation, Oslo, Norway, 1967, *Acta Anaesth Scand,* Suppl. 29, 1968, pp. 1-384.
14. Jackson, F., and Kennemer, C.E. (eds.): *The Role of Medicine in Emergency Preparedness,* US Public Health Service—Department of Health, Education and Welfare, Division of Health Mobilization, Washington, DC, to be published.
15. Nagel, E. L., et al.: Physiological Telemetry System for Fire and Rescue Personnel, *Southern Med J,* to be published.
16. *Report on Accident and Emergency Services,* Copenhagen: Special Committee of the Danish National Health Service, October 1966.
17. Safar, P., and Brose, R.: Ambulance Design and Equipment for Resuscitation, *Arch Surg* 90:343-348 (March) 1965.
18. Gowings, D. (ed.): *Ambulance Attendant Training Manual,* Harrisburg, Pa., Department of Health, 1964.
19. Accidental Death and Disability, Washington, DC: National Academy of Sciences/National Research Council, September 1966.
20. Safar, P.: "Intensive Care Unit Organization," in Safar, P. (ed.): *Respiratory Therapy,* Philadelphia: F. A. Davis Co., 1965, Chapter 15, pp. 361-373.
21. Workshop on Intensive Care Units (Hamilton, W. K., Chairman), National Academy of Sciences/National Research Council, *Anesthesiology* 25:192-222 (March-April) 1964.
22. Coronary Care Units, Public Health Service Publication No. 1520, Washington, DC: United States Public Health Service, October 1964.

20. Survey Discovers What Is Wrong With Hospitals' Emergency Service*

J. Cuthbert Owens, M.D.

Findings from a survey of emergency departments in 72 general hospitals in Colorado, conducted over a two-year period, suggest how many problems exist in emergency care in the United States.

Any survey, especially if it is an incomplete study of an area, will find both good and bad organization in some of the institutions. This report would confirm this, since comments have been chiefly on the negative aspects and of an obviously critical nature in an attempt to stress the need to improve the quality of emergency medical care.

The largest hospital surveyed had 475 beds, the smallest had 14 beds. Seventy-one percent (51) of the hospitals had less than 100 beds, 53 percent (38) had less than 50 beds, and 42 percent (30) had less than 35 beds. Forty-four of the hospitals had only general practitioners on the staff, 18 had interns and/or residents, 18 had complete coverage by all types of specialists, and 10 had partial specialty coverage.

*Reprinted from *The Modern Hospital,* Vol. 106, No. 1, January 1966.

In 66 of the hospitals 179,152 emergency patients had been seen in 1958. However, by 1963 the yearly total had risen more than 70 percent to 314,810 patients.

Many judgmental factors are involved in deciding what is an emergency case. The average percentage of patients considered to be true emergencies was reported to be 64 percent, the smaller hospitals having a higher average percentage (70) than the larger ones (40). After reviewing the records, however, the survey team felt that the number of cases that were interpreted as true emergencies was too low.

Demonstrating a measure of the emergency department's importance is the fact that in 14 of the 34 hospitals where both admission and emergency statistics were obtained, more patients were seen in the emergency department than were admitted to the hospital.

Chief sources of information were the administrator, nurses, and—in about one-third of the hospitals—one or more doctors who were present during the interview. Often a staff doctor was contacted later regarding the findings. All hospitals cooperated in the study, as emergency room weaknesses were frankly admitted to the survey team, and advice was welcomed.

Early in the surveys, during the team's visit to one of these hospitals, an administrator stated "Isn't it a shame that with all our present knowledge and equipment to save lives and decrease morbidity we don't take advantage of it?" The thought stayed with the team during the two years of the study.

As the survey team approached the various hospitals, when making its unannounced visits, it was notable that directional signs were seldom adequate. Only six signs were suitably placed with the distance to the hospital indicated.

Since the survey, the state highway department has posted hospital signs in and outside all but the three largest communities. However, throughway exits continue to lack information regarding the availability of emergency medical care, and too few existing signs indicate mileage distance.

At the hospitals themselves, it was found that 10 had no identifying signs at all and 13 had no signs denoting the emergency entrance. Only eight had lighted signs.

Inadequacies in emergency department facilities were generally noted during the survey. Eighteen were considered too small or too antiquated to handle emergency medical care, and in these the level of care was rated as little more than first aid.

However, a 19-bed hospital was rated as one of the finest in providing initial emergency care. Its medical staff does a daily critique on first aid given to emergency cases.

Separate examining rooms for nonemergent patients should be available in every hospital, regardless of size. However, only 19 of the 72 hospitals surveyed had separate examination rooms for nonemergencies. The larger hospitals utilized the outpatient clinic as an adjunct to the emergency department during the peak load after 5 p.m.

A large number of hospitals had no waiting room space containing telephone, toilet, and drinking fountain apart from the working areas of the emergency department.

Many hospitals failed to consider as essential either a wide entranceway to the emergency department or weather doors. Some hospitals provided no marquee at the emergency entrance, for protection from the weather, and inadequate ambulance turn-around space was common.

Poor location of the emergency department was observed in 15 hospitals and in five small hospitals the operating room was used daily as an emergency room.

Twenty-three hospitals were rated as having inadequate emergency equipment and supplies. They were lacking such items as necessary medications, airways, tracheostomy tubes, positive pressure breathing apparatus, defibrillators, and suction machines. Excellent equipment was immediately available in 22 hospitals. In the remaining hospitals the equipment was available but it was kept in other areas such as central supply, operating room, and storage areas.

In an emergency facility, all supplies and equipment should be ready at a moment's notice. Borrowing equipment from the emergency unit never should be permitted, even when duplication of equipment is necessary.

Some of the smaller hospitals lacked certain pieces of equipment they considered too expensive. However, one emergency room in a 39-bed hospital had a defibrillator made by its own personnel at a cost of $40.

The stretcher or examining table should be freely movable to limit the number of times the patient is moved. A patient with a compound fracture may be moved 10 times before diagnostic procedures and treatment are completed. More than two-thirds of the hospitals surveyed overlooked this completely.

Departmental policies should be formulated, put in writing, and executed by the emergency department committee, which should represent the major medical services, hospital administration, and nursing services.

Thirteen hospitals had an emergency department committee but only two of these had the nurse regularly assigned to the department as a committee member. Sometimes, members assigned to the committee had seldom been seen in the department.

Only 12 hospitals exhibited manuals which described the policies and functions of the department. This resulted in haphazard indoctrination when substitute nurses or new employees were required, as well as the tendency for both medical and paramedical personnel to set up their own rules.

The nurse is obviously a vital person in the emergency service. Her decisions must be rapid, she must be able to screen patients, and she must possess knowledge not only of how to assist in all types of emergency care but also how to deal with human beings under stress.

The survey found that indoctrination of nursing personnel was woefully lacking in the majority of hospital emergency units.

Training of nurses in emergency procedures was scanty, and on many occasions was discouraged in the absence of a physician. Some of the nurses queried stated that no nurse should undertake emergency care on her own, contrary to the lay viewpoint concerning policemen, firemen, public service employees, and similar occupations. (The Colorado Nursing Association published an article in its *State Journal* in May 1964, advising all nurses to learn external cardiac resuscitation.)

Few nurses had emergency room training during nursing school and many never had seen a well-organized emergency room. Many lacked knowledge of how to assist the physician in specific types of emergencies or mass casualty care.

Serious study should be directed toward encouraging nurses to add procedures for direct care of the patient to their duties in assisting the doctor, whether he is present or not available. If this void in emergency care is not corrected by allowing nurses to have greater responsibilities in the direct care of the patient, then another type of individual needs to be developed and added to the medical field.

Graduate courses for nurses in emergency care management would be highly desirable.

One emergency department with five rooms had only one nurse in attendance and a census of 1,000 patients per month, or an average of one every 40 minutes.

The survey revealed that nurses wanted to know how to do a better job, and the survey itself helped to stimulate the formation of the Emergency Room Nurses' Association in Denver, which now has some 50 members.

Medical staff coverage of the emergency department should be such that a patient is seen by a doctor within 15 minutes after arrival. A physician should be available on second call if unexpected or unusual situations arise.

Many hospitals provided offices for doctors in or adjacent to the building, apparently following a national trend. When the offices were open, they not only relieved the large census of nonemergencies but also assisted the emergency department, since the doctor on rotation duty could report within 15 minutes.

Every conceivable type of doctors' call system was used in the hospitals surveyed. No system was found to have consistently good coverage for emergency patient care unless a doctor was at the hospital on call.

Short of full-time salaried physicians working in some emergency departments the best systems noted were: (1) in a 350-bed hospital with complete specialty coverage and with only interns on the house staff, 70 general practitioners rotated call in the hospital from

5 p.m. to 8 a.m.; (2) in a 200-bed hospital with complete specialty coverage but with no interns or residents on the house staff, 50 general practitioners rotated call at the hospital on a 24 hour basis; and (3) in a small hospital all doctors had radio communication with the hospital.

Several administrators requested assistance with the problem of physicians refusing to see patients in the emergency room, or being difficult to locate when urgently needed. Hazardous situations were reported because of lack of cooperation among certain members of the profession.

Some mechanism should be available whereby specialty services can be obtained if needed, for the survey found that 32 of the 44 hospitals with no staff specialists were 50 to 200 miles from a specialty consultation. One city was 263 miles, over two mountain ranges, from a neurologist or neurosurgeon. Neither of these specialties was available, other than on a visiting basis, to any hospital in the western half of the state.

Although specialty coverage may be difficult because of distances involved, in the interest of better patient care the specialty fields should investigate methods of improving the present situation. Movement of critical patients from one hospital to another is a serious hazard which should be eliminated.

In contrast to the problem of obtaining specialty coverage, the survey team found that in the larger hospitals specialties—internists, pediatricians, and psychiatrists—heretofore not frequently identified with the emergency unit, have become interested in utilizing observation beds and in the availability of emergency equipment. In one large emergency unit, a psychiatrist and psychiatric social worker were assigned full-time to handle psychiatric problems either as a primary or secondary cause. The census for psychiatry increased from 25 patients to 200 patients per month.

If adequate staffing and facilities are to be provided in the emergency department, the economics of its operation must be considered. For its emergency services the hospital must make a charge, not to make a profit but to be sure costs balance services rendered.

At several large hospitals, where the emergency department was not in the red, the opinion was expressed that departments with 500 or more patients a year should not have a deficit if good business practices were employed.

Although the survey only superficially evaluated economics, a high percentage of deficiencies were noted. Seldom did a hospital include in its emergency department financial records collections from x-ray and laboratory procedures done on emergency patients, even though one-third of the patients had x-rays taken and almost one-half had some lab procedures performed.

In a few hospitals no master record book was available to record the number of patients seen, the length of time they were present, the type of complaints, and the treatment given. Some hospitals had no accurate statistics.

Under such circumstances, it seemed inconceivable that any knowledge of the actual budget necessary to operate the unit could be available, but the administrator invariably stated that it ran at a deficit.

A concern for public relations was reflected in charging practices. No charge was made in 13 hospitals and in 11, charges ranged from $1 to $7.50. One small, poorly equipped, and undermanned hospital attempted to discourage patients from being seen in the emergency room by charging $7, but dropped the fee to $3 when it couldn't collect.

Complaints were reported about emergency room charges although administrators invariably stated that the fees are a many-sided necessity. Patients complained about "double jeopardy" when they had to pay both a doctor's fee plus the emergency department charge when meeting their physician in the emergency room for his convenience.

In one hospital, a sign indicating a $3 charge had been torn down by doctors on eight occasions. This feeling was not observed among most physicians in other communities although some felt the emergency room was a community responsibility as were ambulances, heart pump, and so forth. There was no argument against the hospital receiving a just financial return but there were many instances where the charge was abused by not providing a "courtesy" space for a doctor to see a nonemergent patient he had asked to meet him at the emergency department.

If the level of hospitals' emergency care is to be improved, there must be a frank appraisal of present care and facilities, an open admission of deficiencies, desire for improvement, and dissemination of advice and guidelines.

Hospitals need the help of medical societies, hospital associations, medical schools, and other organizations concerned with emergency care. Such guidance should include all emergency medical services: hospital, ambulance, first aid, and rescue units, all of which are parallel adjuncts needing coordination.

As a result of this and other surveys, a number of events have occurred in Colorado. Ways to provide first aid training for emergency room personnel are being studied. Ambulance construction and method of use are being evaluated. Plans are under way to provide supervision and training for ambulance crewmen. Some hospitals have employed architects to correct physical deficiencies in emergency room construction plans. Administrators are seeking and obtaining aid in combating emergency department problems which result in poor public relations, economic waste, and inadequate personnel coverage. Physicians and nurses are requesting information on newly available equipment and newly perfected procedures used in handling emergency problems.

The Colorado Department of Health has recently published new standards for the emergency department, medical societies are studying means of improving emergency medical care, and both nursing and medical educators are adding courses and training in emergency medical care to the curriculums.

All the facilities, techniques, and systems required to save lives are available, and what is needed is to put them all together and make them work.

All general hospitals, large or small, should at least have personnel and facilities to handle emergencies initially, and then seek specialized care as needed.

21. Moonlighting Policy: The Hospital Proposes but the Chief Disposes*

Resident Physician

High stipends may come and low stipends may go, but moonlighting (apparently) will go on forever. . . .

At least, as was pointed out in the last issue, *Resident Physician's* survey findings show that moonlighting is not necessarily a result of low stipends nor is it necessarily eliminated by high stipends. In fact, a further look at the survey results reveals that there are other factors which exert a stronger influence on moonlighting than stipends. One of these, as might be expected, is hospital policy; another, the chief of service's policy.

One of the questions in *Resident Physician's* questionnaire asked house staff to indicate their hospital's official policy on moonlighting. And, one of the surprises revealed by the survey is that hospital "type" seems to have little to do with hospital policy when it comes to moonlighting.

A little more than half of the interns and residents polled—*regardless of whether they were in university hospitals, city, county or state hospitals, voluntary*

*Reprinted from *Resident Physician*, Vol. 13, March 1967. Third in a series based on a survey of more than 2,000 interns, residents, chiefs, and directors of medical education.

Table 1
HOSPITAL POLICY AND THE MOONLIGHTING RATE AMONG RESIDENTS

Hospital Policy on Moonlighting	Total Residents No.	%	Moonlighting Residents No.	Moonlighting Rate %
PROHIBITS	635	57.2	181	28.5
Enforces ban	(229	38.4)*	(22)	(9.6)
Does **not** enforce ban	(367	61.6)*	(154)	(42.0)
DISCOURAGES	212	19.1	93	43.9
DON'T KNOW	177	15.9	39	22.0
HAS NO POLICY	44	4.0	13	29.5
OTHER**	41	3.7	17	41.5
NO ANSWER	1	0.1	0	0.0
TOTAL	1110	100.0	343	30.9

*Figures do not include 39 residents who did not answer whether their hospital enforced moonlighting ban or not.

**Hospital tacitly approves of moonlighting and/or permits it under certain circumstances and/or on some services.

hospitals, etc.**—reported that, in their hospitals, "moonlighting is strictly forbidden." An additional 20% said their hospitals "discourage" moonlighting and only a very few—another 4%—indicated that their hospitals either tacitly permit moonlighting or, at least, permit it under certain circumstances and/or on certain services (Tables 1 and 2).

But, of the 635 residents in hospitals where moonlighting is forbidden, only 227—little more than one-third—said the ban is actually enforced.

Words, Idle Words

And how does all this affect house staff's moonlighting habits?

**An exception to this were the federal hospitals. Slightly more than ¾ of house staff in federal hospitals reported their hospitals ban moonlighting.

Well, apparently, the hospital's "strict" ban on moonlighting—as long as it is limited to words—doesn't seem to disturb house staff after-hours activities one iota.

True, potential moonlighters among interns may be deterred . . . to some extent . . . by their hospital's *stated* policy: Only 5% of the interns in hospitals where moonlighting is forbidden dare to ignore the interdiction, while the moonlighting rate among interns in all other hospitals is almost twice that.

However, by the time a house officer reaches resident stature, his awe for the Establishment palls—or his needs are greater or his schedule less hectic than during his internship days. Whatever the reason, ban or no ban, 28.5% of our resident-respondents, in hospitals forbidding moonlighting, moonlighted anyway, while the moonlighting rate among residents in all other hospitals was not much different—34%.

Table 2
HOSPITAL POLICY AND THE MOONLIGHTING RATE AMONG INTERNS

Hospital Policy on Moonlighting	Total Interns No.	%	Moonlighting Interns No.	Moonlighting Rate %
PROHIBITS	178	53.5	9	5.1
Enforces ban	(74	43.8)*	(4)	(5.4)
Does **not** enforce ban	(95	56.2)*	(5)	(5.3)
DISCOURAGES	60	18.0	7	11.7
DON'T KNOW	62	18.6	3	4.8
HAS NO POLICY	17	5.1	3	17.6
OTHER**	14	4.2	6	42.9
NO ANSWER	2	0.6	0	0.0
TOTAL	333	100.0	28	8.4

*Figures do not include nine interns who did not answer whether their hospital enforced moonlighting ban or not.

**Hospital tacitly approves of moonlighting and/or permits it under certain circumstances and/or on some services.

However, when a hospital's stated policy is backed up with action, the moonlighting rate plummets. Thus, of those residents in hospitals where the moonlighting ban is enforced, only 22—*less than 10%*—were moonlighting, while the moonlighting rate for residents in all other hospitals was 37%—*almost four times as high!*

Among interns, enforcing policy with action doesn't appear to have any greater deterring effect than that attained by merely issuing a statement of policy: In our survey, the moonlighting rate remained at the same low 5% level.

On the other hand, among interns in hospitals where moonlighting was tacitly permitted, or "ap-

---

THE 'LEGAL' FORMS OF MOONLIGHTING

Over 400 house staff members reported that their hospitals gave them the opportunity to earn extra money by working during their time-off at certain 'hospital-sanctioned' jobs. The following are the most common forms of such 'legal' moonlighting.

	Number of respondents mentioning
EMERGENCY ROOM COVERAGE	228
COVERING CLINICS, WARDS, ETC.	65
STUDENT PHYSICALS	45
LABORATORY WORK	29
OUTSIDE (AFFILIATED) HOSPITAL COVERAGE	27
RESEARCH WORK	23
NURSING	13
ADMINISTERING OB-ANESTHESIA	12
TEACHING STUDENTS AND NURSES	6
AUTOPSIES	5

proved of," the moonlighting rate shot up to 44%—i.e., four out of the nine interns in such broadminded hospitals moonlighted. (But our statistical analyst won't allow us to make much out of this on the grounds that nine is too small a sample on which to base any valid conclusions.)

Among residents (where our sample was considerably larger) the hospital's "liberality" seems to have but slight 'moonlightogenic' effect: 41% of the residents polled took advantage of their hospital's tacit (or open) permission to moonlight—an increase of 10% over the moonlighting rate in other hospitals.

However, a greater inducement to moonlighters came from unexpected quarters.

Some hospitals offer their house staff the opportunity to earn extra money by working on their off hours at jobs sanctioned by the hospital. (See Box 1.)

However, whether the hospitals offer such opportunities out of the goodness of their hearts or largely because they need the extra coverage or added help, is open to question.

At any rate, almost 30% of the house staff polled reported that their hospital—regardless of the type*—offered such stipend-supplementing opportunities. Nevertheless, our survey figures show that, despite their hospital's "largess," many house staffers choose to take their business elsewhere. In fact, the rate of moonlighting—of the *illegal* variety**—seems to be

*Again, federal hospitals seem to be an exception to this. Barely 1% of house staff in federal hospitals reported that their hospital offered them opportunities to earn extra money.

**In our questionnaire, we defined moonlighting as "working outside the home hospital in a job—either medical or non-medical—not specifically sanctioned by the hospital."

considerably higher among house staff of hospitals having such a jobs-available policy than among those who have to go off home base to find ways of supplementing their income.

Why do house staff feel that the pastures are lusher elsewhere?

Possibly one answer may be that they *are*: At any rate, from the complaints of many of our respondents, it was obvious that they at least *believed* the pickings were better in other hospitals. One moonlighter noted sourly: "Sure the hospital offers us a chance to make extra money—donating blood at $25 a pint." Another observed, "We're allowed to work in the E.R.—but the hospital pays outsiders more than they pay their own residents." And still another wrote with exclamation points: "My hospital pays $10 for a 24-hour shift in a busy emergency room!!!"

In many cases, the number of jobs available to house staff is very limited—for example, covering high school football games and other athletic events, perhaps two or three times per year, for $20 or so per game. Often, too, the openings are restricted to senior residents.

Another reason for house staff foraging elsewhere may be that, by offering them the opportunity to take on extra work for pay on home territory, the hospital in effect gives its implicit okay to moonlighting. "After all," as one moonlighter pointed out with irrefutable logic, "if we're allowed to cover our hospital's busy emergency room on our nights off, why can't we do the same thing in another hospital where we're paid more and can get more sleep?" Why, indeed?

On the other hand, a hospital policy of hiring outside moonlighters though officially maintaining a ban on moonlighting is, in house staff eyes, hypocritical, inconsistent, and tantamount to condoning moonlighting. "Moonlighters in our E.R. are only accepted from outside hospitals. Isn't that absurd?!!" asked one resentful resident, not unreasonably.

It was also obvious that many inequities regarding employment opportunities for house staff exist among the different hospitals. For example: one hospital has an outpatient home medical service. Residents are permitted to see these patients regularly, much as a private doctor would, and they are paid a regular fee for each patient seen. Another hospital pays its residents to take night calls for the "private wing" simply because, according to one of its residents, "it benefits members of the hospital staff—but the hospital won't allow any other form of moonlighting." At a third hospital, residents are occasionally called upon to see private patients when their own doctors do not want to come out for emergencies. "The hospital collects the fee without the slightest consideration for a 'house staff fund' or the like," wrote one resident moonlighter. "Hospitals must make a radical change in their attitude towards residents—both professionally and financially. Somebody has failed somewhere, allowing the present situation to have perpetuated itself for so long. Wish the AMA would get wise!"

Big Chief: Him Heap Nice Fella

But if hospital policy struck such a sour note with house staff, not so the policy of chiefs. For the most part, it would seem, chiefs and residents make beautiful harmony.

Slightly less than 30% of the respondents reported that their chiefs of service prohibit moonlighting (Tables 3 and 4). Another 14% indicated that their chiefs try to "discourage" moonlighting but without maintaining a strict blanket ban on it. A surprisingly large number (almost 38% of the interns and 26% of the residents) had no idea what their chief's policy on moonlighting is—an indication that he couldn't be too adamant about it ... or that they, themselves, weren't too interested in moonlighting. And an even larger number of residents—almost 30%—reported a comparatively easy-going attitude towards moonlighting on the part of their chiefs, an attitude which ranges from "disapproves but looks the other way" to downright encouragement.

Of course, to a certain degree, the chief's policy seems to be dictated by hospital policy. However—according to house staff, at least—not all chiefs toe the hospital policy line: Of the more than 600 residents in hospitals prohibiting moonlighting, only 44% reported that their chiefs prohibit moonlighting, too. In fact, an almost equal number of residents in these hospitals—37%—indicate that their chiefs have a more open-minded policy on moonlighting than that of the hospital.

CHIEF'S POLICY ON MOONLIGHTING AND THE MOONLIGHTING RATE AMONG INTERNS

Chief's Policy*	Total Interns		Moonlighting Interns	Moonlighting Rate
	No.	%	No.	%
PROHIBITS	81	24.3	5	6.2
DISCOURAGES	48	14.4	7	14.6
DISAPPROVES BUT LOOKS THE OTHER WAY	52	15.6	6	11.5
OTHER**	13	3.9	2	25.0
DON'T KNOW	125	37.6	7	5.6
NO ANSWER	14	4.2	1	7.1
TOTAL	333	100.0	28	8.4

*As reported by interns.

**Chief either approves of or permits moonlighting or permits it under certain circumstances and/or depending on individual intern.

CHIEF'S POLICY ON MOONLIGHTING AND THE MOONLIGHTING RATE AMONG RESIDENTS

Chief's Policy*	Total Residents No.	%	Moonlighting Residents No.	Moonlighting Rate %
PROHIBITS	333	30.0	53	15.9
DISCOURAGES	156	14.0	40	25.6
DISAPPROVES BUT LOOKS THE OTHER WAY	248	22.3	154	62.1
OTHER**	75	6.8	38	50.7
DON'T KNOW	293	26.4	57	19.5
NO ANSWER	5	0.5	1	20.0
TOTAL	1110	100.0	343	30.9

*As reported by residents.

**Chief either approves of or permits moonlighting or permits it under certain circumstances and/or depending upon the individual resident.

And how does the chief's policy affect the moonlighting rate? Just as you would expect: Among residents whose chiefs prohibit moonlighting, the moonlighting rate was only 16%, while among all other residents (who reported what their chief's policy on moonlighting is), the moonlighting rate was three times as high.

Where the chief merely "discourages" moonlighting, the rate went up to the more or less 'normal' level of 26% and where, though he "disapproves" of it, he "looks the other way," the moonlighting rate hit the all-time record of 62%. Not even among residents whose chiefs actually "approve" of moonlighting does the moonlighting rate—in our survey, 55%—reach that high.

Since policy is not always backed by action, house staff were also asked to indicate what they thought their chief's reaction would be if he were to discover they were moonlighting. Thus, though some 30% of the residents had reported that their chiefs prohibit moonlighting, only 12% felt that their chiefs would do anything so drastic as to fire or suspend them or report them to hospital authorities (Tables 5 and 6). Another 15% thought their chiefs might forbid them from continuing to moonlight and/or warn them that a "next time" meant dismissal. Furthermore, about one-third felt their chiefs would do nothing at all about their moonlighting or, at least, do nothing as long as it did not interfere with their hospital work, and another 19% thought their chiefs would only try to discourage them but not insist that they stop moonlighting.

In fact, their responses to the question "If your chief found out that *you* were moonlighting, what do you

Table 5

EXPECTED REACTION OF CHIEF TO MOONLIGHTING—INTERNS

Expected Reaction of Chief to Moonlighting	Total Interns		Moonlighting Interns	Moonlighting Rate
	No.	%	No.	%
FIRE, SUSPEND, NOTIFY AUTHORITIES	35	10.5	0	0.0
FORBID FURTHER MOONLIGHTING	42	12.6	5	11.9
DISCOURAGE OR REPRIMAND	61	18.3	5	8.2
NOTHING AS LONG AS DOESN'T INTERFERE WITH WORK	19	5.7	1	5.3
NOTHING (UNQUALIFIED)	73	21.9	10	13.7
DON'T KNOW	37	11.1	3	8.1
OTHER (HE KNOWS, ETC.)	1	0.3	0	0.0
NO ANSWER	65	19.6	4	6.2
TOTAL	333	100.0	28	8.4

Table 6

EXPECTED REACTION OF CHIEF TO MOONLIGHTING—RESIDENTS

Expected Reaction of Chief to Moonlighting	Total Residents		Moonlighting Residents	Moonlighting Rate
	No.	%	No.	%
FIRE, SUSPEND, NOTIFY AUTHORITIES	132	11.9	19	14.4
FORBID FURTHER MOONLIGHTING	169	15.2	42	24.9
DISCOURAGE OR REPRIMAND	210	18.9	61	29.0
NOTHING AS LONG AS DOESN'T INTERFERE WITH WORK	76	6.9	28	36.8
NOTHING (UNQUALIFIED)	303	27.3	151	49.8
DON'T KNOW	122	11.0	25	20.5
OTHER (HE KNOWS, ETC.)	6	0.5	1	16.7
NO ANSWER	92	8.3	16	17.4
TOTAL	1110	100.0	343	30.9

think he would do?" covered the range of passions from a hysterical "Scream!" to an amiable "Congratulate me!" But by and large, most house staff believe their chiefs are an understanding (if emotional) lot and would lend sympathetic ears to their tales of financial woes. (See Box 2.)

But how does house staff's *opinion* of their chief's policy on and reaction to moonlighting compare with the Real Thing?

At the same time *Resident Physician* sent out its questionnaire on moonlighting to house staff, it also took a poll of chiefs of service and directors of medical education and *their* opinions on moonlighting. The results indicate that chiefs and DME's are made of sterner stuff than what house staff believe . . . or, at any rate, they think they are.

CHIEFS OF SERVICE: AS HOUSE STAFF SEE THEM

One of the most pleasing revelations of RESIDENT PHYSICIAN'S moonlighting survey has been that low stipends and long hours have not extinguished house staff humor. Despite that strictly American invention, the multiple-choice question (the type used for the most part in RESIDENT PHYSICIAN'S questionnaire), which doesn't allow much room for creative expression, our respondents somehow managed to circumvent the rigid form and e-x-p-a-n-d. They were most expressive when it came to their chiefs of service, whom the majority regard with a kind of acid affection, a feeling somewhat akin to that of a citizen towards his Uncle Sam around the Ides of April. The result: Some smiles amidst a slew of statistics.

The question was: "If your chief found out that *you* were moonlighting, what do you think he would do?" The answers . . .

THESE EMOTIONAL CHIEFS

- Raise hell!
- Have a stroke!
- Rupture his middle meningeal artery.
- Radical neck dissection.
- Throw a tantrum.
- Create a scene.
- Spank my hand.
- Give me a sermon.
- Say, "tut, tut!"
- Be very unhappy. . . .
- Be very philosophical about the whole thing. . . .

THESE PRACTICAL CHIEFS

- Nothing. He moonlights himself.
- Deny it!
- Approve—as long as he doesn't "know" about it.
- Wonder when we sleep.
- Reprimand or dismiss me — depends upon quota of residents!
- Avoid asking direct questions about it.
- Nothing—rather than pay more.
- Nothing—he needs me.
- Nothing he *can* do—all his residents moonlight.
- Advise me to keep quiet so he won't "find out."
- Organize a committee.

THESE REASONABLE CHIEFS

- When he discovered that we were working at another hospital as medical officers, covering only emergencies and deaths, we were able to convince him to allow it on the basis that we could get more sleep there than at our own hospital.
- Make sure that the moonlighting doesn't interfere with my duties. He usually arranges to take calls at home when I am away.
- Try to help me out of my financial emergency with department funds.
- Advise me to try to find an alternative if possible. He's a helluva nice guy.

22. What It Takes To Organize for Service*

Robert H. Kennedy, M.D.

As in many other parts of a hospital, the emergency facility is a combined responsibility of the trustees, administrators, medical staff, and nursing staff. The trustees usually delegate their powers to be carried out by administrators and physicians. Unless the latter two and the nursing profession have defined authority and a written statement as to how it shall be implemented, no emergency department can render service to patients which is of the highest order or even passably effective.

Early in 1963 the Committee on Trauma of the American College of Surgeons recommended certain standards for emergency departments. These were approved by the board of regents. One paragraph receives too little notice: "The following standards are desirable. In certain institutions many of them may be impractical. Under the latter circumstances, they should remain as ideals to be approached as nearly as possible."

This is equally important in any statements in this article. Because we say a thing should be done does

---

* Reprinted from *The Modern Hospital*, Vol. 106, No. 1, January 1966.

not give it legal standing as a requirement. Circumstances in any individual hospital may make any of the standards impractical in that institution.

The minimum components of an emergency department committee should be representatives of each of the major medical services, an administrator, and the emergency department supervising nurse. This should be a standing committee of the medical board or medical staff, reporting to them or even, in special instances, to the board of trustees. Its duty is to recommend all policy relating to the emergency department.

What might some of the problems be which would come before this committee?

To Determine Allowable Work

Will general anesthesia be given?

If this is required, the patient, as a rule, should be admitted to the inpatient service and treated in a hospital operating suite. General anesthesia should not be administered at any place which does not fulfill the following four requirements:

1. A history and examination, including laboratory, should be obtained, as comprehensive as required for any major operative case in the house.

2. The same personnel should administer anesthesia as would do so in the main operating room.

3. The area used must be explosion-proof.

4. A recovery room which is covered every moment until the patient is fully conscious must be available.

Will small operative cases be allowed such as excision of sebaceous cysts?

This is common practice. There is no objection to it if space is planned for this purpose and if adequate personnel is assigned to handle these cases in addition to any serious emergency which may come in.

I have been present when ambulance attendants have brought in a badly injured traffic accident patient and the nurse has asked them to wait, since no examining table was available to put the patient on. I have been in a new $500,000 emergency facility which had six explosion-proof operating rooms and no examining rooms. All could have local anesthesia patients booked from 7:30 a.m. to 3:30 p.m. six days a week and could have listed these three weeks in advance. I could not learn whether, if all tables were occupied, one of the sebaceous cyst patients would be asked to climb off the table.

Further, a lower charge for the same type of case is commonly made in the emergency department than in the operating suite. No wonder the emergency department is often called the "bargain basement."

What nonemergencies will be treated?

Will the emergency department be expected to handle return visits? Return visits after hospital discharge for dressings and so forth at the convenience of the physician? Continued care of hospital employee compensation cases? Pre-employment examinations of hospital personnel? Special examination of hospital inpatients or referrals from physicians' private offices (*e.g.,* bronchoscopies, sigmoidoscopies)?

We have found such nonemergency practice in large hospitals where competent areas in separate outpatient departments were available. We have also visited institutions where all major hospital dressings and even every pelvic examination on hospital inpatients must be done in the emergency department, the patient usually being moved there by stretcher.

Any of these types of cases can be attended in the emergency area but only if the physical set-up is planned for this work and only if there is sufficient personnel to cover it without interfering with real emergency care.

The difficulty is that this department has commonly been made a catch-all without serious thought, a place where groups may go who are wanted nowhere else. At least the area might then be christened with another name, if a major portion of its function is far removed from emergencies.

How long is resuscitation to be carried on in the emergency department?

Since at present 60 percent of the patients are often medical and pediatric cases and less than half usually have any real emergency, the multiple injury case frequently fails to receive the attention he needs and deserves, merely because of the case load.

Intensive care wards have become popular, practical, and lifesaving. Does the patient in serious condition, whether a coronary or a traffic accident, deserve to go almost immediately to an intensive care ward, rather than having free airway assured, laboratory procedures ordered and performed, and specialists consulted in the hectic atmosphere of the emergency department? This should be a responsibility and a recommendation of the committee.

In some hospitals the idea is carried even farther and the seriously injured person goes directly to an operating room reserved in the regular suite for this purpose, not even entering the emergency facility. Lives are thereby saved which might not be by any other method.

To Plan Doctor Coverage

In the 22 percent of acute general hospitals which have interns and/or residents, in what instances must an attending doctor be called?

In the 78 percent without house staff, when a rotation system is used, how can a doctor be relieved of this duty? What penalty follows his not appearing for duty? Is this rule enforced?

In many hospitals one finds the radiologist or pathologist quite noisy in his denunciation of this assignment. On investigation one often learns that most private doctors come in to see their own patients and that the physician on rotation sees no more than one or two patients when on 24 hour call once in four to six weeks. Many hospitals allow an older doctor to pay a younger one to fill his tour of duty, but the older doctor is entirely responsible if the younger does not show.

I have known of hospitals where repeated failure to appear at duty time in the emergency department has resulted in canceled privileges in the only hospital in a community. This is harsh treatment but rules are worthless and the patient suffers unless penalties are stated and punishment carried through.

To Control Observation Beds

These are of great value in many institutions when properly used, worse than useless without definite rules or when these rules are not enforced. I visited one hospital where the cardiologist would not allow any coronary accident to be moved from the emergency department for four days.

With a full house, the observation beds often are used for new admissions. The neurosurgeons are given particular credit for this irregularity. Usually they work at three or four hospitals. They may have a tight schedule and find a reservation cannot be honored and so have the patient sleep in the emergency department. On return from the recovery room all hospital beds may still be full and the patient again be assigned to an observation bed, often for several days.

Better no observation beds than an area without definite written rules which are enforced with justice to all.

To Establish All Procedures

There are frequent personnel changes, and standard operating procedures are needed if any reasonable average of care is to be maintained. The committee must be responsible for preparing and constantly updating both professional and administrative procedures.

Is an x-ray always taken after the reduction of a fracture before a patient is allowed to go home?

If not done, swelling may go down and plaster loosen, or some minor accident might change position, leaving the surgeon and the hospital with no proof that the fracture ever was reduced. In at least some states, an administrator should not allow this to happen since it has been decided that the hospital and the doctor are equally responsible for anything which goes on under the hospital roof.

Are masks worn by all personnel while caring for a fresh wound or is such procedure limited to the operating suite and/or dressing areas?

There has been much discussion regarding the spread of infection in hospitals from the mouths and noses of personnel. Should not the fresh wound be thus protected immediately on arrival in the emergency facility rather than exposing it to staphylococci for a time and later commencing a more aseptic routine?

Are the same criteria used for permission to care for patients in the emergency department as in the operating suite?

We have noted rather large procedures performed in the emergency department by physicians who are not allowed the privilege of doing the same in the operating room. Does the committee believe that the residents of their community deserve a double standard in care according to what floor it is given on? Should not emergency department privileges be stated in writing for all physicians so that everyone may be aware of them?

I came across one hospital where 460 physicians had privileges in the emergency department to work on their private patients. Were they all of the same mental caliber and training? Or should the standard operating procedures and staff action have delineated the limits of each person's scope of care among the local residents?

To Assist Disaster Planning

The committee should determine the relation of the emergency room to the disaster plan. Too often the same committee is given responsibility for each of these. In most institutions the emergency department is the worst possible place for a sorting area in time of disaster. Commonly it is not large enough on an ordinary day at the hours of the peak load, so how can it be expected to deal competently with a disaster?

The triage station established by the disaster plan should be the largest open area available, often the lawn if the weather is good. Otherwise an auditorium in the nurses' home, the hospital lobby, the outpatient department waiting room, or even an open area in the basement may prove the best place.

The emergency department should be used for care of one of the four or five groups divided at triage; e.g., for suture of less extensive lacerations. Sorting should be the function of the most experienced doctor present, not left to residents indefinitely, as is too frequently true.

These are some of the problems which should be settled by the emergency department committee. It is evident that they cover much territory. The aim must always be improved care for the patient. Thus good public relations may be preserved and promoted.

In addition to the committee there should be a single M.D. director of the department. He should be responsible to the committee for the implementation of policy and the supervision of professional services. He would be expected to look in on the facility each day and be available to back up the nurse's action whenever needed.

It is he, not the nurse, who should talk with the physician on rotation who does not respond promptly. If the department is to run smoothly, the nurse in charge must always know there is someone to whom she can appeal promptly. The director should change infrequently, if satisfactory, possibly with at least a one-year tour of duty.

It is notable that directors of medical education too often make little use of the department for teaching. Yet knowledge of shock and tissue reaction is basic in any medical field, and there is no better place to observe and treat shock than the emergency facility.

The age of laissez faire has passed in almost all fields. Physicians working in a hospital must take more responsibility for the community and must be their brothers' keepers.

A good example, which has appeared repeatedly in many of the surveys I have made, is tetanus prophylaxis for the patient coming in with a fresh, contaminated wound. Too often the procedure is determined by each private physician. I know no reason why the staff should not establish a uniform prophylaxis program.

If what goes on under the hospital roof cannot be managed by the doctors for the greatest good of the patient, we will find government at some level taking charge before too long. This is but one example of staff responsibility for their weakest or most careless members and to the community.

For many years physicians have been in the habit of accepting many favors from hospitals, taking these as their due because they did so much charity work in the hospital. Times have changed markedly in the last generation, and it is uncommon for a doctor not to be paid for his work either by the patient, by insurance, or by welfare. There is now little reason why he should be allowed to see any class of patient at any time in the emergency department and then object to that patient's paying the department's basic fee.

The physician can no longer regard the hospital in terms of his personal capitalistic economy. As a member of the staff he is responsible to the hospital and to the community for the actions of his confreres as well as his own. He must support the emergency department committee and the director of the department in the making and implementing of policy for the good of all.

23. Here Are Ways To Use Facts About E.R. To Build Good Public and Press Relations*

Lee Feldman

No aspect of a hospital's operation can create more community relations problems than its emergency department. Both the handling of news of an emergency case which has attracted press interest and the handling of the patient himself can have considerable impact on a hospital's community relations. And if a patient is mishandled, this may also arouse press interest or send a disgruntled person into the community who will become an ambassador of ill-will.

Much of what occurs in a hospital is privileged information.

But hospital information is a two-sided coin, for much of what happens is a matter of public record and is within public domain. Very often you have to call the side while the coin is still spinning in the air. When you guess wrong you know it—the press pounces on you.

It must be recognized that newspapers have regular "beats," the coroner's office, the police and fire de-

*Reprinted from *The Modern Hospital,* Vol. 106, No. 1, Jan. 1966.

partments, and the various courts within the city, county, and state. Some reporters spend their full working days in press rooms of these places, reporting in by phone. Therefore, if a 90-year-old woman slips and falls on the ice, breaks her hip, and dies two or three days after being admitted to the hospital, this becomes a coroner's case and inquiry by the press is almost inevitable.

If a law suit is filed against an institution in one of the courts, chances are the press will know about it before the hospital does, and hospital officials will be receiving telephone calls from reporters asking for comment on the litigation.

Since certain hospital information often is obtainable by the press from other sources, denying what is already available to reporters can accomplish nothing for the hospital except to incur the ill-will of the media. An unfriendly press can be most devastating by either giving one side of a story or by suggesting that the hospital has something to hide.

Can a hospital afford to ignore what is commonly referred to as a "bad press"? No, it cannot. Because, if it does, it will sacrifice the three major public relations objectives of all medical institutions:

1. Enhance the patient's confidence in the hospital and minimize his anxiety about being hospitalized.

2. Convey the image that your hospital is a prestigious place to work to facilitate the recruitment of first-rate professional, paramedical, and administrative personnel.

3. Maintain the confidence and respect of the public to ensure its continued financial support.

This is what you risk losing by being uncooperative, indifferent, or hostile to the press. And this applies to the entire hospital and not to emergency room personnel alone.

Hospitals, by the very nature of their work, must be conservative in the handling of information about their patients. The press, on the other hand, is in the business of ferreting out news and has a long tradition of making exposés of cover-ups, many of them real, others the result of overly active imaginations. But basically, the press must be reassured that there is no cover-up of negligence of any kind. This requires a certain amount of skill; but again, a few pointers can go a long way in disarming and reassuring reporters.

However, the needs of the patient are paramount and always will be. Therefore, if an emergency room supervisor is faced with an emergency situation which requires her full attention and the press calls, she must explain that she has to remain with the patient. She should tell the reporter that she will call him back as soon as the patient is out of danger and no longer needs her immediate attention. In most cases, he will understand; but she should be sure to call him back, or have someone at the hospital call for her.

For most emergency cases, and many of these will be police cases, the kind of information that can be released is as follows:

1. Name, address, marital status, age, sex, occupation, and employer of the patient.

2. A brief description of the nature of the accident whether it was a fire, a shooting, or an automobile collision.

3. General information on the nature of the injury and condition of the patient, such as lacerations of the right arm, smoke inhalation, or what have you, and the usual standard condition report such as critical, serious, fair, or good.

In an incident that may reflect discredit on a patient, or his family, involving alleged circumstances such as suicide or attempted suicide, intoxication, drug addiction, or moral turpitude, hospitals are justified in withholding details as self-protection against damage suits.

In these situations, it's best to use the police officer involved in the incident or the coroner as the preferred source of information. If the body of the decedent is already at a funeral home, you can give the name of the funeral home as an additional contact for details.

Although photographs in the emergency room are permissible, the hospital and the physician in charge must reserve the right to withhold consent under certain circumstances:

1. When the patient's condition does not permit him to be disturbed by photographers.
2. Crisis situations (because of heavy patient load).
3. When discretionary action is deemed advisable.

When you don't have certain information, or when you do have information you feel you cannot reveal, at least try to help the press by giving them something or some source of information. Try to convey the feeling that you want to help the reporter do his job, which is to get news. Reporters must call back to city editors who make deadlines three, four, or five times a day; their business is news. If you help them do their job, very often you will develop a friend, and heaven knows there are times when you really need one.

Being as cooperative as you can will often affect the tone of the articles written about the hospital.

Obviously, you can only go so far. Extreme caution is required when giving out certain types of information and some information should not be released at any time. A list of some important precautions, in releasing news of emergency cases, is presented in the box.

What Should Not Be Released to the Press

While hospitals should seek to cooperate with the various news media in releasing information about persons treated in their emergency rooms, there are various kinds of information which should not be given out. By observing the following rules the hospital will protect the patient and his family, and itself, when dealing with the press.

1. In no case should an opinion be given as to the severity of an injury until the condition has been determined by a physician, and no prognosis should be made. This applies particularly to injuries of the head.

2. In the case of fractures, state only the injured member involved.

3. If there are internal injuries, indicate that there are such injuries and give the location only when determined by the physician.

4. If the patient is unconscious, this fact may be stated if the patient has been brought to the hospital unconscious.

5. The cause of poisoning may be revealed only if known, and no statement concerning motives, accidental or intentional, may be given, and no prognosis should be made.

6. If there is a bullet wound, this may be released, but no comment regarding how the wound was inflicted may be given, that is, by accident, suicide, or a fight.

7. If the patient has a stab wound, this may be indicated but no comment should be made regarding how the wound was inflicted.

8. No statement may be made about whether or not the person was intoxicated.

9. If the patient is burned, this can be released, and the part of his body that is burned may also be stated when known. You may also indicate the severity of the burn; however, as with some of the other causes, you should not discuss how the accident occurred nor should a prognosis be given.

One other suggestion, which cannot be emphasized enough, is to avoid, if possible, using the term "no comment." This term to the press is like waving a red flag in front of a bull. It suggests a cover-up, which in turn implies negligence of one kind or another. If the press suspects a cover-up, it will push harder and, in some cases, will concoct or falsely infer conclusions to get a story. You can give the press information that you know they either have or information you know they can get, or you may plead violation of medical ethics.

When the hospital's emergency room is shown in an unfavorable light by the press, it seems that the public is predisposed to readily accept the propostion that there is something wrong at the hospital. And this leads to consideration of the second major factor in the emergency room's impact on a hospital's community relations—relationships with the persons who are served by the emergency department.

Hospitals have fallen down in properly educating the public on the proper role of the emergency room. After viewing some of the popular literature that has been written on the emergency room, one can understand why the emergency room now has a bad image with the public.

A story in *Redbook* magazine entitled, "The Tragic Inefficiency of Hospital Emergency Wards," charges that: "Emergency medical care in the United States today . . . is almost everywhere an unorganized crazy quilt of miscellaneous bits and pieces that just don't fit together. Hence, things are all too likely to go wrong even in cities where there are excellent hospitals ready to receive you."[1]

There is a growing awareness on the part of the public that the load of the emergency room is mushrooming due to an increase in nonemergency cases, but there is a need for all hospitals to do more to educate the public on the proper role and function of the emergency room.

These major questions, that are faced day after day, must be answered:

1. What is an emergency?
2. What cases should be seen in the emergency room?
3. What is an emergency room?
4. How is the emergency room used?
5. Are only emergencies treated?
6. How soon are patients treated?
7. How are emergency rooms staffed?
8. Can children be treated in the absence of the parents?
9. Does the hospital have ambulance service?
10. How can an emergency patient be admitted to the hospital?
11. How is emergency service paid for?
12. What about insurance?

One of the most important of these, and one which leads to a great deal of awkwardness, is how emergency patients are admitted to the hospital.

When a patient has prepaid insurance or has private financial means and wants to be admitted and you tell her that she cannot be, she may suspect your motives. This is particularly true with members of minority groups, who may, irrespective of what the doctor in charge says about the methods of admission, feel subjected to racial or religious discrimination.

A patient may have had a broken arm and had to wait a long time before someone looked at him. What he may not have known is that the staff may have been working on a case much more critical than the broken arm.

The real question is what can we do about this? A program of education should be undertaken before the situations arise. And one way of doing that is to prepare a pamphlet for distribution to each patient who comes in—a pamphlet which explains how the emergency room operates and answers the questions that I have stated.[2]

If an individual feels that he is being unjustly treated and you show him a printed pamphlet, he then realizes that you are not making this up on the spur of the moment and that this is a matter of standing policy. Many hospitals do have such pamphlets or publications, and they go a long way in reducing misunderstanding and avoiding unpleasant incidents. A pamphlet is certainly not going to solve all of your public relations problems, but it will help.

What is really needed is a full-scale public relations program implemented through local hospital councils in cooperation with member hospitals. The program would include feature stories in the papers, public service announcements and interviews on radio and television, and a speakers' bureau.

The emergency room has been described as the crossroads of the hospital. Scenes of human drama are enacted there every day and few people ever imagine or can possibly envision the range of human experience that takes place there. The emergency room is all this, and more. It is also an open window to the hospital. And although the public may only see one small aspect of what happens, the entire institution is often judged by what is seen and heard through that window.

FOOTNOTES

1. Brecher, Ruth and Edward: The Tragic Inefficiency of our Hospital Emergency Wards, Redbook, September 1964, 123:55.
2. Spencer, James H., M.D., F.A.C.S.: Records and Evaluation of Emergency Department Care. Bulletin of the American College of Surgeons, November-December 1964, p. 358.

24. Hospital Emergency Service and the Open Door*

Leonard S. Powers, J.D.

Compared to its antecedents, the modern hospital is a revolutionary institution. Until this century the community hospital was little more than a rooming house to which the transient sick were taken and from which most never left. It served to isolate, with minimum care, those who could not afford medical treatment at home, especially those with contagious diseases who could be a burden and threat to the well. Today, the hospital is a complex center of activity—a vast assemblage of superbly trained and highly specialized talent and expensive equipment devoted to healing those suffering from accident or disease. No longer is it only for the impoverished sick; all strata of our society come to it and all demand that the very best in medical technology and skill be available to them.[1] And as the complexity and expense of operating the hospitals increased, they began to take on a distinctly business-like appearance much unlike that of the earlier charity-oriented organizations. One sig-

*Reprinted from *Michigan Law Review,* May 1968, Vol. 66, No. 7.

The research assistance of Mr. Carven Angel, senior student at the University of Florida College of Law, is gratefully acknowledged.

nificant aspect of this development was the eventual demise of the charitable immunity doctrine as applied to hospitals.[2]

One department of the hospital subjected to especially rapid change in recent years has been the emergency service. Every section of the country notes a tremendous increase in public demand for emergency room services.[3] That "the public has taken to the emergency department like a duck to water"[4] is certainly no exaggeration; it may be an understatement. While the propriety of such a magnified role for the emergency room in the total treatment context is far from clear, and, indeed, is the subject of a continuing dialogue within the medical profession,[5] the increased emphasis is already with us. Like the shift in hospital practices which led to the rapid demise of the charitable immunity doctrine, so will this development force changes in the law. This article will focus on the emerging duty of hospital emergency rooms to treat patients seeking their aid.[6]

Before discussing that question, it is helpful to examine the changes in emergency room practices in greater detail. The emergency room was originally what its name implies—a place for the treatment of severe injuries and diseases demanding immediate attention.[7] Its location was usually in some remote part of the hospital. It had no organizational status as a department, and the quality of care rendered there was usually below the general standard for the hospital.[8] The emergency room of a modern hospital is a drastically different place.[9] Now the public goes to the emergency room for treatment of all kinds of injuries and illnesses.[10] The number and volume of services demanded have resulted in some emergency rooms becoming, in effect, complete miniature hospitals.[11] The United States Public Health Service predicts 49.3

million annual emergency room visits by 1970 compared to only 32.1 million ordinary hospital admissions. This is a 79 percent increase, per 1,000 population, in the use of the emergency room compared to an 8 percent increase in ordinary admissions over the 1960 figures.[12]

It is quite clear, then, that the public considers the emergency room to be a community medical center.[13] It is the only place where the best equipment and facilities and at least some care are available on any day, at any hour, and without appointment. It does not require the presence of the sometimes unavailable family doctor.[14] In fact, one explanation for this development is undoubtedly the concurrent disappearance of the traditional family doctor and the house call, and the advent of the clinic, regular office hours, and the doctors' days off.

Yielding to the demands of the public and to the changing structure of their profession, some physicians and hospital administrators have challenged the profession to bring about a wholesale expansion of emergency facilities and organization.[15] There are those who feel that no one who comes to the emergency room desiring treatment should be turned away —even if no true emergency exists. There is a feeling that what may not be an "emergency" to the physician may nevertheless be one for the patient and that hospitals must accept the public's conception of the emergency room as a place to get medical aid rapidly with a minimum of administrative complication. Others, resisting extension into nonemergency cases, admonish their colleagues to return the emergency room to its original function. Attempts have been made to re-educate the public concerning the true function of the emergency room,[16] but the public, now accustomed to relying on the hospital emergency room for these vital services, has not been willing to be re-educated.[17]

There is some agreement, however, on what an ideal emergency room should be. First, if there is reasonable doubt whether medical care beyond "first-aid" is required, this judgment should be made by a licensed physician.[18] Some cases are obviously not emergencies and are not presented or claimed to be such. These "first-aid" cases do not require treatment by a licensed physician; anyone can give such aid within the limits of his competency. Whether these cases will be treated by the emergency staff or redirected to more suitable sources of assistance depends on the defined role of that particular center. But where an "emergency" is claimed, at least the determination should never be made by a nurse, orderly, aide, or clerk. Many hospitals in practice go beyond this minimal requirement and require treatment of emergency room cases by a licensed physician.[19] There is general agreement that a patient presenting himself to the emergency room should not be dismissed, discharged, or transferred without the approval of a licensed physician.[20]

Yet it is clear from scattered comments and some reported cases that many emergency rooms do not provide the services of a licensed physician.[21] In three cases that resulted in death, nurses turned people away from the emergency room without being seen by an intern, resident, or staff physician.[22] In other cases, patients were transferred[23] or discharged[24] by interns without examination or approval by a physician. Where a physician was summoned for treatment or decision, there may have been undue delay.[25] Even where a physician ordered discharge, there have been instances in which he was ignorant of the patient's condition.[26]

The most shocking aspect of the emergency room situation, however, is not the inadequate procedure or substandard quality of care provided, but the fact that these vital services are not necessarily available to the stricken patient who presents himself for emergency care. Following the traditional common-law rule that there is no affirmative duty to render emergency aid to another human being who is in peril, private and most public hospitals may legally refuse aid in an emergency case.[27] This rule, rather surprising in this context, is mitigated by the stated standards of the medical profession which are directed toward providing prompt and effective aid to *all* emergency patients.[28]

Surely no emergency treatment has ever been denied solely because of the legal right of the hospital to refuse treatment. It is to be expected, on the other hand, that treatment might be refused if the case is nonemergent or if the emergency facilities are full. There have, however, been other reasons given for failure to give emergency room treatment which do not comport so readily with the physician's creed: lack of referral to the hospital, membership in a disfavored medical insurance group,[29] pre-emergency care by another doctor,[30] or contagious disease.[31] Other grounds of refusal to treat include discrimination on grounds of race, emergency room personnel being unable to locate a physician, or simply that the facility is closed.[32]

Whatever the emergency room's status as part of the hospital organization, the quality of care given, or the procedures followed, most of those charged with the operation of hospitals are aware of the new role thrust upon the emergency room. Many administrators and physicians are motivated by a recognition that the public is entitled to better service than is presently available.[33] Our question concerns how the law will cope with the expectations of the public and the generally sympathetic response of hospital officials and the healing professions. What should the law require as a minimum, with a tort action against the hospital becoming available if that minimum is not met? We begin with the shocking proposition that present law in most American jurisdictions is said to permit a hospital to keep its doors closed to the person seeking emergency medical aid.

PRESENT STATE OF THE LAW

The General Common-Law Rule and its Exceptions

Whether a hospital must render emergency medical services to the sick and injured is a question residing in that branch of tort law relating to coming to the aid of someone in peril. It will be helpful, therefore, to examine briefly some of the general principles that have emerged in this area.

Basic to the older common law was the distinction between action and inaction—between misfeasance and nonfeasance. Liability was imposed for intentional or negligent misfeasance but not for nonfeasance or failure to act. Affirmative action resulting in harm to another was a breach of duty resulting in liability but mere failure to intervene to benefit another—even to save him from serious harm—was not considered actionable since there was no duty to act in the first instance.[34] Justification for this distinction has been found in the individualistic philosophy of the traditional common law; it refused to restrict a man's freedom by imposing a sort of forced labor in the form of a duty to be helpful to those in distress.[35] Charity began and ended at home, and even there, as evidenced by the family immunities, there was very little.

As social institutions and relationships became more complex, the courts were required to reconsider the subtle problem of inaction. Liability slowly developed for nonfeasance under some circumstances; where warranted, judicial exceptions developed to the general rule of no liability for nonfeasance.

One exception developed in cases in which the defendant engaged in some sort of prior affirmative action placing the plaintiff in peril.[36] There had long been a duty to come to the aid of another if one tortiously put another person in peril, but this, of course, could be characterized as misfeasance. The duty has been significantly extended to those who innocently cause such bodily harm to another as to leave him helpless and in danger of further harm.[37] Further, if by one's prior affirmative act a force is innocently set in motion which threatens peril, then he must act to prevent the risk from taking effect.[38] The common thread that knits these situations together is the defendant's connection with the risk that has thrust the plaintiff into a position of peril.

A second exception to the no duty to act rule developed where the defendant undertook to confer a benefit upon another, and that person suffered harm because of his reliance upon the undertaking.[39] Even when there is no prior contractual duty to engage in the undertaking, certain duties are assumed when such a voluntary undertaking begins. To take a well-known example, a railroad which undertakes to maintain a traffic signalman at a street crossing takes on the duty to perform that function with due care.[40] Liability extends beyond misfeasance in affirmative acts undertaken to include liability for negligent failure to perform the undertaking at all when performance was reasonably to be expected. The duty to continue to aid another who is helpless when a discontinuance would leave the other in a worse position than when the defendant took charge of him is within this exception.[41]

A third exception bases a duty to act upon some special relationship—some special dependence—between the defendant and the person in peril. There are duties to aid and protect imposed upon employers,[42] common carriers, innkeepers, and invitors,[43] but other relationships of dependence may also impose a similar duty as, for example, public utility and customer. Most of these special relationships are found where there is a contractual relationship between the parties, or at least a potentiality of contract.

The residual applicability of the general rule after these exceptions have taken their due may be illustrated by the hypothetical familiar to all first-year law students: a man walking along a river bank sees a small child drowning in shallow water but ignores its calls for help even though he is a competent swimmer. This may be cruel and morally wrong, but there is no legal duty to rescue. Here, there is a completely fortuitous chain of events which places one person in a situation where he has the power to alleviate the distress of another. This is the factual situation where the courts and commentators still assert that there is no legal duty to assist the one in peril.

Liability for failure to aid another in peril, then, cannot today be determined without full appreciation of the factual context. Slight variations in facts bring important exceptions into operation; these exceptions, in turn, permit recovery where the general rule would deny it. Therefore, it is important to know how the courts have categorized the encounters between persons suffering medical emergencies and the hospitals maintaining emergency services.

Recent Hospital Cases—An Overview

The general rule has been stated to be that persons do not possess any right to be admitted to a hospital and that a hospital is not obliged to accept a patient not desired by it nor even to assign a reason for refusal to admit.[44] As the rule is stated, there is no exception for medical emergencies or emergency rooms. This rule is said to apply to all private hospitals and to public hospitals in the absence of a statutory duty.

Most of the statutes creating rights to treatment apply only to public hospitals. One exception is the Illinois statute, which imposes a duty—applicable both to public and private hospitals where surgical operations are performed—to give emergency medical treatment or first aid to any person who applies.[45] Most statutes authorizing the creation of governmental hospitals limit hospital use to persons with some defined relationship to the governmental unit supporting the institution.[46] A person coming within the statutory class probably has an implied right to admission although the statutes create no express right. Some statutes provide for waiver of the normal admission requirements for treatment in emergency cases.[47]

If this is so, then absent some statute, it would seem to follow that a hospital cannot be held civilly liable for nonadmittance and consequent nontreatment. Yet, in nine out of eleven recent cases to be discussed below the courts held the hospital liable. Although in three of the nine cases the hospital may have done something it should not have done,[48] in at least six of the cases it appears that the courts found that the hospital should have done something which it failed to do.[49] On one theory or another, exceptions to the general rule were found to exist. The theory most frequently used has been the concept of a voluntary undertaking to render aid. The opinions, unfortunately, generally fail to specify the essential elements which amount to an undertaking or the extent of the duty assumed once an undertaking is found to have occurred. The legal obligations of the hospital confronting a medical emergency, then, have not been adequately formulated.

This sort of conceptual uncertainty is not uncommon where the courts are confronted with seriously conflicting policies. The urge to deny any duty to render aid springs from the individualistic notion that one should be able to set one's own policies for rendering a gratuitous service. The existence of a duty might also impose a tremendous burden on smaller hospitals, draining financial and manpower resources to the point of forcing some of these institutions to abandon the emergency service altogether. While liability insurance might soften the financial blow, the adverse publicity generated by allowing such suits could be equally damaging. On the other hand, ethical and moral pressures to assist another human being in an emergency have strong appeal in such cases. The result of a hospital's lack of treatment is often serious: in all but one of the eleven cases death ensued.

Conceptual difficulties aside, it appears that the general rule of no duty to render aid is not actually shielding hospitals from civil liability in emergency room cases, and this is a reliable indication of judicial dissatisfaction with that rule. A narrow path must be walked if hospital liability is to be avoided. Indeed, there may be no reliable path. In at least one jurisdiction the only sure way to avoid liability is apparently to accept the person in distress who appears at the emergency room and render with due care whatever emergency assistance is necessary.[50] On similar facts one other jurisdiction has reached the same result in substance if not in theory.[51] How close other courts will come to imposing liability for turning patients away at the door is uncertain because few of these cases arise. Hospitals do not ordinarily turn away summarily those who appear asking for emergency aid; thus there are no modern cases for the general rule to operate upon. Each case seems to fit an exception.

Recent Hospital Cases—A Factual Analysis

The eleven recent cases mentioned earlier comprise much of the authority on the subject of hospital liability for nontreatment. Since the facts of each case are critical in determining whether some exception to the general rule is applicable, each case will be discussed in some detail. Certain factual patterns, however, are discernible and form a framework for analysis. The eleven cases, then, fit into five factual patterns.

1. *After the hospital exercised control, it gave some aid to the applicant and then released him with the mutual understanding that he was in no better condition than before.*

Birmingham Baptist Hospital v. Crews[52] A child suffering from diphtheria was taken to a private hospital. The house physician rendered treatment, consisting of a throat swab, oxygen, and two injections of antitoxin. There was a dispute concerning whether the antitoxin temporarily weakened the child's condition. After this treatment the superintendent required the family to take the child home because hospital regulations forbade accepting patients with contagious diseases. Within fifteen minutes after returning home the child died.

Crews, which denied recovery to the plaintiff, was the first important case on the question in the recent past. It is usually cited as the leading case for the general rule that there is no right to be admitted to a private hospital. Because it did not deal with the failure to give emergency aid to a person coming to the emergency room, it is precise authority only on the question of the duty of a hospital to admit a person for ordinary hospital services. In fact, the court found that emergency treatment had been provided by the hospital; the issue was whether the hospital had a duty to provide more than that. While recognizing that a hospital may create a duty to provide even ordinary hospital services by undertaking to act, the court provided no guidelines as to how or when such a duty comes into existence. It merely held that rendering emergency care alone will not create a duty to render ordinary, nonemergency, hospital services, especially when the patient is suffering from a contagious disease.

Crews is an example of rendering aid and sending the patient away with the mutual understanding that he is in no better condition than before treatment. It is completely consistent with the general tort law with respect to the duty to aid one in peril. The hospital provided aid and, although its help conferred no particular benefit, it did not make the condition worse. *Crews* cannot be regarded as a case of failure to admit or failure to render emergency aid; if a wrong was committed, it would be wrongful discharge or abandonment. On the lack of duty to render emergency treatment, the principle for which it has so often been cited, the *Crews* case contains only dicta. Furthermore, in an age of rapidly expanding medical facilities and changing socio-institutional attitudes, *Crews* is thirty-four years old.

It may be, however, that the *Crews* rule of no duty to accept a prospective patient for ordinary hospital services has been extended by other courts to emergency room services. This is not to say that such a rule has been applied to limit hospital liability; rather, it is inferred from the many judicial efforts in emergency room cases to find some exception to the "general rule." In other words, courts have generally dealt with emergency room cases as though the *Crews* dictum were settled law. One reason for this assumption, of course, was that it fit into the lack-of-duty position of nonfeasance cases generally.

2. *After the hospital exercised control, it kept the applicant for some period of time without giving aid and then sent him elsewhere for aid.*

Methodist Hospital v. Ball.[53] A young automobile accident victim was carried to the emergency room of the hospital at 11:45 p.m. Another person, not involved in the accident, was considered by an intern to be more in need of immediate attention and was given the only available bed in the hospital. The intern in charge examined the boy's abdomen and checked his pulse and blood pressure but gave no further medical attention. No licensed physician was called. When the boy attempted to leave his stretcher, several hospital employees assisted in holding him down, with one person applying pressure to his back. After forty-five minutes at the defendant hospital, the boy was taken to another hospital where he died at 1:00 a.m. from a ruptured liver and internal bleeding.

New Biloxi Hospital, Inc. v. Frazier.[54] A man, bleeding profusely from a gunshot wound in the arm, was taken to the emergency room of the hospital. Three nurses saw his condition but did nothing to stop the bleeding. The head nurse called a doctor but did not inform him of the extent of the bleeding. The doctor examined the man but did not stop the bleeding. On learning that the patient was a veteran, the doctor made arrangements for his transfer to a veteran's hospital and left him with the head nurse. The nurse was to advise the doctor of changes in the patient's condition. In spite of shock symptoms, however, she made no report to the doctor. After two hours in the emergency room, the patient was transferred to the veteran's hospital where he died within a half hour from hemorrhage and shock.

Tacit adherence to the *Crews* Draconian principle probably accounts for the conclusion in these two cases that the deceased had been legally accepted as a "patient."[55] Neither opinion, however, offers a satisfactory explanation of how one becomes a patient or why a patient deserves better treatment in a medical emergency than one who, though a nonpatient, is nevertheless physically present. Hospital personnel in both cases exercised control over the patient by accepting him into the emergency room with the obvious intention of rendering some aid, but none was, in fact, rendered. A voluntary undertaking to render service, standing alone, has not been sufficient for other courts to find patient status, or it has not been necessary in order to hold the hospital liable. The only significant difference between these cases and other emergency cases is that here the persons were kept in the emergency room for a substantial time without receiving any aid and were later transferred somewhere else to receive the necessary attention. Except for these two cases, the law appears to be that a person does not achieve patient status until *treatment* starts, except in cases of formal admission for general hospital services.

Perhaps *Ball* and *Frazier* represent attempts to come within the exception of voluntary undertaking-assumed duty. The courts may have been seeking added assurance for their result by finding a hospital-patient relationship, which means a special dependence contract and another possible exception to the general nonfeasance rule. These cases may mean that, if the hospital-patient relationship exists, the hospital has a duty to render whatever treatment the condition requires and that admission may occur without any formalities or any treatment. Consider the following language from the *Frazier* case:

> In an emergency, the victim should be permitted to leave the hospital only after he has been seen, examined and offered reasonable first aid. A hospital rendering emergency treatment is obligated to do that which is immediately and reasonably necessary for the preservation of the life, limb, or health of the patient. It should not discharge a patient in critical condition without furnishing or procuring suitable medical attention.[56]

In neither case was the injured person formally admitted: in *Ball* the deceased received only a superficial examination upon entering the emergency room and was kept forty-five minutes before being transferred; in *Frazier* a doctor was summoned and the injured man's name was recorded, but he remained for two hours. Whether anything less than forty-five minutes would create the hospital-patient relationship is unclear, but if this is enough, then practically anyone in distress who gets through the emergency room door may be a "patient." This may mean that the amazing potency of the dictum in *Crews* has evaporated, just as privity of contract in defective products negligence cases disappeared when Judge Cardozo began to write the opinion in *MacPherson v. Buick Motor Co.*,[57] and for very similar reasons. The common law regurgitates what it cannot digest.

The results of *Ball* and *Frazier* could be rationalized under other tort rules. If an individual undertakes to aid another and should recognize that the aid is necessary for the other's protection, he will be liable for harm resulting from failure to use due care to perform his undertaking if his failure increases the risk of harm to the other.[58] The hospitals in both cases materially increased the time before aid was received. This delay itself might have been a significant factor in causing death; surely it increased the risk of harm. On this theory of liability, however, the existence of a hospital-patient relationship would be unnecessary to liability. Injecting the hospital-patient relationship into the cases makes them appear to be breach of contract or wrongful discharge cases, and this compounds confusion.

3. *After the hospital exercised control, it gave some aid, but then released the applicant giving him reason to believe the emergency had passed, when in fact his condition was the same or had been worsened by the treatment.*

Barcia v. Society of New York Hospital.[59] On the advice of a family physician, the parents of a two-year-old girl took her to the hospital. A physician employed by the hospital gave her an examination, including a chest X-ray, blood count, and throat culture. He decided that her condition was not critical enough to require hospitalization. The child's condition deteriorated after she returned to her home. Again she was taken to the hospital on the family physician's advice. This time she was formally admitted but died several hours later. Another physician at the hospital asked the parents "why didn't you bring her sooner, I might have been able to save her."[60]

Reeves v. North Broward Hospital District.[61] The patient was given a urine test and a blood pressure check by a hospital resident physician. He diagnosed the case as hypertension and gave the man sedatives. A relief doctor came on and signed the release of the patient into the custody of two brothers without seeing or treating the patient. Eleven hours later the man died of a subdural hematoma en route back to the hospital.

Bourgeois v. Dade County.[62] A man was found unconscious in his underwear on the lawn in front of a hotel and was taken by police to the emergency room of the hospital. An intern found his pulse and chest sounds normal. The man was unable to give his name or a history of his condition, and the intern made no other effort to obtain a history. No X-rays were taken. There was conflicting testimony about alcohol on the patient's breath. After a superficial examination, the intern released the patient to the police as a drunk. Several hours later he died in a jail cell from punctures of the thoracic cavity by broken ribs.

Ruvio v. North Broward Hospital District.[63] Plaintiff's husband was taken to the hospital emergency room on a Sunday. Under normal practice the resident physician on duty in the emergency room screened emergency cases. On Sundays, however, although a physician was on call, the emergency room nurses screened patients and called the physician only if there was a question in their minds about the existence of an emergency. Two nurses refused the applicant admission or any treatment without a doctor's order on the ground that no emergency existed. A friend took him directly to an outside physician who found him to be an emergency case and had him admitted to the same hospital. He died two days later of a coronary infarction.

Barcia involves both an undertaking to treat and a negligent diagnosis,[64] but judgment for the plaintiff was rendered simply on the basis of negligence—without any discussion of duty to treat. The case is an example of aid given without due care which unreasonably increases the risk of harm to another by creating a false sense of security and preventing the person from seeking aid elsewhere. The delayed admittance due to the initial inaccurate diagnosis was apparently crucial to the patient's chances.

In *Reeves* there was both negligent diagnosis and negligent treatment.[65] The Florida appellate court reversed a directed verdict for the defendant on the grounds that the evidence presented a jury question as to whether the hospital "did not exercise such reasonable care toward the deceased as his known condition required."[66] Perhaps this means that a hospital taking a patient into the emergency room may not terminate treatment until it does whatever the patient's true condition reasonably requires. Reading the case more narrowly, it may mean that the treatment and diagnosis constitute actionable neglect only because they created a false sense of security in the patient and deterred him from seeking other aid. As in *Barcia,* the hospital's intervention may have left the patient in a worse condition than he was before. Had the hospital given no aid, he would perhaps have received the necessary and proper care at another facility.

Bourgeois[67] was also a case of negligent diagnosis. In fact, the staff pathologist and emergency room supervising physician testified that improper procedures were followed. Again, recovery for the plaintiff may be rationalized on the basis of an intervenor who puts his potential beneficiary in worse condition than he was before. The hospital personnel not only caused movement and handling by the police which aggravated the patient's condition, but they also prevented other proper care. In *Ruvio*,⁶⁸ however, a directed verdict for defendant was affirmed on appeal. Here the time period before death was substantially longer than in the cases previously discussed. Affirmance was on the grounds that plaintiff failed to prove that any action or inaction by the hospital staff was the proximate cause of death or that the hospital staff had breached any duty. There was no indication, however, that the court thought that no duty to the deceased existed.

4. *After the hospital exercised control, it gave some aid to applicant and sent him elsewhere for further treatment.*

*LeJeune Road Hospital, Inc. v. Watson.*⁶⁹ A mother took her son to the hospital for a scheduled appendicitis operation. The boy was examined, given medication, and dressed in a hospital gown. After waiting two hours the boy and his mother were required to leave because the mother could not produce 200 dollars in cash. Although there was evidence that the boy was violently ill at the time of leaving the hospital, they were obliged to go to another hospital where the operation was performed.

*Jones v. City of New York.*⁷⁰ The patient suffered an abdominal stab wound. After examining her and cleaning and dressing the wound, an emergency room intern arranged for her transfer from the charitable hospital to a city hospital for further treatment. She died there during an exploratory operation.

In this factual pattern, unless the examination and treatment given are negligent, it seems more difficult in legal theory to hold the hospital liable than in the prior three factual categories. The voluntary undertaking-assumed duty rule in nonhospital contexts is that the intervenor may terminate his services at any time as long as he does not leave his intended beneficiary in a worse position. He is neither required to continue his assistance indefinitely or to do everything it is within his power to do.[71] Both of these cases, nevertheless, held the hospital liable.

Watson, which is relevant even though not an emergency room case, avoided the rule of no duty to continue treatment by finding that the plaintiff had been accepted as a patient. Once patient status is achieved, a dependent contractual relationship exists and the patient may not be discharged if the removal aggravates his condition or increases the risk of harm. The extent of control by the hospital necessary to create the hospital-patient relationship was not discussed.

In *Jones* the hospital was held liable on the theory that the deceased was denied necessary treatment at the emergency stage and that the transfer contributed to her death. The court did not find that the deceased was a patient. Perhaps the court was saying that after exercising some control the hospital should have done everything within its power to minister to the person's needs and that it did not successfully shift that duty to the second hospital. Again, this seems to be a different voluntary-undertaking rule than that which applies in the nonhospital context.

5. The hospital refused to exercise control over the applicant and did not give any aid. The applicant was turned away at the door.

O'Neill v. Montefiore Hospital.[72] Plaintiff's husband awoke at 5:00 a.m. experiencing severe chest and arm pains and breathing difficulties. He dressed and walked with his wife three blocks to the hospital emergency room. The wife explained to the nurse in charge that he was very ill, and she thought he was suffering from a heart attack. Upon discovering that the applicants were members of a particular insurance plan group, the nurse explained that the hospital did not treat members of that group but offered to call a physician who was associated with the plan. The husband spoke with that doctor. Exactly what transpired is unknown, but the doctor did not come to check him or seek his admission to the hospital. At this point plaintiff requested that her husband be treated by a hospital doctor since it was an emergency. The nurse disregarded the request with the explanation that he could see his own physician later in the morning. The husband died while undressing after returning home.

Wilmington General Hospital v. Manlove.[73] Plaintiff's child had been under a doctor's care for three days. By the fourth day the child had not begun to improve. Knowing their physician was not in his office on that day, the parents took the child to the hospital emergency room. They explained to the nurse that the child had had a continuously high temperature, diarrhea, and two sleepless nights. The nurse responded that the hospital could not give any treatment because of the danger of conflict with the attending physician's medication. The nurse did not examine the child in any way, but did make an unsuccessful effort to reach the family physician. She suggested that they return the next day when the pediatric clinic opened. The child died from bronchial pneumonia that afternoon at home.

In these cases, the hospital, rather than exercising any control or giving any treatment, refused to treat the applicant. One might think that the argument still open under the general rule of no duty to act would permit the hospital to escape liability in such circumstances. None of the general exceptions is applicable here. First, no innocent or negligent conduct of the hospital has caused the peril to the sick person, and no force threatening peril is under the hospital's control. Second, there has been no undertaking to aid the person in peril. Third, there is no special relationship of dependence between the hospital and prospective patient since by all the tests there is no patient. In both *O'Neill* and *Manlove,* as may be guessed from this elaborate preface, the courts found the hospitals liable.

Both cases had these facts in common: (1) the person seeking aid was refused examination as well as treatment; (2) the nurse called a physician for the person; and (3) the individual died shortly after leaving the hospital. The intermediate New York appellate court in *O'Neill* split three to two in reversing a dismissal of plaintiff's claim. The court found that the evidence was sufficient to create two issues which should have been submitted to the jury: Did the nurse's actions amount to a voluntary undertaking-assumed duty by the hospital to provide medical care, or did she merely perform a personal favor? And, if the hospital assumed such an obligation, was it reasonably fulfilled? An effort was thus made to bring the case within the orthodox voluntary undertaking principles. The plaintiff's case cannot be made to fit this bed, however, without changing the requirements for this exception as established in nonhospital contexts. The opinion maintained that after exercising *any* control the hospital must do everything within its power to minister to the needs of the person. If any control was exercised, it was certainly minimal.

The *Manlove* case more squarely presents the question at issue here.[74] The complaint itself was based on the hospital's refusal to treat in an emergency case. The Delaware court did not find that the sick child was a "patient." The court emphasized that it was not treating the case as one in which the hospital "assumed" to treat the applicant. It treated the issue as being whether the hospital had a duty to treat the person at all, and not whether the hospital was negligent in the treatment it gave. Making its views quite clear, the court held that a hospital cannot refuse aid in a medical emergency and remanded for a determination of whether an unmistakable emergency existed.

In taking this position, the Supreme Court of Delaware rejected the holding of the lower court, which held for plaintiff on the theory that receipt of public funds and an exemption from taxation converted the defendant private hospital into a public hospital. Clearly then, in Delaware the *Crews* rule is limited to provide only that a hospital owes no duty to accept patients to cases of acceptance for *ordinary* hospital services. In emergency cases, the applicant seeking medical aid in reliance upon a well-established custom of the hospital to render emergency care has a right to receive such aid and the hospital a corresponding duty. Duty and the resulting liability, according to the Delaware court, rests on the existence of an unmistakable emergency and reliance by the prospective patient on the hospital's custom to treat emergency cases.

This formulation may present difficulties in proving reliance upon a custom. Perhaps fewer doctrinal difficulties would be encountered if *Manlove* were regarded as an expanded voluntary undertaking case. Though the court initially rejected this approach—no doubt to emphasize its rejection of prior cases—it later admitted the analogy of the facts to cases of negligent termination of gratuitous undertakings, citing the predecessor of section 323 of the *Restatement (Second) of Torts.* Such a rationale involves an expansion of the voluntary undertaking concept as applied in prior cases. Prior cases, especially the *O'Neill* case, went to great lengths to find an undertaking to provide aid to the particular prospective patient. In *Manlove,* the term means an undertaking to provide aid in all emergency cases in general for which a refusal in any particular case would constitute a breach of duty. There could be no reliance on an undertaking under the prior cases until the particular prospective patient presented himself for treatment and the hospital in some way indicated an intention to treat him. This explains the attempts of courts to find that the hospital exercised some kind of control over the person or that the person had legally become a patient. Clearly, *Manlove* goes further.

Such an expanded concept of undertaking may be a step other courts would be reluctant to take, but it is also true that few cases have arisen that could not be neatly fitted within an orthodox exception to the old rule of no duty. The *Manlove* court's emphasis upon an established custom is most likely an attempt to state a requirement of reasonable reliance by the prospective patient upon the general undertaking. The *Restatement (Second) of Torts* makes liability for harm caused by an undertaking to provide aid depend upon increased risk or reliance.[75] And, reasonable reliance must be based upon a sufficient undertaking by the defendant. Reliance may be thought reasonable in a case like *Manlove,* because the expense required to open an emergency room is sufficient indication of serious intent to undertake to render aid in medical emergencies. Opening an emergency facility, however, hardly amounts to either contract or a gratuitous promise when viewed from the position of the hospital, and it is certainly not an "undertaking" as that term is used in the *Restatement*.

THE LAW AND SOCIETAL ATTITUDES

There is a striking divergence between the general rules of law relating to the provision of emergency medical service by hospitals and the general consensus of lay and professional opinion. The rationale supporting the general rule that there is no duty to act is in conflict with the generally accepted conception of the role of the modern hospital. Further, the result permitted by the rule is felt to be shocking and morally reprehensible by all, apparently, except the legally trained. We have already noted that some courts, reflecting this dissatisfaction, have been able to permit recovery by skirting but still rendering homage to the rule.

The most convincing justification for the general rule is the protection of individualism. The common-law courts, following their highly individualistic philosophy, refused to force men to be unselfish or to require them to be Good Samaritans.[76] Individualistic values are undeniably basic to Anglo-American law, but more important to contemporary American society is the value and worth of human life. The development of modern American hospitals has been spurred more by this human concern than by selfishness or profit.[77]

Such motives as philanthropy, sympathy, charity, and compassion are almost universally accepted as underlying the founding and operation of hospitals. The hint of a profit motive in hospital operation has been particularly subject to criticism from members of the medical profession.[78] Considering hospitals as created for service to society, one doctor wrote that "(t)he public servant, institutional or individual, who reveals for an instant a selfish aim is instantly discredited. . . . Surely we may look forward to the day when all hospitals shall present to society harmonious, united service, adopted with the greatest care and in absolute unselfishness to the needs of the time."[79] If most hospitals are motivated by such ideals, as experience would suggest, it is peculiarly inappropriate to attribute to them a desire to refuse emergency medical aid to those in need of care.

There are factual differences between hospitals and other business institutions which may support a different legal rule in medical emergency situations. The profit motive—incorporating a notion of absolute managerial discretion to deal with all parties so as to maximize profits—is at the heart of private enterprise and is the great stimulus to efficiency and improved service. When a business enterprise ceases to be profitable, it generally liquidates and retires from the business scene. A hospital cannot quit so easily. Its worth to the community is not measured by net earnings, but by the quantity and quality of services which it renders.[80] While some would argue that profit-seeking would force hospitals to be more efficient, it has been deplored as an organizational objective for hospitals and criticized as an obstacle to improvement in the quality of medical care.[81] The plain fact is that not even the private hospital operates or is regarded as an ordinary private business where unfettered managerial discretion is required. If unable to support itself with income from patients who pay for their services, even the private hospital does not usually close; it is supported by the community through private and public assistance. With the profit motive and its concomitant need for managerial discretion inapplicable, then, the way is open to impose upon hospitals some sort of duty to act in emergency situations.

More indicative of the special role which the hospital plays in the community is the position of many members of the medical profession who speak in terms of the public's *right* to a coordinated, community-wide program for the best possible medical services, including adequate provision for emergency patients.[82] To speak in these terms is to recognize the overwhelming importance to our society of emergency medical services. Indeed, because of this important role, there has been some consideration given to the suggestion that hospitals be regulated as public utilities.[83] Hospitals certainly possess some of the characteristics of public utilities: they characteristically enjoy monopolistic positions in many communities and provide services in which the public has a tremendous interest. A recent sociological study of community hospitals concluded that effective hospital medical care and treatment is possible only with the mobilization of total community effort.[84] As the authors suggest, this effort may be better mobilized in the form of public-utility-style regulation of striking differences in practices among hospitals.

It appears, then, that the values associated with the origin of hospitals as well as the best principles of their operation are in conflict with the values traditionally thought appropriate in the context of a fortuitous encounter between two men, one in need of emergency aid and the other having power to give it. Today, the hospital, particularly the emergency room, is vital to the community; it cannot be characterized as the locus of a chance encounter. A rule which evolved in the context of independent medical practitioners—and which today is criticized even in that context—should not be applied to hospitals automatically and without consideration.

Beyond these criticisms of the no-duty rule's rational underpinnings, many, especially those without legal training, feel that the rule permits a morally reprehensible result. It permits hospitals arbitrarily to refuse aid in emergency cases, even though the hospital personnel recognize that they have a moral duty to provide facilities and care in such cases.[85] Surely it is the general recognition and discharge of this duty by the hospitals that accounts for the relatively few reported cases on denial of treatment. Hospital officials and administrators are acutely aware of the censure they face if their doors are closed to those in need. Aside from the risk of potential litigation,[86] any such denial of emergency service may have a substantial adverse effect on the hospital's public image.[87]

More than half a century ago, Professor Bohlen wrote that "it should not be forgotten that a system of law which lags too far behind the universally received conceptions of abstract justice, in the end must lose the sympathy, the confidence, perhaps even the respect of the community."[88] The fact that not only the public, but also those most intimately concerned with the operation of hospitals, feel that hospitals should provide emergency aid to those in distress argues eloquently for imposing a legal duty. At times, it seems the only ones who have anything to say for the no-duty principle are the lawyers and judges. Further, if it is true, as Holmes wrote, that the law is a prediction of what judges will do, then the no-duty rule may no longer be the law in the hospital emergency room context. All modern cases fall into the exceptions, and the only support for the no-duty principle is in dicta and secondary authorities.

SOME ALTERNATIVE PROPOSALS

Many years ago, one of the great men of American law proposed a general rule—to be enforced by criminal penalties as well as civil liability—requiring that aid be given to those in peril.[89] The liability would attach to anyone failing to interfere to save another from imminent death or great bodily harm when he might do so with little or no inconvenience to himself, if death or great harm did follow as a consequence of his inaction. Although American jurisdictions have failed to adopt this proposal,[90] it is significant that other countries, especially in Europe, have created such statutory duties, generally enforceable by criminal penalties.[91]

In the United States, only Illinois has imposed a specific statutory obligation on both public and private hospitals to render emergency aid.[92] The Illinois statute imposes a fine on the defendant hospital for each offense.[93] The selection of criminal over civil sanctions reflects the strong policy considerations favoring such a duty to render aid. The duty created is specifically and narrowly limited to hospitals where surgical operations are performed; it arises only when emergency treatment or first aid is needed in case of injury or acute medical conditions. This limitation deserves special note.

Unlike Professor Ames' proposal—discussed at the outset of this section—or the European laws, the Illinois statute does not create a general affirmative duty upon all citizens to aid those in peril. The duty to aid created by this statute avoids some of the objections that have been raised to a general affirmative duty: (1) that it is too difficult to single out which person should be liable when many people could have assisted; (2) that it is too difficult to delineate all the circumstances in which a duty to aid would arise; (3) that the law should not enforce unselfishness; and (4) that such a duty would impose a form of slavery and infringe on individual freedom, which is fundamental in our society.[94]

The first objection is obviously inapplicable to the Illinois statute. There is only one possible defendant: a hospital which refuses emergency aid. The second objection is similarly inapplicable. The concern is not with all circumstances in which a duty may arise, but only with a "medical emergency" in the hospital emergency room. It is no real objection that this will require the courts to distinguish between emergencies and nonemergencies: courts make analogous distinctions in almost every case on the docket. In fact, medical evidence should make performance of this task more precise than in many other types of cases and the traditional reasonable man standard so familiar to the courts in so many other negligence situations would seem apt. The third and fourth objections seem inappropriate as applied to corporate or governmental enterprises, which most hospitals are. In the hospital context these two objections amount to a claim of the right to absolute managerial discretion that is certainly open to dispute.

The general rule that the hospital owes no duty to aid in a medical emergency undoubtedly emanated from the companion principle that a physician is under no duty to give medical aid even in an emergency.[95] The third and fourth objections are more tenable when directed to the question of whether an individual physician is to be regarded by the law as a public utility who must enter into contracts and render his services irrespective of his own wishes. There are many distinctions that may properly be made between a hospital that maintains an emergency room and the typical physician, even when he is in his own office. We need not enslave practicing physicians in order to require hospitals to be the Good Samaritans their emergency room signs and public image proclaim them to be.

Such a narrowly limited statute, then, seems to stand up well against the traditional arguments and has a good deal to recommend it. In the absence of this sort of statute, however, can the hospital be found liable within the rubrics of common-law tort? To hold a hospital liable for failure to confer a benefit may seem to violate the generally accepted definition of tort: an injury inflicted upon one person by the act of another, which act was intended or could reasonably be calculated to result in harm.[96] This definition, however, is today not exclusive; the law of torts already requires that some acts be done. Because of this dual nature of tort law, it is important to review the relationship between affirmative legal duties and misfeasance torts in considering whether the law should require hospitals to render emergency treatment.

The early English common law had no logical classification of legal rights and obligations. Litigants were compelled to fit their claims into the procedural forms of trespass or trespass on the case. Many rights and duties with logically different attributes were, consequently, indiscriminately classified as torts. Only because of their commercial importance did the affirmative duties today classified as contracts become a distinct branch of law. Bohlen felt that many other affirmative duties should likewise have been separated from the body of tort law.[97] This would have avoided the confusion and unfortunate decisions resulting from the failure to identify the salient features of different legal rights and obligations and the considerations underlying them. Professor Bohlen proposed that at least the duties to take positive action be given the status of a distinct class within tort law. This class would be subdivided into four groups: (1)

obligations created by statute; (2) obligations arising from family relationships; (3) obligations attached by custom as an incident to tenure of real estate, or incumbency of office; and (4) obligations "annexed by the policy of the law as necessary incidents to a relation voluntarily assumed. . . ."[98] Any common-law duty upon hospitals to provide medical aid in emergencies must be "annexed by the policy of the law," and, therefore, falls in Bohlen's last category.

Affirmative duties created by legal policy share important characteristics that serve to distinguish the group and to limit its expansion. First, they are similar to contract duties. Although not specifically agreed to by the parties, volition at some stage on the part of the obligated party is essential to the creation of the duty. The voluntary relationship of master and servant, for example, imposes upon the master an obligation to provide a safe place to work and safe equipment to use.[99] Significantly, the employer is also obliged to render emergency medical assistance to employees injured on the job and unable to care for themselves.[100] Similarly, a voluntary intervention to render emergency aid may impose a duty to render all the aid needed by the imperiled victim, as where the intervention causes the victim to forego other sources of aid.[101] Second, a necessary basis for the duty is always the ability of one to afford the protection and the helpless inability of the other to protect himself.[102] Consequently, the potential beneficiary of the duty necessarily relies upon the obliged party—"necessarily" either as a result of the beneficiary's inability to help himself or of his failure to help himself because of ignorance of facts known to or controlled by the party obliged.[103]

The relation of hospital and emergency patient seems "voluntarily assumed" by the hospital when one considers the total context. The hospital has voluntarily established an emergency facility and voluntarily made its existence known to the public. While this may not be the degree of specific volition required in some other relationships, it is done with the knowledge of the common understanding and growing belief that the emergency room is there for the benefit of the public—that there may be a *right* to such care. Further, the "policy of the law" would be served by creating a legal obligation for hospitals with emergency rooms to care for those who seek aid. It translates into law a moral obligation that is almost unanimously recognized. It would give legal support to the importance of the individual human being by preventing needless loss of life or needless impairment of productive capacity.

It seems altogether appropriate, then, to propose that a duty should be imposed by law upon hospitals that maintain emergency rooms to render treatment to all persons seeking emergency aid. Any hospital negligently failing in this duty should incur civil liability to the extent of the damage caused by the failure to treat. The standard for this negligence liability ought to be that emergency aid which ordinary, reasonable, and prudent hospital employees would have provided.[104]

Lawyers, however, require a theory acceptable under common-law principles that will accommodate this duty. The absence of the duty at the present time only reflects the traditional inertia of the law and not a lack of legal theories to supply an acceptable solution.[105] Indeed, *Manlove* suggests two theories which could support the duty to treat: the public utility theory and the reliance theory.[106]

The lower court in *Manlove* followed the first approach, basing a quasi-public character upon tax exemptions and state subsidies to the private hospital. The public character would obviously be present in a public hospital. Once this status is conferred, it is an easy step to find a duty to serve all members of the public desiring their public or private hospital emergency room services.[107] But there are several problems with this theory. The test for "public utility" status generally has not been dependent upon public financial support but upon whether or not the business is sufficiently impressed with a public interest.[108] While there is some correlation between public support and public interest, many subsidized groups such as farmers, churches, and charities are not public utilities, and some public utilities are not subsidized, such as telephone and telegraph companies. More important, however, is the objection that the public utility theory would create conceptual difficulties in the application of other rules of hospital law; these difficulties could be avoided by alternative theories.[109]

Probably the most appropriate legal theory is reliance upon a voluntary undertaking. The Delaware Supreme Court in *Manlove* used this theory, expanding it in the process to permit mere reliance upon a custom of treating all emergencies. Perhaps the element of custom was included because the early case of *Erie R.R. Co. v. Stewart*[110] indicated that reliance must be upon an established custom. A more desirable formulation, however, would require only "reasonable reliance."[111] In the hospital emergency room context reasonable reliance should not require proof of a custom of treating *all* emergencies. The allocation of scarce hospital resources to an emergency service should be sufficient to induce any prudent man reasonably to believe that the emergency room would perform and not refuse the service for which it was established.

Other theories which might appear to be appropriate, such as the invitor-invitee principles of tort law[112] or the contract doctrine of promissory estoppel, have significant conceptual limitations. The former requires the occupier of land to come to the aid of a business invitee needing emergency assistance.[113] This duty to an invitee is usually justified on the basis of the economic benefit that the occupier expects to gain from the association.[114] The overriding aspect of the relationship between emergency room and prospective patient that calls for a similar rule, however, is not the probable benefit to the hospital, but the potential detriment to the patient growing out of his reasonable reliance. Not many emergency services can be regarded as a potential bonanza of economic benefit. On the other hand, it might be argued that a hospital with medical facilities should be under no less an obligation than a department store with little or none.

The promissory estoppel theory has even less appeal. It is essentially a contractual mechanism for shifting the burden of loss.[115] When invoked, promissory estoppel functions as a substitute for consideration, not as a substitute for a promise. Thus, it holds a promisor to an actual promise and is not used to imply a promise for the sake of creating liability.[116] In emergency room situations like those in *O'Neill* and *Manlove*, the need to imply a promise to give the service negates the applicability of this doctrine.

Selecting the appropriate theory does not, however, answer all the questions. Should there be strict liability for failure to treat an emergency? This would mark a radical shift from the present state of the law. If not strict liability, what kind of effort will satisfy the duty and avoid liability based on negligence principles? The proposed duty involves the treatment of medical emergencies only. If there is no duty to treat nonemergencies, there must be some legally acceptable procedure for distinguishing emergency from nonemergency cases. Another legal problem is to decide what due care requires to satisfy the duty to identify and treat the emergency cases. Obviously, the large general hospital in an urban center is in a different situation than a small local hospital, but how much should the law take individual circumstances into account? Are there not minimum requirements that due care demands from all hospitals maintaining emergency rooms?

Because of the tremendous importance emergency medical care has among the total array of medical services, the law should not sanction any degree of care below that generally prevailing for other medical services. Perhaps hospitals should be required to adopt that procedure which will assure that emergency cases are handled with the degree of care and skill which an ordinary, reasonable, and prudent licensed physician would exercise under similar circumstances. The standards for emergency departments formulated by the medical profession itself call for diagnosis of emergency room cases by licensed physicians only.[117] It would be entirely appropriate for the courts to apply this as a legal standard.[118] There is also much to be said for creating this proposed duty by statute. The process of adjudication is too slow, and the uncertainties need to be removed.

CONCLUSION

There is no longer any basis for failing to require that emergency medical aid be rendered by hospitals with emergency facilities to those in need of such care. Not even the old cases cited in support of a lack of duty really support that position, and all the newer cases have found detours around the obstacle easily. Hospital personnel quite generally assume that there is a duty, and the public makes the same assumption. The law should not continue to honor such an outworn, unpopular, and barbaric dictum as the one permitting the professional "Good Samaritan" to keep its doors closed to the victim of a medical emergency.

FOOTNOTES

1. *See* Hospitals, Doctors, and the Public Interest 293 (J. Knowles ed. 1965); Davis, *The Hospital's Position in American Society,* in Modern Concepts of Hospital Administration 7-16 (J. Owen ed. 1962).
2. For a detailed analysis of the status of the doctrine in the various states *see* Annot., 25 A.L.R.2d 29 (1952); 3 A.L.R.2d Later Case Service 741 (1965). The reasons for the change undoubtedly arise from the changing pattern of financial support for hospitals. *See* Haynes v. Presbyterian Hosp. Ass'n, 241 Iowa 1269, 45 N.W.2d 151, 154 (1950); President and Directors of Georgetown College v. Hughes, 130 F.2d 810, 824 (D.C. Cir. 1942); Davis, *supra* note 1, at 11.
3. In an Ohio study over an eight-year period, the increase per year ranged from 10% to almost 20%. *See* Seifert & Johnstone, *Meeting the Emergency Department Crisis,* 40 Hospitals 55 (1966). The American Hospital Association found a 175% increase in emergency room visits between 1954 and 1964. A.M.A. Department of Hospitals and Medical Facilities, *The Emergency Department Problem—An Overview,* 198 J.A.M.A. 380 (1966) [hereinafter 198 J.A.M.A.] The increase for some hospitals has been as high as 600% in six years. *See* Stichter, Medical Staffing of Emergency Rooms: Legal and Ethical Considerations, 62 The Ohio State Medical J. 600 (1966); Foster, *Public Dis-*

covers Where Care Is: Emergency Rooms, 106 The Modern Hospital 77 (1966).
4. Blalock, *Emergency Care,* 40 Hospitals at 51 (1966).
5. For example, *see* Bergen, *Legal Aspects of Emergency Departments,* in Emergency Department 109 (1966): "Emergency medical care might be defined as care necessary to sustain life or maintain health that cannot be delayed"; Letourneau, *Legal Aspects of the Hospital Emergency Room,* 16 Clev.-Mar. L. Rev. 50 (1967).
6. "Private Hospital" as used herein means any hospital which is not a public hospital. A public hospital is one owned, operated, and supported by government. Van Campen v. Olean Gen. Hosp., 210 App. Div. 204, 205 N.Y.S. 554, *aff'd,* 239 N.Y. 615, 147 N.E. 219 (1924). The responsibility of public hospitals will be treated to the extent not governed by statute since the common-law duties are, in general, the same for both public and private hospitals except where changed by statute. While some statutes creating public hospitals do not specifically grant persons the right to be admitted, they do state requirements that may by implication create rights of admission to such hospitals. Such admission requirements typically relate to residence and financial status of the person seeking admission. An occasional statute provides that governmental hospitals are for "the benefit of the inhabitants of such county and of any person falling sick or being injured or maimed within its limits." Fla. Stat. § 155.16 (1965). Under such provisions, hospitals may be under a duty to admit persons for emergency treatment.
7. Stichter, *supra* note 3, at 600.
8. Meyer, *The Hospital Emergency Department—New Functions and Responsibilities,* 40 Postgrad. Medicine 374 (1966). For many years it has been the weakest and most neglected department in the hospital. 198 J.A.M.A. 380. For a comparison of inpatient and outpatient services *see* Seifert & Johnstone, *supra* note 3,

at 57.
9. The change has been expressed as follows: "From a single room with one or two treatment tables, a few intravenous stands, and perhaps a cabinet of drugs, the 'emergency room' has now expanded into a many-chambered area with facilities for many types of examination and treatment." Noer, *Critical Surgery Belongs in O.R., Not E.R.,* 106 The Mod. Hosp. 92 (1966).
10. Blalock, *supra* note 4, at 51-52.
11. Noer, *supra* note 9, at 92.
12. U.S. Dep't. of Health, Education, and Welfare, Hospital Outpatient Services: Facts and Trends, Public Health Service 14-15 (No. 930-C-6 1964).
13. This development has caused some to characterize the emergency room as a "neighborhood drop-in clinic." Stichter, *supra* note 3, at 600.
14. Many explanations for the new pattern of emergency room use are given. Stichter feels the major reason is "the public's general acceptance . . . of the idea that hospital facilities . . . should be available for all kinds of illnesses and injuries—the idea that the hospital emergency room should be a sort of community medical center." Stichter, *supra* note 3, at 601. For other explanations, *see* Modern Concepts of Hospital Administration, *supra* note 1, at 330; Vaughan & Gamester, *Why Patients Use Hospital Emergency Departments,* 40 Hosps. 59 (1966); 198 J.A.M.A. 380; Seifert & Johnstone, *supra* note 3, at 58.
15. Foster, *supra* note 3, at 78. Faced with overwhelming demand, many hospitals have been modifying their emergency room physical plants, staff arrangements, and technical services. While the quality of care has been improved, there is as yet no generally accepted procedure for rendering emergency care. The immediate concern of the patient centers on the competency, efficiency, and speed of the service rendered to him, particularly if he has a true emergency. His welfare depends directly upon the emergency room procedure, *i.e.,* whether it calls for care or evaluation by a

nurse, intern, or licensed physician and whether it provides for rapid and efficient rendition of service.
16. A Maryland hospital used radio announcements, newspaper stories, and brochures. Foster, *supra* note 3, at 78. For an account of another attempt to cope with the problem *see How One Small Hospital Enlarged Emergency Room,* 106 The Mod. Hosp. 87 (1966); T. Flint, Emergency Treatment and Management 3 (3d ed. 1964): 'the ratio between urgent and nonurgent cases is as high as ten to one.... As a result, facilities designed, equipped and staffed for handling emergency conditions have been swamped with nonurgent patients at times when care of true emergencies suddenly and unexpectedly has become imperative."
17. The reason for the public's attitude has been compared to the thief's reply to why he robbed banks: "Because that's where the money is." Foster, *supra* note 3, at 78.
18. *See* Bergen, *supra* note 5, at 110.
19. Stichter, *supra* note 3, at 604; Modern Concepts of Hospital Administration, *supra* note 1, at 333; Letourneau, *supra* note 5, at 57; T. Flint, *supra* note 16, at 88.
20. E. Hayt, Law of Hospital and Nurse 112 (1958); Modern Concepts of Hospital Administration, *supra* note 1, at 333. One emergency treatment system development is the type instituted in the Yale-New Haven Hospital in 1963. This "medical triage" system emphasizes the screening of true emergencies from cases in which time is not of the essence by physicians. This system appears successful in increasing efficiency and the quality of patient care, [Weiner, Rutzen, & Pearson, *Effects of Medical "Triage" in Hospital Emergency Service,* 80 Pub. Health Rep. 389 (1965)] but it has not been adopted as standard procedure on a national scale by hospitals nor has it been required by law.
21. Seifert & Johnstone, *supra* note 3, at 58: "[T]he physical presence of competent, licensed physicians in hos-

pital emergency departments currently is in the process of changing the community standards of emergency medical service in hospitals."
22. Wilmington Gen. Hosp. v. Manlove, 53 Del. 338, 169 A.2d 18, *aff'd on other grounds,* 54 Del. 15, 174 A.2d 135 (1961); Ruvio v. North Broward Hosp. Dist., 186 S.2d 45 (4th Dist. Ct. App. Fla. 1966); O'Neill v. Montefiore Hosp., 11 App. Div. 2d 132, 202 N.Y.S.2d 436 (1960).
23. Jones v. City of New York, 134 N.Y.S.2d 779 (Sup. Ct. 1954), *modified,* 286 App. Div. 825, 143 N.Y.S.2d 628 (1955); Methodist Hosp. v. Ball, 50 Tenn. App. 460, 362 S.W.2d 475 (1961).
24. Bourgeois v. Dade County, 99 S.2d 575 (Fla. 1957).
25. The standard established by the American College of Surgeons calls for treatment by a physician within 15 minutes after arrival in the emergency room. *Standards for Emergency Department in Hospital,* 48 Bulletin of the American College of Surgeons 112 (1963). In Huffman v. Lindquist, 37 Cal. 2d 465, 234 P.2d 34 (1951), nine hours elapsed before the physician first saw the patient who had suffered a fractured skull in an automobile wreck.
26. Reeves v. North Broward Hosp. Dist., 191 S.2d 307, 308 (4th Dist. Ct. App. Fla. 1966): "Dr. Moorhead . . . did not see or treat Eddie but signed his discharge slip."
27. Birmingham Baptist Hosp. v. Crews, 229 Ala. 398, 157 S. 224 (1934); Olander v. Johnson, 258 Ill. App. 89 (1930); McDonald v. Massachusetts Gen. Hosp., 120 Mass. 432, 21 Am. R. 529 (1876).
28. Letourneau, *supra* note 5, at 51, notes that all statements of standards seem to agree that emergency room arrangements should insure promptness or immediacy of care. The standards of The Joint Commission on Accreditation of Hospitals require that the emergency service provide "adequate medical and nursing personnel available at all times." American Hospital Association, Hospital Accreditation Refer-

ences 137 (1964).
29. O'Neill v. Montefiore Hosp., 11 App. Div. 2d 132, 202 N.Y.S.2d 436 (1960).
30. Wilmington Gen. Hosp. v. Manlove, 53 Del. 338, 169 A.2d 18, *aff'd on other grounds,* 54 Del. 15, 174 A.2d 135 (1961).
31. Birmingham Baptist Hosp. v. Crews, 229 Ala. 398, 157 S. 224 (1934).
32. Horty, *Emergency Care—or Lack of It—Can Make a General Hospital Liable,* 96 The Mod. Hosp. 106 (1961). Statutory prohibitions against racial and religious discrimination prohibit exclusion from admission on such criteria, but do not in themselves create a right to be admitted.
33. Churchill, *The Development of the Hospital,* in The Hospital in Contemporary Life 68 (N. Faxon ed. 1949); Stichter, *supra* note 3, at 601.
34. W. Prosser, Handbook of the Law of Torts 334 (3d ed. 1964); Restatement (Second) of Torts § 314 (1965).
35. Note, *The Failure To Rescue: A Comparative Study,* 52 Colum. L. Rev. 631 (1952).
36. For a classification similar to that presented here *see* 2 F. Harper & F. James, The Law of Torts § 18.6 (1956).
37. Restatement (Second) of Torts § 322 (1965).
38. *Id.* § 321; W. Prosser, *supra* note 34, at 338.
39. Restatement (Second) of Torts § 323 (1965).
40. Erie R.R. v. Stewart, 40 F.2d 855 (6th Cir. 1930), *cert. denied,* 282 U.S. 843 (1930).
41. Restatement (Second) of Torts § 324 (1965).
42. Restatement (Second) of Torts § 314(b) (1965).
43. Restatement (Second) of Torts § 314A (1965).
44. Birmingham Baptist Hosp. v. Crews, 229 Ala. 398, 157 S.224 (1934). Opinions in other emergency room cases usually begin with a statement that this is a general rule.
45. Ill. Rev. Stat. ch. 111½ §§ 86-87 (1966). Although the statute contains only a criminal penalty for failure to comply, a duty to provide care could be based upon it so as to result in civil liability on a defendant hospital

violating it.
46. Colo. Rev. Stat. Ann. § 124-4-3 (1953); Fla. Stat. Ann. § 155.16 (1965).
47. Ariz. Rev. Stat. Ann. § 11-297A (1956); N.Y. Unconsol. Laws § 7301 (McKinney 1961). This type of statutory provision may imply that the public hospital should treat all emergency cases without screening for the statutory requirements.
48. Bourgeois v. Dade County, 99 S.2d 575 (Fla. 1957); Reeves v. North Broward Hospital District, 191 S.2d 307 (4th Dist. Ct. App. Fla. 1966); Barcia v. Society of New York Hospital, 39 Misc. 2d 526, 241 N.Y.S.2d 373 (Sup. Ct. 1963).
49. Wilmington Gen. Hospital v. Manlove, 53 Del. 338, 169 A.2d 18, *aff'd on other grounds,* 54 Del. 15, 174 A.2d 135 (1961); Le Jeune Road Hospital, Inc. v. Watson, 171 S.2d 202 (Ct. App. Fla. 1965); New Biloxi Hospital, Inc. v. Frazier, 245 Miss. 185, 146 S.2d 882 (1962); O'Neill v. Montefiore Hospital, 11 App. Div.2d 132, 202 N.Y.S.2d 436 (1960); Jones v. City of New York, 134 N.Y.S.2d 779 (Sup. Ct. 1954), *modified,* 143 N.Y.S.2d 628 (App. Div. 1955); Methodist Hospital v. Ball, 50 Tenn. App. 460, 362 S.W.2d 475 (1961).
50. *See* Wilmington Gen. Hosp. v. Manlove, 53 Del. 338, 169 A.2d 18, *aff'd on other grounds,* 54 Del. 15, 174 A.2d 135 (1961).
51. O'Neill v. Montefiore Hosp., 11 App. Div. 2d 132, 202 N.Y.S.2d 436 (1960).
52. 229 Ala. 398, 157 S. 224 (1934).
53. 50 Tenn. App. 460, 362 S.W.2d 475 (Ct. App. 1961).
54. 245 Miss. 185, 146 S.2d 882 (1962).
55. Cases cited in notes 53 and 54 *supra.*
56. 245 Miss. 185 at 197, 146 S.2d 882 at 887 (1962).
57. 217 N.Y. 382, 111 N.E. 1050 (1916).
58. Restatement (Second) of Torts § 323 (1965).
59. 39 Misc. 2d 526, 241 N.Y.S.2d 373 (Sup. Ct. 1963).
60. 39 Misc. 2d at 527, 241 N.Y.S.2d at 375.
61. 191 S.2d 307 (4th Dist. Ct. App. Fla. 1966).
62. 99 S.2d 575 (Fla. 1957).

63. 186 S.2d 45 (4th Dist. Ct. App. Fla. 1966), *cert. denied*, 195 S.2d 567 (Fla. 1966).
64. Barcia v. Society of N.Y. Hosp., 39 Misc. 2d 526, 241 N.Y.S.2d 373 (Sup. Ct. 1963).
65. 191 S.2d 307 (4th Dist. Ct. App. Fla. 1966).
66. 191 S.2d at 309.
67. 99 S.2d 575 (Fla. 1957).
68. Ruvio v. North Broward Hosp. Dist., 186 S.2d 45 (4th D. Ct. App. Fla. 1966), *cert. denied*, 195 S.2d 567 (1966).
69. 171 S.2d 202 (3d Dist. Ct. App. Fla. 1965).
70. 134 N.Y.S.2d 779 (Sup. Ct. 1954), *modified*, 143 N.Y.S.2d 628 (App. Div. 1955).
71. Restatement (Second) of Torts § 323 (1965).
72. 11 App. Div. 132, 202 N.Y.S.2d 436 (1960).
73. 53 Del. 338, 169 A.2d 18, *aff'd on other grounds*, 54 Del. 15, 174 A.2d 135 (1961).
74. *Manlove* is discussed in Recent Development, *Duty To Admit Emergency Patients Imposed on Private Hospital Maintaining Emergency Ward*, 62 Colum. L. Rev. 730 (1962); Recent Development, *Private Hospital Must Admit Unmistakable Emergency Cases*, 14 Stan. L. Rev. 910 (1962); Note, *Torts—Hospitals—Undertakings—Duty of Private Hospital Maintaining Emergency Ward To Treat in Case of Unmistakable Emergency*, 40 Texas L. Rev. 732 (1962); Recent Case, *Torts—Liability of Private Hospital—Refusal of Treatment in Emergency Ward*, 31 U. Cinc. L. Rev. 183 (1962); Case Comment, *Torts—Private Hospitals—Liability for Refusal To Provide Emergency Treatment*, 64 W. Va. L. Rev. 234 (1962). For a general discussion of this issue *see* Note, *Must a Private Hospital Be a Good Samaritan?*, 18 U. Fla. L. Rev. 475 (1965).
75. Restatement (Second) of Torts § 323 (1965). If reliance is the basis of the duty and consequent recovery, some nasty complications may be lurking as to the amount of damages recoverable. Awards may be limited to the harm actually caused by the reliance only. A similar problem is presented when a promise is enforced un-

der § 90 of the *Restatement of Contracts,* where a recovery may be limited to the reliance damage. 14 Stan. L. Rev. 910, 915 (1962).
76. *See* Note, *The Failure To Rescue: A Comparative Study.* 52 Colum. L. Rev. 631 (1952).
77. M. MacEachern, Hospital Organization and Management ch. 1 (1957); Modern Concepts of Hospital Administration ch. 1 (J. Owen ed. 1962); Faxon, *The Place of the Hospital in the Social Order,* in The Hospital in Contemporary Life ch. 8 (N. Faxon ed. 1949); Goldwater, *Concerning Hospital Origins,* in The Hospital in Modern Society ch. 1, § 1 (A. Bachmeyer & G. Hartman eds. 1943).
78. *See* Hospitals, Doctors, and the Public Interest 293-94 (J. Knowles ed. 1965).
79. *The Hospital in Modern Society, supra* note 77, at 17.
80. *Id.,* ch. 1, § 4.
81. Hospitals, Doctors, and the Public Interest, *supra* note 79, at 293-94.
82. *Compare* Stichter, *Medical Staffing of Emergency Rooms: Legal and Ethical Considerations,* 62 The Ohio State Medical J. 600-601, *and* Faxon, *supra* note 77, ch. 8, *with* Hospitals, Doctors, and the Public Interest, *supra* note 78, at 293.
83. Horty, *When Hospital Has Emergency Room It May Be Required To Give Treatment,* 96 The Modern Hospital, 103 (1961).
84. I. Belknap & J. Steinle, The Community and Its Hospitals (1963).
85. Modern Concepts of Hospital Administration 330 (J. Owen ed. 1962).
86. 2 University of Pittsburgh Health Law Center, Hospital Law Manual 7-8 (1961): Since the risk of incurring liability is much greater than the inconvenience or cost of furnishing such treatment, it is suggested that the hospital furnish the necessary care routinely so as to insure the exercise of reasonable conduct and not aggravate the condition. . . . It is in the hospital's interest to prevent suits from arising out of emergency

room situations by furnishing routine care to minimize injury and prevent harm.
87. Davis, *Hospitals Neglect Public Relations Aspects of Emergency Department,* 102 The Modern Hospital 10 (1964); Horty, *supra* note 83, at 106, 159; Seifert & Johnstone, *Meeting the Emergency Department Crisis,* 40 Hospitals 55, 57 (1966).
88. Bohlen, *The Moral Duty To Aid Others as a Basis of Tort Liability,* 56 U. Pa. L. Rev. 316, 337 (1908).
89. Ames, *Law and Morals,* 22 Harv. L. Rev. 97, 113 (1902).
90. W. Prosser, Handbook of the Law of Torts 336; Seavey, *I Am Not My Guest's Keeper,* 13 Vand. L. Rev. 699 (1960).
91. Criminal penalties in the form of a fine or imprisonment are the normal sanction, though in some instances civil remedies are available. *See* Note, *Failure To Rescue: A Comparative Study,* 52 Colum. L. Rev. 631 (1952); Note, *Must a Private Hospital Be a Good Samaritan?,* 18 U. Fla. L. Rev. 475 (1965). Belgian, Danish, Dutch, French, German, Italian, Norwegian, Polish, Portuguese, Rumanian, Swiss, and Turkish codes contain or have contained such statutes. *See* Dawson, *Negotiorum Gestio: The Altruistic Intermeddler,* 74 Harv. L. Rev. 1073 (1961).
92. Ill. Rev. Stat. ch. 111½, §§ 86-87 (1966). Section 86 reads as follows: No hospital, either public or private, where surgical operations are performed, operating in this State shall refuse to give emergency medical treatment or first aid to any applicant who applies for the same in case of injury or acute medical condition where the same is liable to cause death or severe injury or serious illness. It was first enacted in 1927 and amended in 1963. A Pennsylvania statute requires all hospitals to have at least one licensed physician or resident intern on call at all times, but neither emergencies nor any duty to render aid is mentioned. The sanction is the withholding of funds by the Department of Public Welfare. Pa. Stat. Ann. tit. 35, §§435-36

(1964).
93. The fine is small: "not less than $50.00 nor more than $200.00." Ill. Rev. Stat. ch. 111½, § 87 (1966). Presumably civil liability could also be founded upon a breach of the duty. The only case citing this section was a civil case in which a hospital successfully sued a township for services provided an indigent, the court citing this statute as creating a duty to provide the services, thereby making prompt payment by the governmental unit proper under another statute. St. John's Hosp. v. Town of Capitol, 75 Ill. App. 2d 222, 226, 220 N.E.2d 333, 335 (App. Ct. 1966).
94. The arguments are summarized in Note, *Moral Challenge to the Legal Doctrine of Rescue,* 14 Clev.-Mar. L. Rev. 334, 350 (1965). For a discussion of arguments for and against general affirmative duties *see* Note, *Must a Private Hospital Be a Good Samaritan?,* 18 U. Fla. L. Rev. 475, 486 (1965).
95. *E.g.,* Butterworth v. Swint, 53 Ga. App. 602, 186 S.E. 770 (1936); Hurley v. Eddingfield, 156 Ind. 416, 59 N.E. 1058 (1901); Childers v. Frye, 201 N.C. 42, 158 S.E. 744 (1931); McCoid, *The Care Required of Medical Practitioners,* 12 Vand. L. Rev. 549 (1959).
96. Prof. Bohlen suggested that the term "tort" should have been limited to acts of this nature. Bohlen, *The Moral Duty To Aid Others As a Basis of Tort Liability,* 56 U. Pa. L. Rev. 217, 221-22 (1908).
97. *Id.* at 222-226.
98. *Id.* at 226.
99. *E.g.,* Palmer v. Julian, 161 Kan. 619, 170 P.2d 813 (1946).
100. *E.g.,* Szabo v. Pennsylvania R.R., 132 N.J.L. 331, 40 A.2d 562 (Ct. Err. & App. 1945).
101. Restatement (Second) of Torts § 323, comment c, at 137 (1965).
102. Bohlen referred to the obliged party as the one "having exclusive control of the cause of harm." Bohlen, *supra* note 96 at 233. In a strict sense the hospital has no relation to the cause of harm in a typical emer-

gency room case. As in other cases of detrimental reliance, however, there is a refined sense in which the hospital does have control over harm from aggravation: but for the hospital's false inducement of reliance the harm from aggravation might have been avoided.
103. The two characteristics mentioned here are discussed by Bohlen. *Id.* at 228-29.
104. The tort liability of hospitals ordinarily depends on agency principles, with the employee being primarily liable for his breach of duty, and the hospital being secondarily liable. In many hospitals the physician in the emergency room may be a member of the medical staff who is not an employee of the hospital and whose tortious conduct may not be imputed to the hospital. This may mean in such cases that the physician alone and not the hospital will be liable for breaching the proposed duty. If the governing board of the hospital had adopted a policy resulting in violations of the proposed duty then this would be a so-called "corporate" tort, though the distinction seems meaningless when it is considered that the principal (hospital corporation) is still being held liable for the acts of its agents (directors or trustees) on the basis of what must be an imputation.
105. It was suggested earlier that nearly all emergency room cases can be explained by the rule imposing liability upon one who negligently performs a voluntary undertaking to provide emergency care and thereby increases the harm or risk of harm to the patient.
106. Wilmington Gen. Hosp. v. Manlove, 53 Del. 338, 169 A.2d 18, *aff'd on other grounds,* 54 Del. 15, 174 A.2d 135 (1961).
107. *Cf.* Town of Wickenberg v. Sabin, 68 Ariz. 75, 200 P.2d 342 (1948).
108. *E.g.,* Austin Bros. Transfer Co. v. Bloom, 316 Ill. 435, 147 N.E. 387 (1925).
109. For example, why should the duty to treat be limited to the emergency room under this theory? Other matters of policy now controlled by the hospital board of

trustees would be subject to the same analysis.
110. 40 F.2d 855 (6th Cir. 1930), *cert. denied,* 282 U.S. 843 (1930).
111. Requiring emergency rooms to treat all emergencies should not cause undue concern among hospital administrators over their normal operating practices. With a reasonable reliance limitation it would be permissible to operate an emergency room on a limited schedule if limited resources prohibit twenty-four hour coverage. Horty, *When a Hospital Starts Emergency Care It Must Provide the Best Service It Can,* 96 The Modern Hospital 116, 165 (1961). The hospital, however, would be responsible for informing the public of its limited operation by posting emergency room hours on entrance signs, in telephone listings, and in other public advertisements. Any restrictions on the type of emergency service provided should be clearly publicized to prevent the public from relying upon the hospital for general emergency room services. A specialty hospital providing emergency service only in its medical specialty, for example, should take reasonable steps to make this known to the public. Horty, *supra* note 83, at 105.
112. This approach has been mentioned in 2 University of Pittsburgh Health Law Center, Hospital Law Manual 7 (1961) and Note, *Must a Private Hospital Be a Good Samaritan?,* 18 U. Fla. L. Rev. 475, 482 (1965).
113. L. S. Ayres & Co. v. Hicks, 220 Ind. 86, 40 N.E.2d 334 (1942); Restatement (Second) of Torts § 314(A)(3) (1965); W. Prosser, *supra* note 90, at 337.
114. W. Prosser, *supra* note 90, at 396.
115. Restatement of Contracts § 90, illustration 2, at 111 (1932).
116. Bard v. Kent, 19 Cal. 2d 449, 112 P.2d 8 (1942); 1A A. Corbin, Corbin on Contracts § 200 (1963).
117. *Standards for Emergency Department in Hospital,* 48 Bull. of Am. College of Surgeons 112 (May-June 1963). The same standard is clearly implied in T. Flint, Emergency Treatment and Management 88 (3d ed.

1964).
118. In Darling v. Charleston Hosp., 33 Ill. 2d 326, 211 N.E.2d 253 (1965), the Illinois Supreme Court gave legal recognition to the Standards of the Joint Commission on Accreditation of Hospitals.

25. Planning Community Emergency Health Care Services: Fitting Together the Fragments

Martin D. Keller, M.D., Ph.D.

William R. Gemma, M.H.A.

The emergency health care system encompasses the distribution and determinants of medical emergencies, the manner in which they are treated, and their health outcomes. A medical emergency, from the point of view of the seeker for service, may be defined as an unexpected or unforeseen condition or change of status, in which someone perceives an urgent need for medical attention. The need may be felt by the individual requiring attention or by an observer, and this may lead to a call for help or direct approach to a source of medical care. In any case, the nature of the condition can only be determined after appropriate examination by a qualified person. Therefore, the eventual designation of any given event as a "true" medical emergency is a professional task and it is retrospective.

Emergency *medical* care is concerned primarily with the response to a call for help and service to the individual seeking aid at emergency rooms or other sites of medical care. Emergency *health* care is also concerned with situations prior to and subsequent to the entry of the individual into emergency medical care. What sorts of problems activate the system? Where, when, and to whom do they occur? How may they be prevented or reduced in number and severity? Who is receiving care and who is not? Are there alternative means of coping with the demands for care? How does the system operate and how does each part of the system affect health outcomes? How may the system and its components be improved? All of these are health care questions.

Each community has its own history of emergency services and its unique setting that makes up the context of this aspect of health care. The utilization of community emergency medical services is determined by:

a. Characteristics of the area and the population;
b. Nature and distribution of events leading to medical emergencies;
c. Knowledge and attitudes of the people served and their experiences in the health care system;
d. Access to providers of health care;
e. Organization of the emergency response system.

For the planner these elements form the basis for understanding the nature of the emergency health care system, assessing its quality, and considering the possibility and efficacy of change.

The components of the system do not fall into place by themselves. Each is governed by a culture of its own. The public have their perceptions. The communication and transportation systems grow up along lines of their own. The personnel are selected and trained by organizations that have special interests and perceptions. Vehicles and equipment are selected by still others on the basis of a variety of standards.

Medical manpower and hospitals enter the system in many diverse ways, frequently with no coordination with the other components. Who puts the whole thing together? For a start, one might consider the hospital emergency room. For the most part, the emergency room is "nobody's baby." Medical practice in the United States, particularly in hospitals, is governed along traditional specialty lines. How does emergency medicine fit? It seems to be best defined in negatives. It is not medicine; it is not surgery; it is not pediatrics; it is not obstetrics-gynecology; it is not psychiatry; and so on and on. Yet, it is a bit of all. One might say that it is the ultimate realm of the generalist, but this has not been an item of emphasis in general practice or family medicine. More recently, attempts have been made to define the "emergency physician" and to designate specific areas of knowledge and technique that constitute his realm of specialty. The American College of Emergency Physicians and a number of new residency programs in emergency medicine are making a contribution in this effort. However, they still find it difficult to fit into the constellation of traditional specialties.

There is another and more serious problem inherent in the usual definition of the emergency physician. For the most part, his realm of activity is defined as the emergency room, with occasional inpatient care. He rarely, if ever, steps out of the hospital door and considers the linkage of the emergency medical facility to the community emergency response system. Consequently, in most cases the prehospital emergency medical response system and the hospital emergency medical facility coexist, more or less peacefully, but show little evidence of mutual involvement in the comprehensive job of emergency health care. Moreover, even in the rare instances where there is some integration in the total system, there appears to be relatively little attention to the natural history of the conditions that activate the system. Who takes the time to examine the factors that are associated with the causation and distribution of the events leading to medical emergencies; the dynamics of the entry of a call for assistance; the effectiveness of the response system in terms of personnel, training, and equipment; the linkage of prehospital to hospital care; and the manner in which the actions taken are reflected in health outcome? Who has the responsibility for putting the scenario together and playing it back to the actors, so that they may examine their roles and the structure and effectiveness of the program? With a few rare exceptions, none of this is being done. The proven value of the clinical-pathological conference or case review as an educational tool and a way of monitoring the system has yet to be introduced effectively in emergency medicine.

Let us consider the prehospital emergency medical response system. In general, this responsibility is vested in the fire department or in special volunteer groups. As a rule, emergency health workers serve with devotion and many have received good training in first aid and rescue techniques. However, there are startling differences in organization, training, and response capabilities. One of the most common organizational formats, the fire department emergency service, faces a number of serious problems. Recruitment and the ladder of promotion remain within the traditional fire-fighting line. In short, one must be a fireman to enter the emergency service and one must continue to qualify, serve, and pass examinations in fire-fighting in order to gain advancement. This mode predominates despite the fact that, in most instances, emergency units are far busier than fire-fighting units and generally deal with conditions of greater import to life and health. One need but compare the massive response, in terms of equipment and personnel, to a fire alarm with the modest response to an emergency medical call. Perhaps it is time for the development of an emergency service with multiple pathways of personnel entry and advancement, where not all of the emergency workers need be firemen, and where the fire unit is but one segment of the over-all service.

How does all of the above relate to the planning of an emergency health care system? It is precisely the difficulty in assigning responsibility for the over-all system and the fragmentation of the system into loosely related components that interferes with planning. Reviewing plans that have been submitted for funding to various agencies at local, state, and federal levels, it becomes apparent that no one assumes the authority to speak for the system. Consequently, the plans reflect mostly the particular component to which the individual or agency relates. The system, thus, is pushed ahead in a very uneven way, in which the benefits of advance in one component may be inhibited by the inadequacy of other components to respond or coordinate with this change. It becomes apparent that a first step in planning an emergency health care system is the assignment of the task to an individual or organization whose scope encompasses the entire system and who has acceptability and authority to enter into all its components. Suggestions have been made of the need for a new type of medical specialist, an emergency health systems specialist, whose concern would extend to the entire field. Such a physician would address the causes of medical emergencies; the perceptions of the populations served; emergency response in terms of personnel and equipment; and the linkage of initial care to definitive care and health outcome.

An alternative, and perhaps a supplement to the emergency health system specialist, is an organization that has been generally termed an "emergency medical services advisory council." In a study currently being conducted at the Ohio State University, 135 councils were identified in the United States at the beginning of 1972, and it appears that the number is increasing rapidly. These councils are variously constituted and many of them have broad enough representation to involve at least the major components of the emergency health care system. The council offers a forum for the interaction of representatives of the specific components and allows them to find areas of mutual concern and to develop the habit of cooperative endeavor. Many of these councils include representation from comprehensive health planning agencies and regional medical programs. For the most part, such agencies are not linked exclusively with any particular component of the system, and it is this comprehensive view that is vital to the evolution and development of the emergency health care system.

Given the appropriate individuals or organizational structures for planning, the tasks may be defined as: assessment of the current status of the system; setting goals in a realistic time frame; and the articulation of policy and plans aimed at achieving these goals. If this is done in terms of the system as a whole, there will generally be more than one pathway, depending in part on priorities and in part on the knowledge and ingenuity of the planners. One of the constraints that must not be neglected is the necessity for mobilizing public support. It may be necessary to give priority to the achievement of changes that can be clearly shown to be valid improvements that can be achieved in a short time. However, while increase in the number of ambulances and decrease in waiting time in emergency rooms are desirable and unquestionably enhance some aspects of service, the system as a whole may still function poorly. The appearance of progress is important, but it is no substitute for critical examination of the system.

An appropriate start for the planning effort could be a listing of the system variables. These may be differently perceived by planners with varying backgrounds, but this type of classification fosters a comprehensive approach. Such a listing of variables follows.

EMERGENCY HEALTH CARE VARIABLES

The Setting
1. Geography and
   Demography of Area
2. Prior Experience:
   Incidence of specific types of "Emergencies" and operation of the local EMS system
3. Levels of General Education:
   Self-Help and Awareness of EMS System
4. Resources:
   Personnel, Equipment, Facilities, Finances

The Action

A. *Initial Actors:*   Person in Need of EMS
Others on Scene

Variables: Time
Place
Nature of Event
Resources at Site

B. *Possible Initial
    Actions:* Self-Help/First Aid
    Decision to Call for EMS

    Variables: Perception of Urgency
    Knowledge of First Aid
    Knowledge of Techniques of Activation of EMS System
    Experiences and Expectations
    Communication System
    Proximity to Emergency Medical Facility (EMF)

C. *Responses to
    Call for EMS:* Communication of Advice
    Dispatch of Help

    Variables: Recipients of Call
    Location
    Communications
    Nature of Described Event
    Resources Nearby or at Distance
    Distance from and Access to EMF

D. *When Help is
    Dispatched:* Travel Time
    Location of Squad Base
    Location of Site of Event

    Variables: Roads
    Distances
    Weather Conditions
    Highway Traffic
    Communications Enroute to Site

E. *Actions by EMS Personnel at Site of Event:* Assessment of Patient Status
First Aid/Resuscitation Techniques
Communication with Consultants (Telemetry, if available)
Decision to Transport
Stabilization and Preparation for Transport
Selection of Receiving Facility

Variables: Training of Personnel
Equipment
Condition of Patient
Number of Potential Patients at Scene
Communication System
Categorization of EMF's

F. *Treatment Enroute:* Life Maintenance
Supportive Treatment
Preparation for Action in ER
Communication with Consultants

Variables: Condition of Patients
Distances and Transit Time
Architecture of Vehicle
Equipment
Training of Personnel
Communications Enroute to EMF

G. *Delivery to Receiving EMF:* Approach to EMF
Transfer of Patient
Transfer of INFO to EMF Staff

Variables: Accessibility

H. *Actions in ER:* Assessment
Emergency Care
Decisions on Further Care

Variables: Condition of Patient
EMF Personnel
Equipment
Availability of local
Consultants
Communication
Linkage with other
Medical Centers
Admission Policies

I. *Subsequent Treatment:* Continuity of Care

Variables: Availability of Specialized Services
Coordination of Patient Care Services

The Outcome

Relating definable and measurable health variables to actions taken, and assessing the contribution of each component and the impact of the system as a whole.

Consideration of the above variables and any others that may interest the planners can lead to an approach to the acquisition of information to define the current status of the emergency health care system and reveal possible avenues of intervention. Utilizing census data, a demographic-geographic atlas of the area may be prepared and the emergency events that activate the system may be mapped in relation to the location of emergency squads, hospitals, and other elements of the response system. It is usually necessary to obtain information on "walk-ins" to emergency rooms, since they generally far outnumber the cases transported by emergency vehicles. It is most instructive to determine where the walk-ins come from, the nature of their medical problems, and the reasons for their utilization of the emergency room in preference to other providers of care. These data may form a basis for the study of demand for service. It could reveal over- or under-utilization and the possibilities of developing alternative methods of providing the desired medical care. However, it is still necessary to go outside the health care delivery system to discover the instances where service was needed and not received. This is much more difficult and calls for surveys of the knowledge, attitudes, and practices of the population and their experiences in the system.

The details of the operation of the emergency health care system are best ascertained by a participant-observer moving through the system and recording events and actions. It is not uncommon to find that no person working in the system has such experience. A detailed display of the operation, thus obtained, is frequently a revelation to all. It serves as a suitable introduction for planning and the consideration of change. Utilizing a list of EMS system variables, such as that presented above, it is possible to assess the characteristics of each component in a given community and to decide whether intervention is feasible and desirable. Such decisions are based on predictions of the impact of a proposed change and cost, in terms of expenditure and missed opportunity for investment in other items. In a sense, this is a simulation model of a rudimentary sort. More sophisticated, computerized models have been developed, but they have not as yet been adequately tested to demonstrate their utility in planning or monitoring the system.

There is clearly a need for public input into the planning process. While it is generally agreed that the consumer has a role in planning, the nature of this role is difficult to define. The consumer is qualified to indicate how he feels about the service available to him and what he would like to have, but the actual planning to achieve desired goals requires considerable expertise. There is also little evidence of consumer unanimity and, for the most part, no mechanism for ascertaining consensus. Consumer input may be approached through a mechanism for determining consumer grievances and questions regarding the system. A type of ombudsman, readily available to the public, who would record, classify, and analyze questions, complaints, and demands, might constitute a very useful source of data for planning.

The planner cannot help but be an evaluator as well. He must first evaluate the existing system, and build into his plan a means of evaluating the impact of change. This requires acquisition and maintenance of uniform data that will lend itself to analysis. Therefore, any plan must include development and field-testing of standardized forms for recording the activities in each component of the system. To continually monitor the validity of these data, a sample of events calling for emergency response may be drawn. These can be investigated in detail to obtain information regarding the variables that are of interest. This sampling of events, if well chosen, can also be made to serve as the material for educational conferences involving the providers of service, including all the personnel who have contact with the actions that constitute the operation of the system. The contribution of each designated action to definable health outcomes may be assessed as a guide to future action. This type of education is particularly important, since it is exceedingly difficult to introduce changes in the system unless they are consonant with perceptions of the providers.

Planning community emergency health care services is an integral part of general health care planning, but it offers a number of unusual opportunities. It is these very opportunities that have stimulated the surge of interest that has recently marked this aspect of health care. Beyond the clear validity of an emphasis on service to people with urgent need for medical care, the following special properties should be taken into consideration in planning:

1. The high visibility of emergency services and the ease with which people can relate these services to their perceived needs offers a special opportunity to generate public interest and support. Planning should, therefore, include provision for the dissemination of information through the communications media to mobilize public sentiment. It is perhaps easier to do so in this aspect of health than in most others.

2. Physicians and hospitals can be enlisted in the development of the community emergency health care system. They generally do not perceive this as an area of competition. Few physicians offer emergency care outside of their usual places of work and hospital services generally do not extend outside the hospital door. There are few service programs in health care in which there is so little vested interest among medical professionals. In communities that have well-developed private programs of emergency transport, planning should be directed to reconciling public and private interests and the development of a coordinated service that best meets community needs.

3. Paramedical personnel are most likely to be accepted as providers of critical medical services,

without direct supervision by physicians, in emergency situations. Their actions do not generally encroach on the domain of the physician of a hospital, and the urgency of the situation calls for rapid decision and action. Therefore, the "emergency medical technician" may stand as the prototype of a class of relatively independent paramedical personnel. Planning should take this into account in education of personnel and staffing of the system and in terms of the implications for the allocation of tasks in other facets of health care delivery.

4. The setting of end points or dependent variables that may be related to changes introduced into the emergency health care system is crucial to evaluation of the impact of these changes. In only a few instances is it possible to say with assurance that a given service prevented death or disability. However, it can be clearly demonstrated that certain changes in the system will allow prompt response to a call for help. Trained personnel with appropriate equipment will arrive on the scene rapidly and act effectively. Such services are clearly appreciated by the public and a consensus can be obtained from medical specialists regarding the probable contribution to health. By setting reasonable end points, based on both public and professional perceptions, there is little doubt that enhanced emergency health services will show demonstrable gain in a short period of time.

5. Enhanced emergency health care services may also have an important influence on the over-all health care delivery system.

   a. Distance and time factors that are so evident in emergency health care can be utilized as a basis for definition of health service regions and subregions. The need for prompt response without regard to jurisdictional boundaries is a stimulus to cooperative endeavor among neighboring political jurisdictions, health planning organizations, health departments, hospitals, and other organizations associated with health care. This can constitute a new approach to the rationalization of health service marketing areas.

b. The development of communication and transportation services that are effective in urgent situations can be the beginning of an over-all communication and transportation system for general health care delivery. Alternative and more economical means can be utilized for movement of patients to and from home and hospitals and between facilities; transport of health personnel; and transport of equipment and materials from one site to another. The emergency dispatching center can also serve as a general health advisory center, with some augmentation of personnel and equipment. This type of elaboration of the changes introduced in emergency health services can have a profound effect on health care delivery in general.

c. Emergency health services cannot be encompassed entirely by one agency or one segment of the community. It is, therefore, an excellent template for bringing together many community groups concerned with health. It is a common ground for the public and the private sectors, official and voluntary agencies, representatives of several levels of government, and the wide array of health manpower. Considered comprehensively, emergency health service is an excellent subject for area-wide health planning. For the most part, it is relatively untouched and it welcomes attention. It is a subject around which a community can develop the habit of cooperative action to meet mutual goals. Planning, implementation, and evaluation can lead to demonstrable benefits in a time frame that will show the value of planning and mobilize community support.

INDEX

Age
  of ambulance patients
    Los Angeles, Cal.,
      296-302
  of emergency patients,
    33, 89, 90
    Chicago, Ill., 106-109
    New Haven, Conn.,
      192-204
    New York, N.Y., 141
    San Francisco, Cal.,
      43-44
Alabama
  Birmingham Baptist
  Hospital v. Crews,
    521-523, 524, 525, 533
Alcohol related
  emergencies, 45, 46, 48,
    49, 50, 51.
Aldrich, Carole A., 281-304
Alpert, Joel J., 165-180
Ambulance attendants,
  10, 24
  patient management,
    55, 57, 60, 331,
    426-429
  standards, 444-445, 447
  training, 69-70, 443,
    446-448
Ambulance patients
  SEE Patients:
    ambulance patients;
    nonambulance
    patients
Ambulance runs
  Boston, Mass., 316, 318
  Los Angeles, Cal.,
    302-303
  San Francisco, Cal., 50,
    52, 53-54, 58, 59
Ambulance services,
  10-13, 23, 41, 50-55,
  330-343
  administration,
    329-343, 345-371
  Boston, Mass., 316-326
  automobile accidents,
    317-318, 321-323
  illness, 317, 321-323
  call frequency, 50, 52,
    356-371
  dispatching of
    ambulances, 52, 446
  fees for service, 283,
    292, 303
  level of service given,

345-371
Los Angeles, Cal.
automobile
accidents, 297-298
cardiac cases, 300
demand for service,
282-304
illness, 301-302
poisoning cases, 301
number of ambulances
needed, 354-371
prediction of demand
for, 282-304, 318-326,
355-368
private ambulances,
316-321
public ambulances,
282-304, 316-322
response time, 287, 331,
346-354, 363-368
response time
SEE ALSO
Ambulance
services: service
time
rural, 363-366
service time, 331, 347,
348-371
size of area served,
346-354, 363-368
standards, 444-457
SEE ALSO
Emergencies:
prehospital response
systems
Ambulances, 11

communications
systems
SEE
Communications
systems and
equipment:
ambulance services
design, 450-451
equipment and
supplies, 55-56, 58, 67,
68, 70-71, 425-429,
450-457
location of dispatch
center, 346-354, 367
oxygen equipment, 453
physician-staffed,
449-450, 455-457
physician-staffed
SEE ALSO
Physicians:
ambulance
supervision
resuscitation
equipment, 453-454
splints, 455
standards, 445, 450-457
stretchers, 451
suction equipment, 452
American College of
Emergency Physicians,
563
American College of
Surgeons, 18, 491
American Red Cross, 444,
447
American Heart

Association, 443, 447
American Hospital
 Association, 18
American Society of
 Anesthesiologists
 Committee on Acute
 Medicine, 441-465
Analytic Sciences
 Corporation, The 427
Anesthesia, 461, 492-493
Assault victims, 43, 45, 46
Automobile accidents,
 9-10, 45, 297-298,
 317-318, 321-323

Ball v. Methodist
 Hospital, 523, 524-526
Barcia v. Society of New
 York Hospital, 526,
 527-528
Bellotti, Carole, 305-326
Billing of patients, 29-30,
 41, 150-151, 152, 255,
 476, 499
Blacks SEE Negro
Boston, Mass.
 Beth Israel Hospital,
  254, 255, 270, 313,
  316-317, 318-321, 323
 Children's Hospital
  Medical Center, 165,
  166, 313, 317, 318-321,
  323
 Peter Bent Brigham
  Hospital, 313, 317,
  318-321, 323

 Police Department, 313,
  317, 318-323
Bourgeois v. Dade
 County, 527, 528

Cardiac cases
 defibrillation by
  nurses, 465
 defibrillation by
  paramedical
  personnel, 429, 444
 Los Angeles, Cal.
  demand for
  ambulance
  services, 300
 Miami, Fla., 427
Cardiac compression,
 443, 444
Cardiopulmonary arrests
 in-hospital, 394-397,
  399, 412-423
Cardiopulmonary
 resuscitation
 techniques,
 training in, 443,
 447-448, 465
Chase, Robert C., 73-84
Chicago, Ill.
 emergency medical
  service system, 89,
  94, 95, 106-110
Climate
 SEE Weather and
  climate
Clinical selectivity of
 hospital emergency

departments, 98-100,
116-117, 158-160, 181,
232-248, 513-515,
523-536
SEE ALSO Triage
systems
Clowers, Walter, 38
Colorado
Department of Health,
478
Hospital emergency
departments, 469- 478
Communication
doctor-patient
communication,
207-226
Communications
systems and equipment
ambulance services,
70-71, 426, 428-429
in-hospital, 389-424
standards, 446
telemetry, 428-429, 446
Contagious diseases
admissions policies,
521-522
Continuity of care
hospital emergency
departments, 118, 239,
248-249
Cornell Trauma Research
Group, 18
Coronary care units,
mobile units, 427, 428
Coronary surveillance
units, 464
Cost-effectiveness studies

ambulance services,
338-343, 345-371
Costs
emergency medical
care, 115, 380, 476
San Francisco, Cal.,
41
specialized emergency
care facilities, 426
Crews v. Birmingham
Baptist Hospital, 521-
523, 524, 525, 533

Defibrillation
by nurses, 465
by paramedical
personnel, 429, 444
Delaware
Wilmington General
Hospital v. Manlove,
531, 532-534, 543-545
Demographic
characteristics of
patients
SEE Patient
characteristics
SEE specific
characteristics, i.e.,
Age, Income, etc.
Dentists
training in
emergency care, 443
Disposition of patients on
discharge from
emergency facility,
61-62, 65, 94, 150, 151,
239, 243

Index 581

SEE ALSO Continuity
of care: hospital
emergency
departments
Du Val, Merlin K., 9-16
Duhl, Frederick J.,
227-249

Educational level of
emergency patients, 89,
91, 107, 185, 187, 198
Elevators in hospitals
SEE In-hospital
emergencies:
mobility of personnel
and equipment
Emergencies
definition of, 561
prehospital response
systems, 564
SEE ALSO Ambulance
services
Emergency Care
Research Institute, The
389, 427
Emergency medical care
advisory councils, 566
communications
systems, 70-71,
390-424, 426, 428-429,
446
components of, 13-15,
76-78, 561-570
hospitals
SEE Hospital
emergency
departments
SEE In-hospital
emergencies
planning, 562-564,
565-576
standards, 442-465
Emerency Medical
Technical Assistants,
426, 429
SEE ALSO
Paramedical
personnel
Emergency rooms
SEE Hospital
emergency departments
Employment
of ambulance patients
Los Angeles, Cal.,
296-302
Erie Railroad Co. v.
Stewart, 544
Ethnic background of
emergency patients
Boston, Mass., 171
effect on diagnosis and
treatment, 207-212
SEE ALSO Race of
emergency patients

Families as patients
SEE Patients: family
groups
Family medicine
SEE Hospital
emergency
departments: as

community medical
  centers
Feldman, Lee, 501-509
Finances
  SEE Costs
  SEE Income
Financial assistance to
  emergency patients
  New York, N.Y., 143
First aid courses, 444
Florida
  Bourgeois v. Dade
    County, 527, 528
  Le Jeune Road
    Hospital, Inc. v.
    Watson, 529, 530
  Reeves v. North
    Broward Hospital
    district, 526-527, 528
  Ruvio v. North
    Broward Hospital
    District, 527, 529
  Frazier v. New Biloxi
    Hospital, 523-526

Gemma, William R.,
  73-84, 561-576
Geographic accessability
  of emergency medical
  care, 115, 171, 236,
  570-571
Gibson, Geoffrey, 85-124
Great Britain
  emergency health care,
  111-113

Haggerty, Robert J.,
  165-180
Hall, William, 329-342
Hanitzsch, Erik, 329-342
Heagarty, Margaret C.,
  165-180
Health and hospital
  insurance, 113-114, 123,
  144, 152, 173, 531
Helicopters
  use in emergency care,
  373-387, 450
Highway accidents
  SEE Automobile
  accidents
Hisserich, John C.,
  281-304
Hospital Emergency
  Command System,
  390-424, 427
Hospital emergency
  departments
  administration, 27-35,
    148-151, 157-160,
    218-219, 221, 238-242,
    324-326, 472, 491-499
  administrative commit-
    tees, 27, 442-443, 492,
    498
  as community medical
    centers, 103, 105, 117,
    152-154, 157-160,
    176-180, 258-263,
    513-514
  as entry point in the
    health care system,

Index 583

94, 98-100, 110-124,
  157-160, 237, 242,
  247-249
backup services,
  461-462
billing of patients
  SEE Billing of
    patients
Chicago, Ill., 89, 94-95,
  106-110
civil disasters, 389, 497
Colorado, 469-478
continuity of care, 118,
  239, 248-249
  SEE ALSO Patients:
    disposition on
    discharge from
    emergency facilities
equipment and
  supplies, 25, 26,
  460-461, 472
  SEE ALSO
    Ambulances:
    equipment
    and supplies

follow-up care
  SEE Hospital
    emergency
    departments:
    continuity of care
  SEE Patients:
    disposition on
    discharge from
    emergency
    facilities

in-hospital emergencies
  SEE In-hospital
    emergencies
laboratory tests,
  148-150, 461
legel responsibility to
  provide treatment,
  515-547
  Illinois, 519, 539, 540
manuals of policies and
  functions, 28, 473,
  492, 508
  SEE ALSO Hospital
    emergency
    departments:
    standards
medications
  prescribed, 149-150
moral responsibility to
  provide treatment,
  535-538
New Haven, Conn.,
  181-205
New York, N.Y. 135-164
nonemergent use,
  26-28, 32-33, 94-96,
  100, 107-109, 159-160,
  176-180, 181-206,
  207-226, 470-471,
  493-494, 513-514, 546
  SEE ALSO
    Hospital
    emergency
    departments: as
    community
    medical centers

SEE ALSO
    Hospital outpatient
    departments
observation beds,
    495-496
physical facilities, 24,
    25, 28-29, 426, 461,
    471-472
    effect on
      doctor-patient
      relationship,
      218-219
policy statements
    SEE Hospital
      emergency
      departments:
      manuals of policies
      and functions;
      standards
population served
    SEE Patient
      characteristics
    SEE Patients
    SEE entries for
      particular
      characteristics, i.e.,
      Age, Income, etc.
quality of care, 18,
    118-119, 496-497
release of information
    to reporters, 503-506
rural hospitals, 19-20,
    23, 27
San Francisco, Cal.,
    37-72
specialized facilities,
    426
staff, 27-28, 40, 324-325,
    482, 484
    SEE ALSO Nurses
    SEE ALSO
      Paramedical
      personnel
    SEE ALSO
      Physicians
    SEE ALSO Social
      workers
standards, 457-465, 478,
    491-499
    SEE ALSO Hospital
      emergency
      departments:
      manuals of policies
      and functions
surgery, 28-29, 492-493
systems, analysis,
    73-84, 85-125
types of cases, 28, 32,
    232, 234, 235
    New York, N.Y.,
      144-147
    San Francisco, Cal.,
      43, 45-48
    United States, 17-35,
      85-93, 111-115
utilization
    SEE Hospital
      emergency
      departments:
      workloads
    SEE Utilization: of
      hospital emergency

Index 585

departments
workloads, 33, 46-50, 308-311
days of week, 46, 140, 309, 319-323
effect of weather, 309-326
holidays, 319-320
time of day, 51, 139-140, 237-238, 308-309
wound treatment, 29, 496, 498
x-rays, 148-150, 461, 496
Hospital emergency rooms
SEE Hospital emergency departments
Hospital insurance
SEE Health and Hospital insurance
Hospital outpatient departments, 253-271
patterns of use, 258-261, 263-271
staff
SEE ALSO Hospital emergency departments: staff
SEE ALSO Nurses
SEE ALSO Paramedical personnel
SEE ALSO Physicians
SEE ALSO Social workers
attitudes toward patients, 254-271
Hospital residents
moonlighting, 479-490
Housing
SEE Residence: of ambulance patients; of emergency patients
Housing density
SEE Land use

Illinois
hospital's legal responsibility for treatment, 519, 539, 540
Illness
SEE ALSO specific types of illness, i.e., Cardiac cases
Boston, Mass.
demand for ambulance services, 317-318, 321-323
Los Angeles, Cal.
demand for ambulance services, 301-302
San Francisco, Cal., 45, 46, 48
Income
of ambulance patients
Los Angeles, Cal., 296-302

of emergency patients,
  89, 91
 Boston, Mass.,
  170-171, 173
 Chicago, Ill., 106-109
 New Haven, Conn.,
  186, 192-197, 200
 New York, N.Y., 143
In-hospital emergencies,
  389-424, 427
 communications
  equipment, 392, 398,
  405-406
 detection and
  reporting, 394-396,
  405, 415, 416, 420
 dispatching of
  personnel, 397-401,
  406-408, 415, 416, 420
 medical equipment,
  394, 399-400
 mobility of personnel
  and equipment, 394,
  399-400, 401, 407-408,
  412-416, 420
 personnel, 392, 394,
  397-399
 response time, 390-424
Injuries
 SEE ALSO Automobile
  accidents
 accidental injuries
  Los Angeles, Cal.,
   299
  San Francisco, Cal.,
   43, 45, 46

Intensive care units,
  462-465, 494
Interns
  moonlighting, 479-490
Italians as emergency
  patients, 208-209

Jacobs, Arthur R.,
  373-387
Jones v. City of New
  York, 529, 530
Jurkowitz, Maeda,
  253-271

Keller, Martin D., 73-84,
  561-576
Kennedy, Robert H.,
  491-499
King, Barry G., 37-72
Kosa, John, 165-180

Land use
  and demand for
   ambulance services,
   296-302, 364-368
Lave, Lester B., 281-304
Lavenhar, Marvin A.,
  181-206
Lawsuits, 502, 504,
  521-535
Laymen and emergency
  care, 442-443
Lee, Sidney S., 253-271
Legal responsibility for
  treatment
  hospitals, 515-547

Illinois, 519, 539, 540
  physicians, 540
Levine, Stephen A.,
  389-424
Los Angeles, Cal.
  ambulance service,
    283-304
  Central Receiving
    Hospital, 284

McCarroll, James R.,
  17-35
McLaughlin, Curtis P.,
  373-387
Manlove v. Wilmington
  General Hospital, 531,
  532-534, 543-545
Marital status
  of ambulance patients,
    296-302
  of emergency patients,
    89, 92, 185, 192-198,
    200
Medical students
  intensive care training,
    465
Methodology
  studies of ambulance
    patients, 38-40
  studies of ambulance
    services, 284-295,
    313-315, 333-340,
    357-368
  studies of effect of
    weather on
    emergency
    department
    workload, 313-315
  studies of emergency
    care services
    simulation models,
      75-8, 333-340,
      363-371, 375,
      381-387, 392-424
    systems analysis,
      85-125, 333-340,
      375-387, 392-424
  studies of emergency
    communications
    systems, 392-424
  studies of emergency
    department
    equipment, 18-23
    facilities, 18-23
    patients, 38-40,
      137-140, 166-167,
      182-184, 188-192,
      200-203, 230-231
    staff perceptions,
      256-258
    workloads, 38-40,
      313-315
  studies of helicopter
    emergency services,
    374, 379-387
  studies of psychosocial
    complaints, 230-231
  studies of urgency of
    presenting
    complaints,
    182-184, 188-192,
    200-203

Mississippi
  New Biloxi Hospital, Inc. v. Frazier, 523-526
Mobile Emergency Medical Care, 425-429
Models
  of emergency care systems
    SEE Methodology: studies of emergency care services; simulation models
Moonlighting by house staff, 479-490
  in emergency rooms, 482, 484
Moral responsibility for treatment, 535-538

Nagel, Eugene, 427
National Academy of Science—National Research Council, 426
National Center for Health Statistics
  Health Interview Survey, 89
Negro emergency patients
  Boston, Mass., 170, 173
  New York, N.Y., 142
  San Francisco, Cal., 41-42
New Haven, Conn.
  hospital emergency departments, 181-205
  Yale-New Haven Hospital, 181-206
New York, N.Y.
  Barcia v. Society of New York Hospital, 526, 527-528
  emergency health care, 135-164
  Jones v. City of New York, 529, 530
  O'Neill v. Montefiore Hospital, 530, 532, 534, 545
  St. Luke's Hospital Center
    Community Health Studies Unit, 137
Nobel, Joel, 427
Noble, John H., Jr., 305-326
Nonemergent use of emergency departments
  SEE Hospital emergency departments: nonemergent use
Nurses
  attitudes toward outpatients, 256-271
  emergency department administration, 498
  intensive care units, 464-465
  training in emergency care, 443, 473-474

Index 589

Occupation of emergency patients
  New Haven, Conn., 186, 192-197
  Ohio State University emergency services advisory council study, 566
O'Neill v. Montefiore Hospital, 530, 532, 534, 545
Operations Research, Inc., 75
Oregon
  Board of Medical Examiners, 429
Oriental emergency patients
  San Francisco, Cal., 42-43
Outpatient care
  SEE Hospital emergency departments: nonemergent use
  SEE Hospital outpatient departments
Owens, J. Cuthbert, 469-478
Oxygen equipment
  ambulances, 453

Paramedical personnel, 219-220, 426, 428, 429, 573-574
  SEE ALSO Ambulance attendants
  training, 443, 445, 449
Patient characteristics, 89, 90-93, 570
  SEE ALSO specific categories of characteristics, i.e., Sex, Race, Income, etc.
  Boston, Mass., 170-180
  Chicago, Ill., 106-110
  Los Angeles, Cal., 284-302
  New York, N.Y., 141-144
  San Francisco, Cal., 41-44
Patient management, 148-150
  by ambulance attendants, 55, 57, 60
Patients
  ambulance patients, 41-49, 51, 53, 54, 55, 58, 60-62, 148, 295-302, 457
  billing of
    SEE Billing of patients
  disposition on discharge from emergency facility, 61-62, 65, 94, 150, 151, 239, 243
  disposition on discharge from emer-

gency facility
SEE ALSO
Continuity of care:
hospital emergency
departments
duration of emergency
department stay, 61,
64, 65
environmental reasons
for seeking medical
care, 102-104, 236, 571
family groups, 165-180
with a private physician, 167, 170-180
with an established
hospital relationship, 168-180
follow-up care
SEE Patients:
disposition on
discharge; from
emergency facility
SEE Continuity of
care: hospital emergency departments
hospital staff attitude
towards, 254-271
medical care prior to
emergency, 147, 152-153, 236
SEE ALSO Patients:
usual source of
medical care
nonambulance patients, 41-49, 51,
62-64, 148

perception of
emergency medical
system, 572
physicians' perception
of patients' complaints, 207-217,
232-242, 245-246
presenting problem
duration, 146, 235
New York, N.Y., 144-147
psychosocial origin,
213-217, 232-233,
239-242
San Francisco, Cal.,
43, 45-48
"shopping around" for
health care, 263-266
site of physician visits,
89-94, 152-153
source of referral to
emergency department, 172, 237
transportation to
emergency room
SEE Patients: ambulance patients
SEE Patients: nonambulance
patients
SEE Ambulance
services
SEE Helicopters
usual source of medical
care, 90-93, 105-109,
153, 167-180, 194-200,

258-261
Physicians
  ambulance
    supervision, 24, 35,
    444, 449-450, 455-457
  availability for
    emergency care of
    patients, 30, 106-110,
    115, 474-475, 494-495,
    514
  billing of emergency
    patients
    SEE Billing of
      patients
  chiefs of service
    opinions of moon-
    lighting, 486-490
  emergency health
    systems specialists,
    565
  intensive care units,
    465
  legal responsibility to
    provide treatment,
    540
  perception of patients'
    complaints, 207-217,
    232-242, 245-246
  perception of patients'
    use of outpatient ser-
    vices, 254-271
  perception of
    psychosocial origin
    of patients' com-
    plaints, 213-217, 232-
    233, 239-242, 245-246

  site of patient visits,
    90-94, 152-153
  specialists, 475
  specialty-orientation,
    238-239
  effect on perception
    of presenting
    problem, 212-213,
    217
  training in emergency
    care, 443
Poisoning cases
  Los Angeles, Cal.
    demand for am-
    bulance services,
    301
  San Francisco, Cal., 45
Police vehicles as ambu-
  lances, 62, 63, 148,
  316-317, 319, 321, 323
Population density
  SEE Land use
Powers, Leonard S.,
  511-547
Press and public
  relations, 501-509, 566,
  573
Privacy, 218
Psychiatric problems
  diagnosis, 231-249
Psychosocial origins of
  patients' problems,
  207-226, 228-233,
  247-248
Public relations
  SEE Press and public

relations
Puerto Rican emergency patients
   New York, N.Y., 142-143

Race
  of ambulance patients
   Los Angeles, Cal., 296-302
  of emergency patients, 89, 91
   Boston, Mass., 170, 173
   Chicago, Ill., 106-108
   New York, N.Y., 142
   San Francisco, Cal., 41-43
Ratner, Robert S., 181-206
Record keeping, 35, 39
Reeves v. North Broward Hospital District, 526-527, 528
Religion of emergency patients
   Boston, Mass., 170
Residence
  of ambulance patients
   Los Angeles, Cal., 295-302
  of emergency patients, 92-93
   Chicago, Ill., 106-109
   San Francisco, Cal., 42
Resident Physician, 479-490
Response time
  SEE Ambulance services: response time
  SEE In-hospital emergencies: response time
Responsibility for treatment
  SEE Legal responsibility for treatment
  SEE Moral responsibility for treatment
Restatement (second) of Torts, 534
Resuscitation
  SEE ALSO Cardiopulmonary resuscitation
Resuscitation equipment
  ambulances, 453-454
Resuscitation techniques, 443-444, 447-448, 465, 494
Resuscitation training standards, 442-444
Robertson, Leon, 165-180
Rural hospital emergency care
  SEE Ambulance services: rural
  SEE Hospital emergency departments: rural hospitals

Ruvio v. North Broward Hospital District, 527, 529

San Francisco, Cal.
  Alemany Hospital, 41, 53
  Central Hospital, 41, 52, 53
  Department of Health, 37
  emergency medical service system, 37-72
  hospital emergency departments, 37-72
  General Hospital Mission Emergency, 39-41
  Harbor Hospital, 41, 52, 53
  Park Hospital, 41, 53
Satin, David George, 227-249
Sex
  of ambulance patients
    Los Angeles, Cal., 296-302
  of emergency patients, 90
    New York, N.Y., 141
    San Francisco, Cal., 43
Sheps, Cecil G., 253-271
Sickness
  SEE Illness
Signs, 24, 470-471

Skudder, Paul A., 17-35
Social class
  SEE ALSO entries for Income, Residence, Educational level, etc.
  of ambulance patients
    Los Angeles, Cal., 295-302
  of emergency patients, 165-166
    Boston, Mass., 171
    New Haven, Conn., 182-206
    New York, N.Y., 141, 142, 155-156
Social workers
  attitudes toward outpatients, 256-271
Solon, Jerry, 253-271
Sox, Ellis D., 37-72
Spanish emergency patients
  Boston, Mass., 173
Staff
  SEE Ambulance attendants
  SEE Hospital emergency departments staff
  SEE Hospital outpatient departments staff
  SEE Nurses
  SEE Physicians
  SEE Paramedical

personnel
SEE Social workers
Standards
  SEE Ambulance services: standards
  SEE Ambulances: standards
  SEE Hospital emergency departments: standards
  SEE Resuscitation training: standards
Stewart v. Erie Railroad Co., 544
Strayer, Daniel E., 73-84
Stretchers, 472
  ambulances, 451
Struxness, E.B., 425-429
Suction equipment
  ambulances, 452
Suicides and attempted suicides, 45, 46
Systems analysis
  ambulance services, 331-343, 363-371
  emergency communications systems, 392-424
  emergency medical care systems, 37-71, 73-84, 85-125, 566-572
  helicopter emergency services, 375-387

Telemetry, 428-429, 446
Temporal accessability of emergency medical care, 115-116
  SEE ALSO Ambulance services: response time
  SEE ALSO In-hospital emergencies: response time
  SEE ALSO Physicians: availability for emergency care of patients
Tennessee Methodist Hospital v. Ball, 523, 524-526
Tetanus toxoid administration, 29, 498
Third party payment, 151-152
  SEE ALSO Health and hospital insurance
Torrens, Paul R., 135-161
Tracheal intubation, 443, 456, 461
Traffic accidents
  SEE Automobile accidents
Transportation to hospitals
  SEE Ambulance services
  SEE Ambulances
  SEE Helicopters
Triage systems, 159, 181, 230, 239, 240-241, 248, 376-379, 462, 497
  SEE ALSO Clinical selectivity of hospital

emergency departments

United States
  hospital emergency departments, 17-35, 85-94, 111-115
  Public Health Service Injury Control Program, 37
Urban hospital emergency care
  SEE names of particular cities, i.e., Chicago, Ill., New York, N.Y., San Francisco, Cal., etc.
Utilization
  of ambulance services
    prediction of use, 282-304, 318-326, 355-368
  of community emergency medical services
    determinants of, 562
  of hospital emergency departments
    environmental reasons for use, 96-105, 165, 172, 308-326, 571
    increase in use, 18, 31-32, 87-89, 165, 305-308, 512-513
    New York, N.Y., 135-163
    prediction of use, 105-110, 182, 188-192, 200-206, 324
  of hospital outpatient departments, 258-261, 263-266

Wade, Preston A., 17-35
Watson v. Le Jeune Road Hospital, Inc., 529, 530
Weather and climate
  effect on demand for ambulance services, 309-326
  effect on workloads at hospital emergency departments, 309-326
Wechsler, Henry 305-326
Welfare assistance to emergency patients, 143, 173
Workloads
  SEE Hospital emergency departments workloads
Wound treatment, 29, 496, 498

X-rays, 148-150, 496

Yedvab, Donna G., 135-161

Zola, Irving Kenneth, 207-224

ABIGAIL E. WEEKS MEMORIAL LIBRARY
UNION COLLEGE
BARBOURVILLE, KENTUCKY